Outpatient Urologic Surgery

Outpatient Urologic Surgery

KEITH W. KAYE, M.D., F.C.S.(S.A.), F.R.C.S.

Department of Urologic Surgery
University of Minnesota
School of Medicine
Minneapolis, Minnesota

Judith Gunn Bronson, M.S., Technical Editor
Douglas (Britt) Hanson, Art Editor

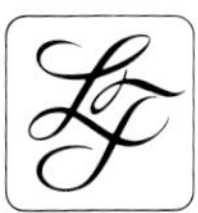

LEA & FEBIGER · *Philadelphia*

1985

Lea & Febiger
600 Washington Square
Philadelphia, PA 19106-4198
U.S.A.
(215) 922-1330

Library of Congress Cataloging in Publication Data
Main entry under title:

Outpatient urologic surgery.

Bibliography: p.
Includes index.
1. Genito-urinary organs—Surgery. 2. Surgery, Outpatient. I. Kaye, Keith W. [DNLM: 1. Urogenital system—Surgery. 2. Ambulatory surgery. WJ 186 094]
RD571.93 1984 617'.46 84-4411
ISBN 0-8121-0907-4

PRINTED IN THE UNITED STATES OF AMERICA

Print No. 3 2 1

To my mother, Helga, and my father, the late Professor Josse Kaye, for their example, everlasting support, and encouragement, and to my wife, Valda, and children, Jessica, Deborah, and Maxine, for making everything so worthwhile.

Preface

Radical changes are occurring in healthcare delivery systems. One of the most exciting is the realization that many surgical procedures, which previously were thought to necessitate hospital admission, can be performed safely on an outpatient basis.

This is advantageous to all parties concerned. Patients benefit because the experience is much more pleasant and positive than being admitted to the hospital. Because outpatient surgical units are geared toward elective operations on healthy patients, the atmosphere generally is one of hope and anticipation, and several studies show that patients greatly appreciate the convenience, efficiency, and dignified manner with which they have been handled in such units. Procedures are less disturbing psychologically, and patients find it more pleasant to recover in the familiar environment of their own homes. They tend to require fewer drugs and laboratory investigations and to become ambulatory much more rapidly, and many are able to return to work sooner. Patients also benefit from the financial aspects of outpatient surgery, particularly when elective procedures are being performed that are not covered by their medical insurance.

Surgeons benefit by working in an environment designed for basically healthy patients so that there is no longer the frustration of having one's local anesthesia or outpatient cases postponed because some emergency or major case takes precedence. This enables the surgeon to make better use of his time, without having to rush or to compromise surgical technique. Contributing to this efficiency is that fact that with experience, operating times for particular procedures in such settings usually become nearly constant, thus permitting cases to be more closely scheduled. Further, there are usually few cancellations, and, of course, postoperative rounds are eliminated. Paper work, the bane of effective time management, is also reduced.

Nurses benefit because of the efficient, but more relaxed, atmosphere of the outpatient operating room, and they appreciate the regular hours.

Finally, medical administrators, insurance companies, and economists in general are realizing the tremendous financial benefits and cost-effectiveness of outpatient surgery: it is estimated that 30 to 40% of all procedures that have been performed on inpatients will, in the near future, be done on an outpatient basis, and outpatient surgery costs 40 to 60% less than the same procedure performed on hospital inpatients. With approximately 20 million surgical procedures being performed in the United States each year, it is apparent that this shift to outpatient surgery would save approximately $5 billion annually.

Insurance companies initially were reluctant to cover outpatient procedures; however, largely as a result of the efforts of Wallace A. Reed, M.D., and the success of his Surgicenter in Phoenix, Arizona, most are encouraging this approach. In January 1981, the Blue Cross and Blue Shield Association issued a policy statement recommending that operations be performed in the "least costly manner enabling delivery of safe high quality patient care" and encouraging "appropriate growth of ambulatory surgery and more selective use of inpatient care for surgery."[1]

At present, urologic surgeons are just beginning to realize the suitability of many aspects of their specialty to the outpatient setting. Many procedures are performed on basically healthy patients, and much of the work involves areas of the body particularly suitable for local or regional anesthesia. This book, therefore, describes principally those conditions that are currently being managed safely on an outpatient basis. Wherever possible, it encourages the use of local or regional anesthesia. Most procedures described are already being performed on outpatients; however, a few chapters cover procedures suitable for local anesthesia or which necessitate only a short hospital stay. Some of these latter operations are on the brink of being done on outpatients, although not enough experience has yet been gained to advocate this approach generally. Naturally, individual urologists will have to decide according to their experience, facilities, and wishes just which procedures can safely be done without admitting the patient to the hospital.

Finally, it is hoped that this book will stimulate further thought and action in this exciting new field.

I am grateful to all those who have helped create this book. In addition to the contributing authors, these people are: Dr. Elwin E. Fraley for his inspiration, encouragement, faith, and friendship; Britt Hanson and the staff of the Medical Media Production Services at the Minneapolis Veterans Administration Medical Center, with whom it has been a pleasure to work through the years; Marlene Lindquist, for patiently and meticulously typing the manuscripts; my secretary, Patti Lien, for so cheerfully and efficiently performing the numerous tasks set her; and finally, Samuel A. Rondinelli, Constance Marino, and Frederic H. West, Jr., of Lea & Febiger, for their help and cooperation.

[1] Detmer, D.E. and Buchanan-Davidson, D.J. Ambulatory surgery. Surg. Clin. North Am., 62:685, 1982.

Minneapolis, Minnesota

Keith W. Kaye, M.D.

Contributors

Kurt Amplatz, M.D.
Professor of Radiology,
University of Minnesota School of Medicine,
Minneapolis, Minnesota

Alfonso Campos, M.D.
Assistant Professor of Pediatric Nephrology,
Tampa General Hospital,
Tampa, Florida

Wilfrido R. Castañeda-Zuñiga, M.D.
Associate Professor of Radiology,
University of Minnesota School of Medicine,
Attending Radiologist,
University of Minnesota Hospitals,
Minneapolis, Minnesota

Ralph V. Clayman, M.D.
Assistant Professor of Urology,
University of Minnesota School of Medicine,
Minneapolis, Minnesota

Boyden L. Crouch, M.D.
Executive Director,
Staff Anesthesiologist,
Surgicenter Systems,
Phoenix, Arizona

David M. Cumes, M.D.
Urologist, Private Practice,
Santa Barbara, California

Naomi, Epstein, M.D., M.B.B.Ch., B.Sc., F.I.A.C.
Pathologist,
Johannesburg, South Africa

Elwin E. Fraley, M.D.
Professor and Chairman,
Department of Urologic Surgery,
University of Minnesota Health Sciences Center,
Minneapolis, Minnesota

George L. Fraley
Business Manager,
Department of Urologic Surgery
University of Minnesota,
Minneapolis, Minnesota

Ciril J. Godec, M.D.
Associate Professor of Urology,
Downstate Medical Center,
State University of New York;
Director of Urology,
Long Island College Hospital,
Long Island, New York

Robert W. Goltz, M.D.
Professor and Head, Department of Dermatology,
University of Minnesota School of Medicine;
Attending Physician,
University of Minnesota Hospitals,
Minneapolis, Minnesota

Ricardo Gonzalez, M.D.
Associate Professor,
Director, Pediatric Urology,
University of Minnesota School of Medicine,
Minneapolis, Minnesota

David H. Gordon, M.D.
Professor of Radiology,
Director of Interventional Radiology,
Downstate Medical Center,
Brooklyn, New York

Keith W. Kaye, M.D., F.C.S.(S.A.), F.R.C.S.
Clinical Assistant Professor,
Department of Urologic Surgery,
University of Minnesota School of Medicine,
Minneapolis, Minnesota

Valda N. Kaye, M.D., F.C. Path.(S.A.)
Department of Dermatology and Dermatopathology,
University of Minnesota School of Medicine,
Minneapolis, Minnesota

Paul H. Lange, M.D.
Professor, Department of Urologic Surgery,
University of Minnesota School of Medicine;
Chief, Urology Section,
Veterans Administration Medical Center,
Minneapolis, Minnesota

Gary E. Leach, M.D.

Assistant Clinical Professor UCLA Medical Center;
Direct of Urodynamic Laboratory and Staff Urologist,
Kaiser Foundation Hospitals,
Los Angeles, California

J. Keith Light, M.D.

Assistant Professor of Urology,
Baylor College of Medicine;
Deputy Chief of Urology,
The Institute for Research and Rehabilitation,
Houston, Texas

Larry I. Lipshultz, M.D., F.A.C.S.

Professor of Urology, Department of Urology,
Baylor College of Medicine;
Attending Physician,
The Methodist Hospital,
St. Luke's Episcopal Hospital,
Hermann Hospital,
Texas Medical Center,
Houston, Texas

Josephine N. Lo, M.D.

Assistant Professor of Anesthesiology,
University of Minnesota Hospitals,
Minneapolis, Minnesota

Harold P. McDonald, Jr., M.D.

President,
McDonald Urology Clinic,
Atlanta, Georgia

Robert P. Miller, M.D.

Assistant Professor of Radiology,
University of Minnesota;
Chief of Special Procedures,
Veterans Administration Hospital,
Minneapolis, Minnesota

Ahmad Orandi, M.D., F.A.C.S.

Clinical Professor of Urologic Surgery
Univeristy of Minnesota;
Attending Urologist,
Lake Region Hospital
Fergus Falls, Minnesota

John W. Pender, M.D.

Emeritus Professor of Anesthesia,
Stanford University;
Anethesiologist,
Palo Alto Medical Foundation,
Palo Alto, California

Jose Amado Perez, M.D., F.A.C.S.

Chairman, Urology Department,
American Hospital,
Miami, Florida

Jean Pitfield-Marshall, B.Sc., M.B., Ch.B., Edin., D.M.R.D., F.R.C.R.

Consultant Radiologist,
Peterborough Hospital, and
Devonshire Hospital,
London, England

Konald A. Prem, M.D., F.A.C.O.G.

Professor and Head, Department of Obstetrics and Gynecology,
University of Minnesota School of Medicine,
Minneapolis, Minnesota

Shlomo Raz, M.D.

Associate Professor of Urologic Surgery,
University of California School of Medicine,
Los Angeles, California

John H. Redpath, M.D.

Anesthesiologist,
Palo Alto Medical Foundation and Surgicenter of Palo Alto, California;
Clinical Assistant Professor of Anesthesia,
Stanford University,
Stanford, California

Rodney J. Repko, Esq.

General Counsel,
Guthrie Clinic Ltd.,
Guthrie Square,
Sayre, Pennsylvania

Gaylan L. Rockswold, M.D.

Associate Professor of Neurologic Surgery,
University of Minnesota School of Medicine;
Head of Neurologic Surgery,
Hennepin County Medical Center,
Minneapolis, Minnesota

F. Brantley Scott, M.D.

Professor of Urology,
Baylor College of Medicine;
Chief, Urology Service,
St. Luke's Episcopal Hospital,
Houston, Texas

Arthur D. Smith, M.D.

Chief, Division of Urology,
Long Island Jewish-Hillside Medical Center;
Associate Professor of Urology,
State University of New York at Stony Brook,
New Hyde Park, New York

Thomas A. Stamey, M.D.

Professor and Chairman,
Stanford University Medical Center,
Stanford, California

Richard Turner-Warwick, B.Sc., D.M.(Oxon), M.Ch., F.R.C.P., F.R.C.S., F.A.C.S., F.A.R.A.C.S.

Senior Consultant Urologist,
The Middlesex Hospital, and St. Peters Hospitals;
Senior Lecturer,
London University Institute of Urology,
London, England

P.J.P. van Blerk, B.Sc.(Med.), M.B.B.Ch., Dip. Surg.

Professor of Urology, Division of Urology,
Department of Surgery,
University of the Witwatersrand Medical School;
Chief Urologist of Johannesburg Hospital,
Johannesburg, South Africa

Robert L. Vernier, M.D.

Professor of Pediatrics,
University of Minnesota,
Minneapolis, Minnesota

Robert M. Weissman, M.D.

Assisant Professor, Division of Urology,
Department of Surgery;
Director of Urologic Oncology,
University of North Carolina,
Chapel Hill, North Carolina

Robert H. Whitaker, M. Chir., F.R.C.S.

Consultant Urologist,
Addenbrooke's Hospital;
Associate Lecturer,
University of Cambridge,
Cambridge, England

Anthony D. Whittemore, M.D.

Assistant Professor of Surgery,
Harvard School of Medicine;
Surgeon, Brigham and Women's Hospital,
Boston, Massachusetts

Contents

SECTION I INTRODUCTION

SECTION II SPECIAL ANESTHETIC AND INVESTIGATIVE TECHNIQUES

SECTION III UROD YNAMICS

Section I

Introduction

1

Hospital-Based Outpatient Surgical Units

KONALD A. PREM, M.D., F.A.C.O.G.

Hospital-based outpatient (ambulatory) surgery centers are rapid-turnover, high-volume facilities designed to provide high-quality minor surgical services. Patients who utilize these centers (variously described as "In-and-Out," "Short-Stay," "Same-Day," "Not-for-Admission," "Day," and "Outpatient" surgery units) free beds for inpatient care and avoid one to three days of hospitalization and the need for many laboratory, pharmacy, and central services. Although the patient appears to gain the most, surgeons, insurance carriers, and hospitals also benefit. Because 20 to 40% of the operations performed on inpatients could be done as ambulatory surgery,[1] ambulatory surgery centers contribute significantly to health-care cost containment.

HOSPITAL-BASED VERSUS FREE-STANDING UNITS

Although both hospital-based and free-standing units can function successfully, the immediate backup provided by the hospital in the event of serious complications allows a wider variety of procedures to be performed in the hospital-based unit. Also, the utilization of the hospital's laboratory, pharmacy, and central services eliminates duplication of equipment and staff.

Before the Ambulatory Surgical Center was started at the University of Minnesota, the inpatient operating facilities had become seriously inadequate. Because the hospital is a referral and tertiary-care center, many of the operative procedures are long and complicated, leaving little time for minor procedures. Increasingly, operations were being performed at nearby private hospitals to reduce the frequency of cancellations, which are embarrassing for the surgeon and upsetting for the patient. Therefore, the University established an ambulatory surgery center in the Outpatient Department that is connected to the main hospital by a skyway and a tunnel. This physical arrangement has the advantages of both the free-standing and hospital-based units and is used, not only by outpatients, but also by some inpatients who require minor surgery.

REQUIREMENTS FOR A SUCCESSFUL HOSPITAL-BASED UNIT

For a hospital-based ambulatory surgery unit to succeed, there must be (1) a demand for its surgical procedures, (2) suitable space for patient and staff dressing rooms and operating and recovery rooms, (3) an anesthesia office, (4) scheduling services, and (5) third-party payers who agree to cover procedures performed in the unit.

DESCRIPTION OF THE UNIT AT THE UNIVERSITY OF MINNESOTA

Procedures Performed

An initial list of 73 procedures was compiled and approved by the Chiefs of the University's various surgical services for performance in the Ambulatory Surgical Center. In the ensuing three-and-a-half years, the list has expanded to more than 190 procedures (Table 1–1).

Floor Plan

The unit has three similarly equipped operating rooms, a postanesthesia recovery room (PAR) combined with an outpatient treatment center and soundproofed treatment room, clean and soiled linen rooms, a storage room, a patient locker and dressing room with three individual cubicles, a lobby and reception area, an administrative office and registration desk, an anesthesiologist's office, and a small employee lounge (Fig. 1–1). Several of these features are illustrated in Figures 1–2 through 1–5.

Staff

According to Patterson et al., an anesthesiologist is the most suitable person to ensure the safety and proper running of an ambulatory surgery program.[2] The University of Minnesota Ambulatory Surgery Center is directed by an anesthesiologist. He is responsible to a policy committee and makes final decisions about accepting patients for surgery in the unit. He is assisted in providing anesthesia by two Certified Registered Nurse Anesthetists (CRNA). Separate nursing staffs, each with a head nurse, manage the operating area and the PAR. The operating area has seven-and-a-half full-time-equivalent registered nurses and a nursing assistant (aide), and the PAR has two full-time-equivalent registered nurses and one nursing assistant. An anesthesia aide and a central supply technician provide autoclaving and tray set-up services. One-and-a-half full-time-equivalent administrative persons attend the registration desk, which is shared with the Colon and Rectal Surgery Clinic (see Fig. 1–2). Initially, persons were employed to staff only two operating rooms, one for general and one for local anesthesia. As utilization of the unit increased, the number of staff was increased to the current level.

The primary responsibility of the CRNA and the anesthesiologist is to provide general or conduction anesthesia. They are not present for local anesthesia procedures unless requested by the surgeon. The PAR staff also manages the Treatment Center, where many outpatient procedures are performed daily (e.g., tranfusions of blood and blood products, paracenteses, pregnancy nonstress tests, removal of Hickman catheters, and postoperative care for cardiac catheterization).

Scheduling

Priority block time for operating rooms for both general and local anesthesia has been allocated to individual surgeons or surgical services that have a predictable weekly caseload of minor procedures sufficient to warrant reserved time and who have shown the most interest in using the facility. The services most active in using the Center have been Gynecology, Otolaryngology, General Surgery, Orthopedic Surgery, Pediatric Surgery, and Ophthalmology, with the Dental, Urology, and Neurosurgery services being the next most frequent users. Scheduling on block time must be completed 48 hours in advance, and the portion of the time not spoken for then becomes available for open scheduling (Fig. 1–6).

Special first-priority scheduling ar-

TABLE 1–1. Ambulatory Surgery Center Procedure List.

Abscess, small, I&D of
Adenoidectomy
Alveolectomy
Amputation, Revision of
Amputation—Digits
Anal Warts, Excision/Fulguration of
Anocirclage
Anoplasty
Anorectal tumor, Biopsy of
Antral Puncture
Apicotomy
Arch bar, Removal or Application of
Artery, Biopsy of
Arthroscopy/possible Arthrotomy, Meniscectomy
Auricular Sinus Tract
Augmentation, Maxillary Ridge
Autologous Bone Marrow Harvest
Bartholin cyst, Marsupialization of
Blepharoplasty
Blomsinger Tube Insertion
Bone Biopsy
Brachial Cleft Cyst, Excision
Breast mass, Excision/Aspiration/Biopsy
Bronchoscopy (in conjunction with other procedures)
Broviac Catheter Insertion
Bunionectomy
Carpal Tunnel Release
Cable graft
Caldwell Luc Procedure
Canalplasty
Cervical Biopsies
Cervical Conization
Cesium Applicator Insertion
Chalazion Removal
Circumcision, Infant
Cleft Lip Revision
Cleft Lip Suture Removal
Cleft Palate Repair/Revision
Cleft Palate Suture Removal
Colostomy Stoma Revision
Colonoscopy—Pediatrics
Conjunctiva, Biopsy of
Curettage of Perianal Wound
Cyst, Excision of/I&D
Cystoscopy (in conjunction with other procedures)
Debridement, Minor
Dental Restorations
Dermabrasion
DeQuerveins Repair
Digital Nerve Repair
D & C
Dressing Changes
Dupuytren's Contracture Release
Ectropion Repair
Entropion
Esophageal Dilatation
Esophagoscopy
Ethmoidectomy
Exam Under Anesthesia
External Skin Tag Excision
Eye Muscle Recession/Resection
Facial Fracture Apparatus, Removal of
Fingernail Removal
Fistulectomy
Fistulotomy
Foreign Body Removal
Fractures, Open/Closed Reduction
Internal Fixation (Nasal, Hand, Foot)
Frenectomy
Ganglion, Excision of
Gastroscopy
Gastrostomy
Granulation, Excision of (sperm)
Gynecomastia, Excision of
Heel Cord Lengthening
Hemorrhoidectomy, External
Herniorrhaphy, Inguinal, Incisional Epigastric, Umbilical
Hickman-Broviac Catheter Insertion
Hydrocele Repair
Hypertrophied Anal Papilla Excision
Hysteroscopy
Intranasal Buttons, Removal of
Internal Anal Sphincterotomy
IUD Insertion/Removal
Iridium Applicator Insertion
Jaw Wiring/Removal
"Joint" Fusion
Joint Manipulation
Joint Decompression
Jones Tube Insertion/Removal
Kidney, Needle Biopsy
Lacerations, Repair of
Lacrimal Duct Probing
Laparoscopy
Laparoscopic Tubal Ligation
Laryngoscopy
Laser Therapy, Cervical, Vaginal Vulvar lesions
Laveen Shunt Insertion
Lesion, Excision/Biopsy of
Lipoma, Excision of
Liver Biopsy—Needle
Lymph Node Biopsies
Lid Repair
Marsupialization Sinus/Cyst
Mammoplasty, Augmentation
Meatoplasty
Morton's Neuroma, Excision of
Motor Point Block
Muscle Biopsies
Nasal Antral Windows
Nasal Polypectomy
Nerve Release
Nerve Repair
Neuroma, Excision of
Neurolysis
Nevus, Removal of
Odontectomy
Orchiopexy
Orchiectomy
Otoplasty
Orbital Wire, Removal of
Penile Prosthesis Implantation
Pessary Placement
Pelvis, Needle Biopsy of
Perianal Abscess, I&D of
Phalloplasty
Pilonidal Cystectomy
Pin Removal
Plantar Wart Excision
Plate Removal
Pulley Thumb Release
PE Tube Insertion
Prosthesis Fitting—Eye
Preauricular Cystectomy
Proctoscopy, Pediatric
Pterygium, Removal
Ptosis, Repair
Retinal Implant Removal
Rhizotomy, Intercostal
Rhinoplasty
Scar Revision-Z-plasty, Excision Keloid
Screw Removal
Sebaceous Cystectomy
Secondary Closure of Surgical Wounds
Septoplasty
Skin Biopsy/Excision of Lesion
Split Thickness Skin Graft
Shunt Revision
Sternal Wire Removal
Strabismus Repair
Spinal Tap
Subcutaneous Lesion, Excision of
Sphincterotomy
Sphincterostomy
Stapedectomy
Suture Removal
Syndactyly Repair
Synovectomy
Symblepharon with Placement of Contact Lens
Tatoo excision
Tarsal Tunnel Release
Temporal Artery Biopsy
Tendon Repair
Tendon Lengthening
Tenotomy, Hand or Foot
Tenosynovectomy
Termination of Pregnancy First Trimester
Transcleralcryoablation
Testicular Biopsy
Testicular Prosthesis Implantation
Tenolysis
Thiersch graft
Trabeculectomy
Toe Nail Removal
Turbinate Procedure/Cautery
Trigger Finger Release
Transplant, Canine Tooth
Tympanoplasty
Tympanomastoidectomy
Ureterostomy, Revision of
Ulnar Nerve Transposition
Ulnar Artery Resection
Vaginal Biopsies
Vasovasostomy
Vesicotomy, Cutaneous
Vulvar Biopsies/Lesions
Vestibuloplasty
Xanthomas of Digits, Removal of

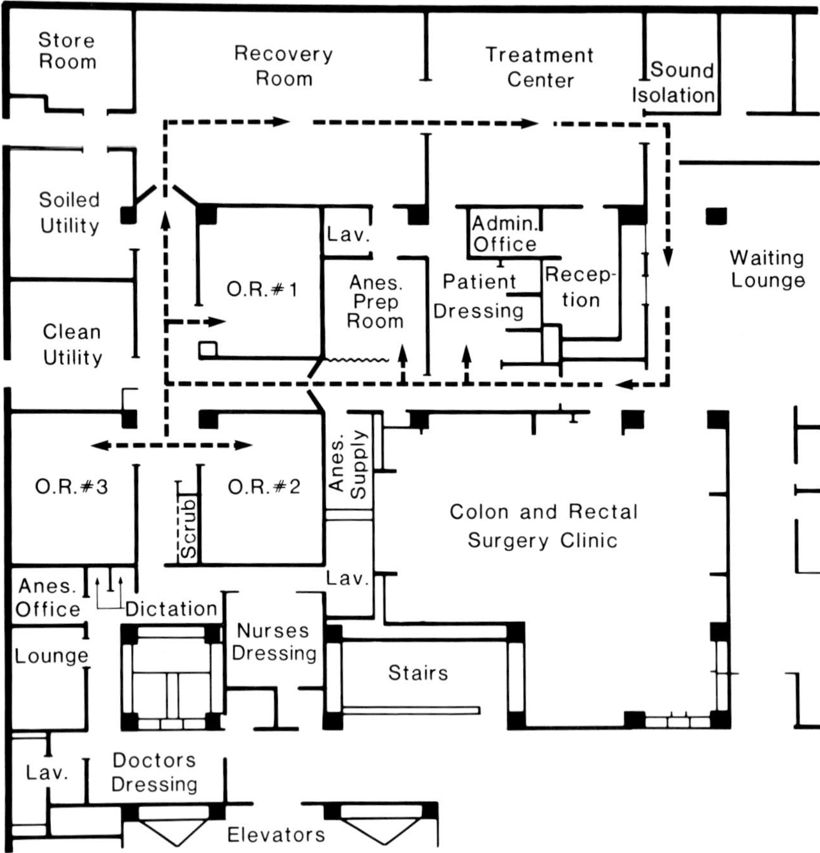

Fig. 1–1. Floor plan of the Ambulatory Surgery Center at the University of Minnesota Health Sciences Complex. Dotted line shows progress of patient during the stay.

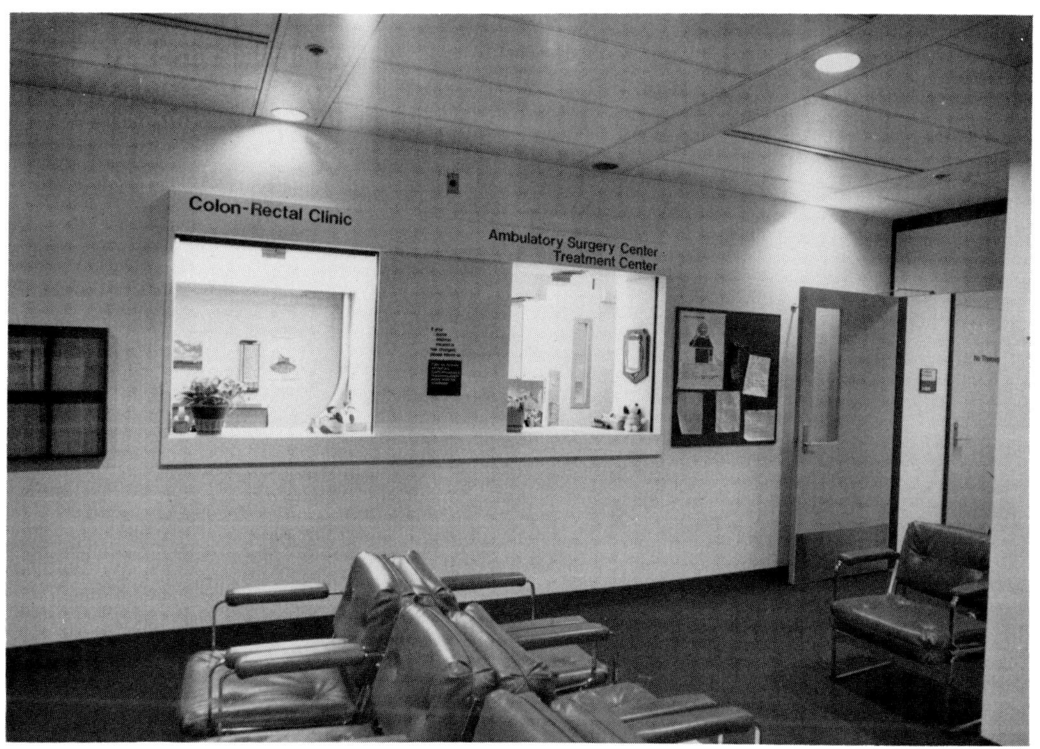

Fig. 1–2. Reception area and waiting room are shared with the Colon–Rectal clinic.

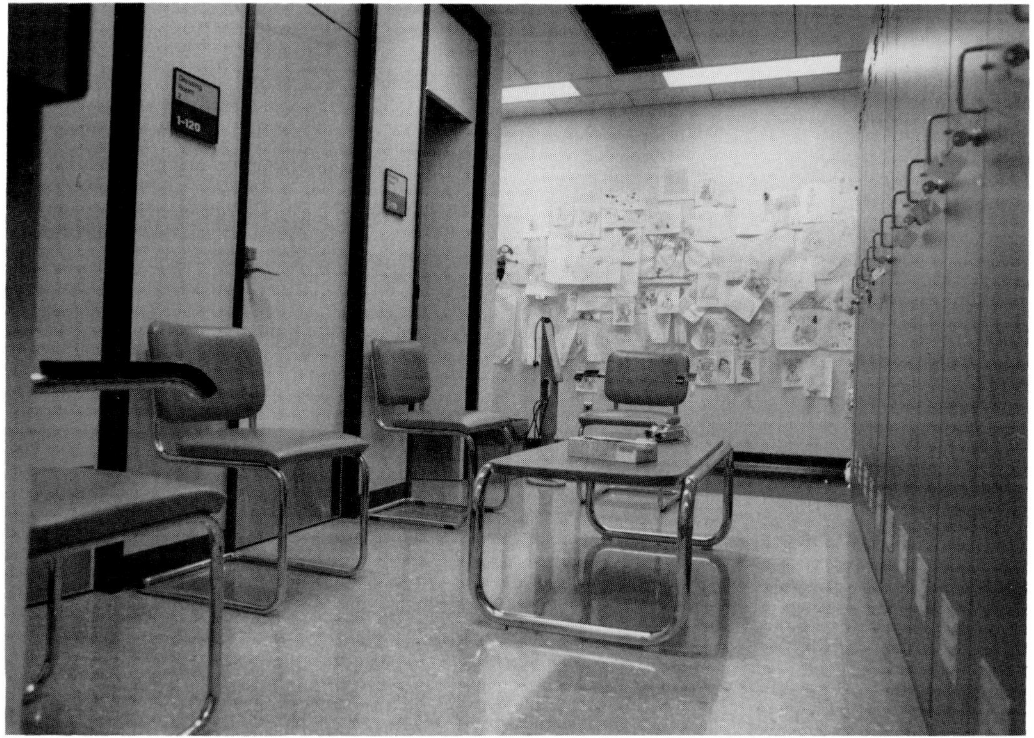

Fig. 1–3. Patient dressing area contains three private cubicles and lockers.

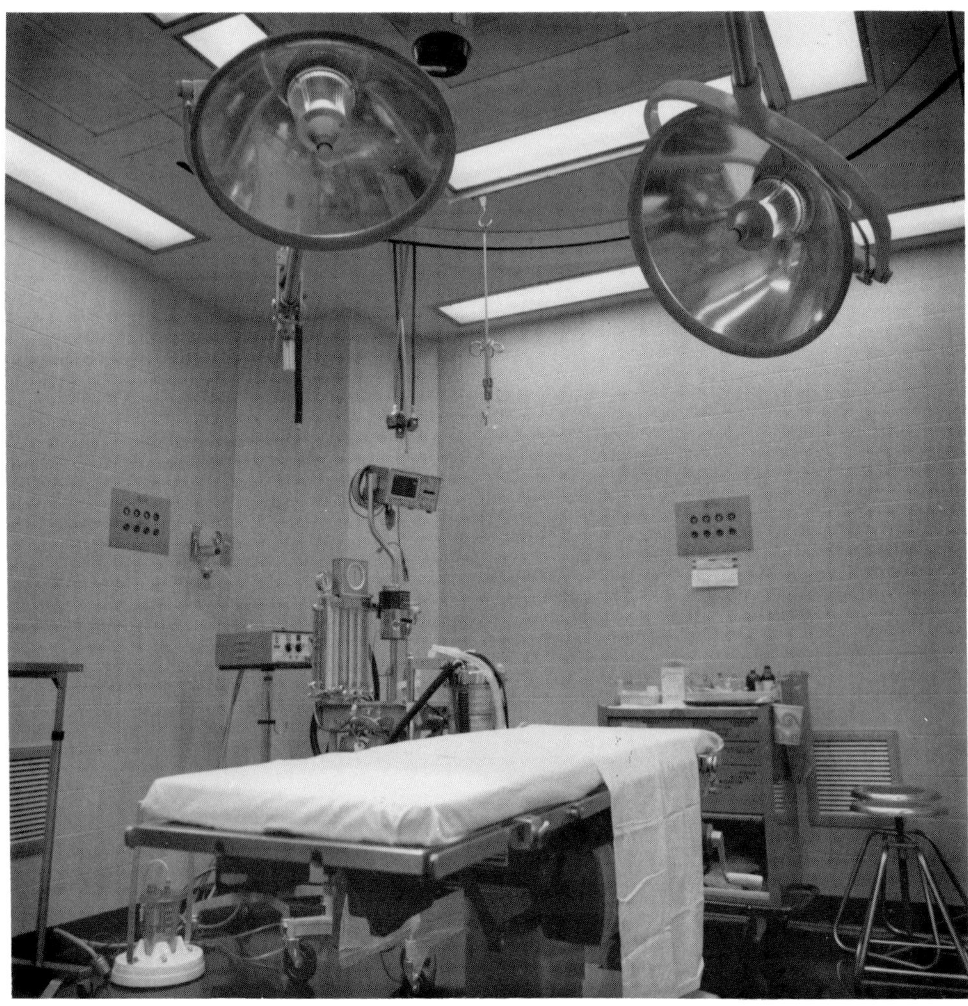

Fig. 1–4. Operating room.

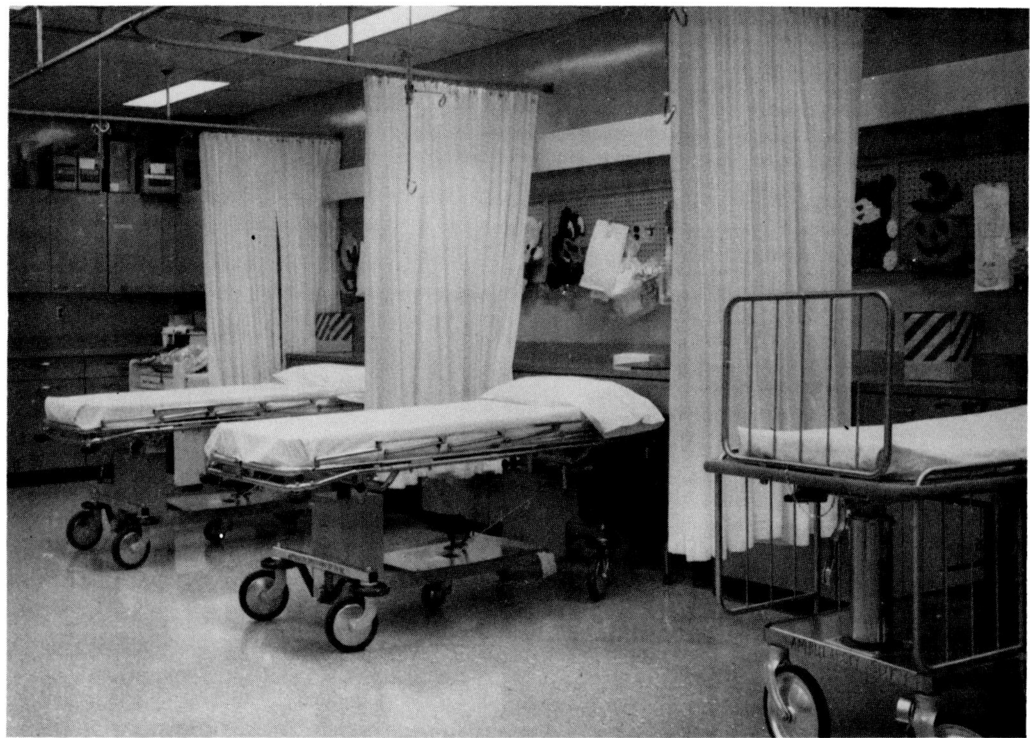

Fig. 1–5. The postanesthesia recovery room (PAR) has seven beds and two reclining chairs.

rangements also have been allowed for surgeons who wish to schedule one or two patients on a specific day and hour each week. If those cases are not scheduled 72 hours in advance, the priority is lost, and the room becomes available for open scheduling. Unallocated time is available each day for open scheduling.

Frozen Sections

Surgeons are discouraged from requesting frozen sections because of the distance between the Center and the Department of Surgical Pathology. When a frozen section is necessary, a surgical pathology resident is assigned to transport the tissues from the Center to the laboratory and to relay the report to the operating room.

PATIENT MANAGEMENT

Scheduling Brochure

At the time a procedure is scheduled the patient is given a brochure that outlines the travel routes to the University Health Sciences Complex and the Ambulatory Surgery Center. The brochure identifies parking areas and the location of various buildings, lists the time for registration and surgery, and contains a detailed set of instructions (Fig. 1–7). The consent form for the procedure is usually signed at the same time and included in the patient's chart.

Preoperative Evaluation

Safe anesthesia and surgery require knowledge of the patient's medical records and physical status even when the procedure is minor with little potential for complications. The medical history, physical examination, and laboratory evaluation (hemoglobin and urinalysis) are usually completed by the patient's personal physician and should be recorded in the patient's hospital chart at least 24 hours before the procedure to

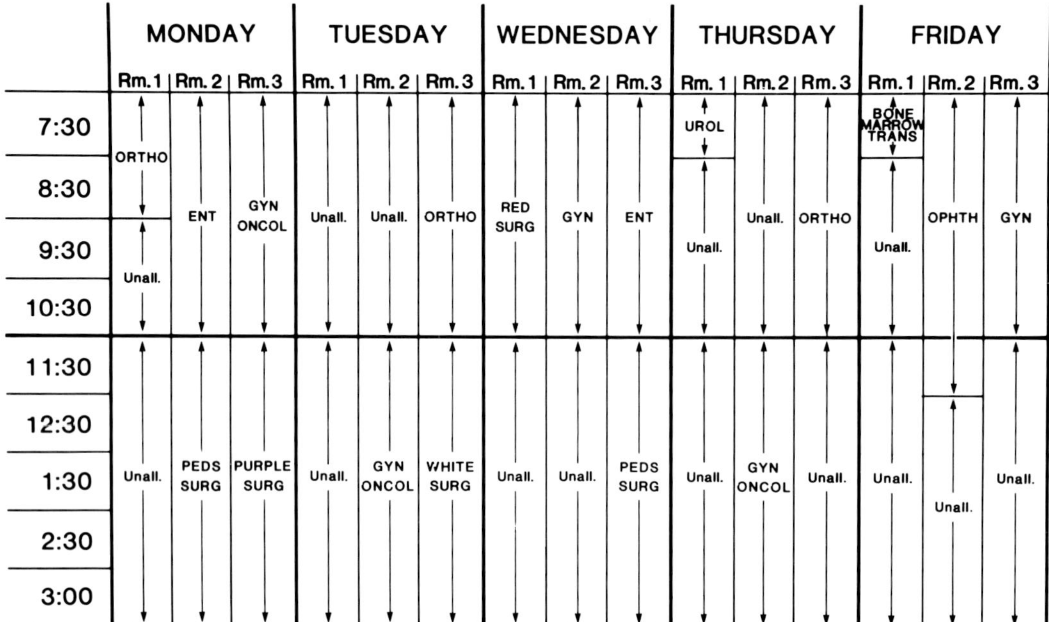

Room 1 is Available for Cases Requiring Local Anesthesia Administered by Surgeon Except First Care Priority Assigned to Bone Marrow Transplant, Fridays with General Anesthesia

Rooms 2 and 3 are Available for Cases Requiring General or Regional Anesthesia Administered by Anesthesiology

Fig. 1–6. Block schedule for the Ambulatory Surgical Center.

permit review by the anesthesiologist. A chest radiograph made within 30 days preceding the operation also must be available at that time, and an electrocardiogram is required for all patients over 50 years of age. The preoperative evaluation for local anesthesia is at the discretion of the surgeon.

Admission

The patient, who has been fasting since midnight, reports to the Center one hour before the scheduled time of surgery. If the laboratory evaluation, medical history, and physical examination were attended to by an outside physician and the records were not sent earlier, they must accompany the patient.

After registration, the patient is escorted to the dressing room, where a cubicle and locker are assigned and a surgical gown is provided. In the anesthesia holding area adjacent to the dressing room, the patient is interviewed by the anesthesiologist, the records are reviewed, and if necessary, a physical examination is done. The patient is given preoperative medications when the assigned operating room becomes available and then is taken to the room and prepared for surgery. Members of the family or friends who accompanied the patient may remain with him or her until that time.

Postoperative Management

After surgery, the patient is transferred to a litter and wheeled to the PAR, from which he or she will eventually be discharged. After the patient is awake, family members or friends may rejoin the patient. When the patient is alert and vital signs are stable, refreshments may be given.

Ambulatory Surgery Center

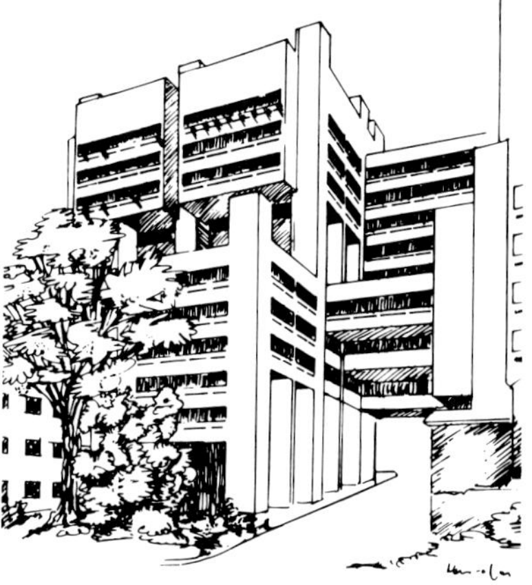

University of Minnesota
Hospitals and Clinics

Your surgery has been scheduled for:

day/date time

You must arrive at the surgery center by:

A

Fig. 1–7. Scheduling brochure. *(A)* Cover. *(B)* Text.

things to remember

Before Surgery

1. DO NOT EAT OR DRINK ANYTHING AFTER MIDNIGHT—NOT EVEN WATER.
2. Notify your surgeon or Ambulatory Surgery Center as soon as possible before your surgery if you develop a cold, temperature, sore throat or other abnormal physical symptoms.
3. Plan to arrive at the Ambulatory Surgery Center at least ONE HOUR before your surgery is scheduled.
4. Please leave money, jewelry and other valuables at home. Wear comfortable clothes, minimal make-up and no fingernail polish.
5. Arrange for a responsible person to accompany you before and after surgery.
6. Please bring the phone number where you can be reached after surgery. A nurse will call you about your condition 24 hours following the operation.

After Surgery

1. The usual recovery period in the Surgery Center is from one to four hours.
2. DO NOT DRIVE A CAR, DRINK ALCOHOLIC BEVERAGES OR OPERATE COMPLEX MACHINERY FOR 24 HOURS AFTER YOUR SURGERY.
3. Important decision making should be delayed until you have made a complete recovery.
4. If you require further observation you may have to be admitted to the hospital.

Consent

You will be required to sign a consent form before surgery is performed.

Minors must be accompanied by a parent or legal guardian who will be responsible for signing the consent form.

Insurance

If you have any questions about your health insurance coverage, contact the subscriber benefits department of your insurance company, or the insurance section of your personnel department if the coverage is through your employer. Some insurance policies do not cover surgical procedures conducted on an outpatient basis. Please feel free also to contact a patient/financial representative in the outpatient registration office on the second floor of the University Hospital Outpatient Facility, or call 376-3095. A Patient Financial Representative will attempt to answer your questions and can explain the credit policy of the Hospitals and Clinics.

Parking Locations

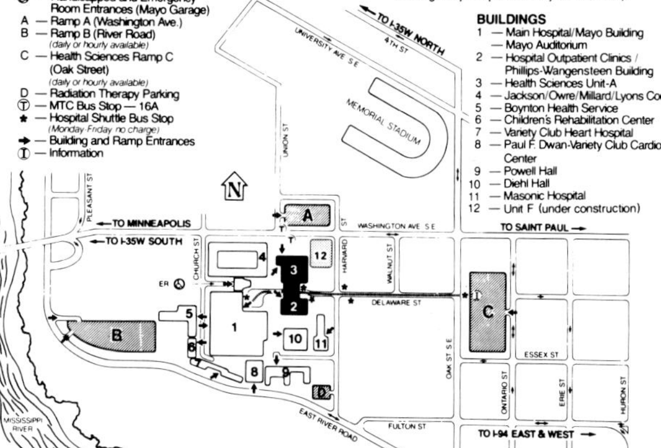

Transportation

Three bus routes (via Washington Avenue and Delaware Street stop) are accessible within the metro area from 7 a.m. to 11:30 p.m., Monday through Friday. The buses are:

Franklin Avenue Crosstown	#2
Franklin Avenue	#8B
University Avenue	#16

For detailed route schedules and fare information, call the Metropolitan Transit Commission at 827-7733.

Questions

If you have any questions or need more information, please call the Ambulatory Surgery Center at 376-2100 from 7 a.m. to 4:30 p.m., Monday through Friday (after hours call the Emergency Department, 373-8000).

B

TABLE 1–2. Cases Utilizing Ambulatory Surgical Center Per Fiscal Year by Service.

	1979–1980	*1980–1981*	*1981–1982*
General Surgery	614	496	404
Pediatric Surgery	262	210	210
Neurosurgery	41	47	57
Orthopedic Surgery	203	204	396
Urologic Surgery	22	45	52
Ophthalmology	94	106	116
Otolaryngology	281	411	404
Gynecology	311	532	619
Dentistry	10	45	42
Other	77	64	70
	1915	2160	2370

Discharge Instructions

A printed instruction sheet concerning home care is given to the patient for guidance at the time of discharge. Such sheets, which have been prepared for various surgical procedures, include instructions for activity, what to do if there is bleeding, care of dressings, pain control, stitch removal, and the follow-up appointment. The PAR staff checks with the patient by telephone 24 hours after discharge. Few patients have required admission to the hospital for any reason when the PAR closed at 4:30 p.m. Other centers have reported postsurgical hospital admissions in 1 to 1.5% of cases.[2–4]

THREE-YEAR EXPERIENCE

More than 6,500 patients have been operated on in the Minnesota Ambulatory Surgery Center since the unit opened in May 1979 (Table 1–2). For some services, especially Gynecology, Otolaryngology, and Orthopedic Surgery, utilization of the Center has increased significantly each year.

Several studies have shown gynecologic procedures to be the most frequently performed in ambulatory surgery units.[2,3,5] This was not our experience initially, with otolaryngology and several surgical and orthopedic procedures being performed nearly as often. Because removal of skin lesions and some breast biopsies under local anesthesia can be done more economically in the surgery clinic, use of the unit by our General Surgery Service has decreased.

EFFECT OF THE UNIT ON INPATIENT SURGERY

Although the number of cases performed in the inpatient operating suites has decreased since the opening of the Center, there is improved utilization of assigned operating time. Fewer major cases must be transferred to other hospitals, and because there are no minor cases in the inpatient suites, less time is lost in patient turnover.

CONCLUSIONS

Because the hospital provides immediate backup in the event of serious complications, a wider variety of procedures can be performed in a hospital-based ambulatory surgery unit than in a free-standing one. The unit has benefits for the hospital also, as it attracts patients who might otherwise go elsewhere for care because of the long wait for operating room time for minor and elective procedures. Provided there is adequate demand, suitable space, and willingness by third-party payers to cover the procedures, a hospital can enhance its value to the community and help contain medical costs with an ambulatory surgery unit.

REFERENCES

1. Davis, J.E., and Detmer, D.E.: The ambulatory surgical unit. Ann. Surg., *175*:856, 1972.

2. Patterson, J.F., Jr., Bechtoldt, A.A., and Levi, K.J.: Ambulatory surgery in a university setting. JAMA, *235*:266, 1976.
3. Davis, J.E.: Ambulatory surgical care: basic concept and review of 1,000 patients. Surgery, *73*:483, 1973.
4. Bartlet, M.K., et al.: The role of surgery on ambulatory patients in one teaching hospital. Arch. Surg., *114*:319, 1979.
5. Corson, S.L., and Loffer, F.D.: Ambulatory gynecologic surgery. Clin. Obstet. Gynecol., *22*:475, 1979.

2

Free-Standing Outpatient Surgical Units

BOYDEN L. CROUCH, M.D.

The concept of free-standing outpatient (ambulatory) surgical care is centered on a facility that is completely separated from a hospital physically and administratively and designed to serve the surgical needs of patients who are well enough to walk in. The concept is intended to deliver surgical care efficiently and to control costs.

HISTORY

The use of surgery, particularly on an expeditious basis, long antedates the development of hospitals, battlefield operations being a conspicuous example. One of the earliest reports of ambulatory surgery in the contemporary sense dates from 1909, when Dr. J. H. Nichol, of Glasgow, Scotland, told the British Medical Association about 7,320 operations he had performed safely on children on an outpatient basis at the Royal Glasgow Hospital. He wrote, "experience of herniotomy, abdominal section and other operations in young children treated as outpatients is gradually reconciling me to the view that we keep similar cases in adults too long in bed."[1] The term "outpatient," however, is at least a century older, having been used by Dr. Benjamin Waterhouse, who wrote to Benjamin Lincoln, the superintendent of Marine Hospital of Boston, on June 29, 1803: "I have instituted what we call 'outpatient,'—thereby preventing them from becoming boarders." The financial benefits of outpatient treatment were already in evidence, as Dr. Waterhouse continued: "[But] for this expedient we might have had 180 to 200 in the house this quarter instead of 143, and yet our bill for medicine has not been higher than last quarter."[2]

Doctor Ralph Waters was one of the first to publish an article on the concept of outpatient surgical facilities. The anesthesia supplement of the *American Journal of Surgery* for July 1919 described a five-room facility in Sioux City, Iowa, called "The Down-Town Anesthesia Clinic." Waters's positive feeling for this clinic was reflected in his desire that many others would develop ". . . downtown minor surgery and dental clinics of much larger scope." This facility was a free-standing outpatient surgical clinic because it was outside hospital control.[3]

A 1966 report by Doctors Dillon and Cohen of the University of California in Los Angeles on their hospital-based outpatient surgical program suggested that such an approach would achieve savings by eliminating the overnight stay.[4] In 1967, Doctors Marie-Louise Levy and Charles Coakley of George Washington

University Hospital concluded that "the real savings is in room and board; the O. R. charges . . . are the same as those in the main operating room."[5] These are logical conclusions, as there is no justification for a hospital to charge less for an outpatient surgical procedure than for the same procedure performed on an inpatient.

The first free-standing surgical unit may have been that of the Providence, Rhode Island practitioner, Dr. Charles Hill, who wrote a letter to *Medical Economics* in 1968 advocating the performance of minor operations in an office instead of a hospital. He developed a suite with complete operating-room facilities and a recovery room in a medical office building. His facility failed, however, because third-party carriers would not pay for procedures performed there.

THE "WHY" OF FREE-STANDING SURGICAL CARE UNITS

The dominant concern of health-care providers has been sick patients; indeed, it has been difficult for the "well" patient to gain entrance to the system. Hospitals have been designed and developed to care for those who are ill or in urgent need of surgical care, whereas a person who is well but needs elective surgical care often has difficulty because, since there is no bed assignment, there is no orientation in the system. Also, because the surgical procedure is elective, it is frequently cancelled or "bumped" in favor of more urgent operations.

The well patient, therefore, became the victim of hospital protocol and routine. The admitting process often included laboratory and radiologic procedures that were not indicated, and these factors, plus unnecessary overnight stays, added considerable expense in a system that was already experiencing skyrocketing costs. Concern for the problems of financing health care were voiced from all sectors, and physicians were urged to "do something."

Insurance Coverage

At first third-party payers were hesitant to reimburse charges for services performed outside the hospital. There seemed to be a feeling that charges for hospitalized patients were unavoidable, controllable, or both. The need for insurance coverage for operations in a free-standing facility was recognized by patients as well as by those who were developing such facilities. This need is now being met.

Efficiency

Although some hospitals were providing care for "in-and-out" patients, the care was frequently delivered in the emergency theater or in the regular operating arena after "important" cases had been concluded. In contrast, the entire approach in free-standing surgical facilities is optimal for the patient as well as for the medical and surgical staff. Cancellations and delays are minimal, turnover times are short, and the general efficiency is maximal.

Independence

The demands placed on staff physicians by hospitals have increased through the years, with more meetings, more rules, and more regulations. Physicians on a hospital payroll are forced to conform to the standards set by that hospital. Accordingly, many physicians feel that they have lost their professional freedom. The free-standing surgical unit minimizes such constraints.

DEVELOPMENT OF THE CONCEPT

After several years of planning and close consultation with many colleagues, Doctors Reed and Ford opened the Phoenix Surgicenter on February 12, 1969. They managed to remove some of the earlier obstacles before launching their program. For example, certain third-party carriers had accepted the idea, although with some reservations, and the facility also had the support of the State Health Department and the county and state medical societies.

The basic objectives for the Surgicenter project were published at the outset. These were:

(1) To give the ambulatory surgical patient equal status with other surgical patients in the health-care system;
(2) To streamline the care for the ambulatory surgical patient, which led to the definition of an intermediate level of surgical care;
(3) To broaden insurance coverage to include payment for surgical procedures performed outside the hospital;
(4) To limit, where possible, the spiralling costs of surgical care; and
(5) To develop an environment and atmosphere pleasing to the patient, the surgeon, the anesthesiologist, and the facility staff.

An underlying goal for these early planners and those who have worked to develop the concept nationally has been to preserve freedom in medical practice. During the 15 years of the Surgicenter's existence, it has had a favorable impact on the health-care delivery system, and the early apprehensions of its critics have been allayed. The published objectives have been attained, although it remains to be seen whether the hitherto-unpublicized objective of preserving freedom in medical practice will be achieved; whether it is or not depends on how quickly our medical leadership capitalizes on the opportunity.[6]

Challenges

The challenges in developing a freestanding ambulatory surgical facility are similar in every community in which such a project has been launched. Local physicians must understand its goals and accept the idea. They must be contacted directly and involved in its development in appropriate ways. The surgeon's office staff must know the facility, its goals, and its ability to meet those goals. Public acceptance can be promoted through talks to local groups, news releases, and local mailings.

Acceptance by the insurance industry and third-party payers has been slow in some regions. However, the development of accountability and the demonstrated savings by the facilities have brought endorsement by most insurance companies in the United States.

Mandates

Early experience with free-standing ambulatory surgical units proved that the concept was practical. The facilities were few, and most of those individuals who were involved in starting them had relied on the experiences of colleagues with a similar interest in the concept. However, complications proved rare, and more surgeons became satisfied that such facilities brought savings to their patients and that the overall efficiency was a boon for them in their practice.

Quality Control

As facilities began to appear, it was evident that a coherent approach was needed to ensure quality control and promote orderly development. At the urging of concerned individuals, including insurance representatives, a group from across the nation began meeting in Phoenix. During a 1973 seminar, the founding of a national organization was discussed; and in the summer of 1974, a constitution and bylaws were drafted. In November of that year, The Society for the Advancement of Freestanding Ambulatory Surgical Care was incorporated under the laws of the State of Arizona. The organization is now known as the Freestanding Ambulatory Surgical Association (FASA).

The need for quality control was apparent, and by 1975, the Society had developed standards and its own accreditation program. This development was welcomed by many third-party carriers, who came to accept FASA accreditation as the basis for reimbursement.

Effects of FASA

Many early claims by the developers of FASA are being validated by others. One such claim is that there is no reason to send all tissue specimens to a pathologist. The Joint Commission on Accreditation of Hospitals has agreed that this is not necessary. Also, many practitioners are realizing that radiologic and laboratory screening procedures can be greatly simplified without compromising safety. In addition, isolation transformers are no longer a standard requirement for operating rooms. The Orkand Corporation Report concluded in 1977 that surgical care can be delivered in a free-standing facility at lower cost than in the hospital without sacrificing quality.[7]

The Society now has a central organization with a board of directors who are involved with the functioning of free-standing ambulatory surgical units on a daily basis. The Society sponsors annual meetings that promote the concept and offer a forum for the development of new approaches to outpatient surgical care. Members of the Society also have worked effectively with Congress; and in 1980, Public Law No. 96–499 was passed, which, when funded, will include the Medicare program as part of the savings now enjoyed by nongovernmental insurance carriers.

The Society's devotion to the primary tenets of cost control and high-quality medical care serves as its basis of identity as an advocate in the health-care delivery system. In 1970, few hospitals claimed to have an outpatient surgical program; as of 1984, there are only a few hospitals that do *not* claim to have such a program. Thus, the Society as an independent organization has favorably influenced the health-care delivery system. It is the aim of the Society to preserve its independent stature devoted to the free-standing care center concept.

Accreditation

Before The Accreditation Association for Ambulatory Health Care was formed, the general consensus was that these new outpatient units were not hospitals, but that their capabilities were beyond those of the surgeon's office.

Organizations such as The American Group Practice Association, The National Association of Community Health Centers, Inc., The Medical Group Management Association, and The American College Health Association began to appear in ambulatory health care. In an effort to understand the needs of, and to provide an accreditation program to serve such outpatient facilities, The Accreditation Association for Ambulatory Health Care, Inc. (AAAHC) was incorporated on March 22, 1979, and conducted its first survey on May 7, 1979. The FASA also recognized its responsibilities for maintaining quality control in a new intermediate level of care; appropriately, it was active in the founding of this accreditation program, which marked the beginning of a new era of quality control.

The surveyors for AAAHC are physicians or administrators who are acquainted with the daily problems of the organization to be surveyed; thus they are able to survey as critics and counselors and to approach problems directly. A facility that does not meet AAAHC standards becomes a direct concern of the surveyor. This approach has been refreshing to many physicians who are accustomed only to signing charts in preparation for a survey. The AAAHC has developed its own training program and relies on surveyors who serve without compensation. The summary conference at the end of a survey procedure is an open meeting, to which all staff of the facility are invited. This allows evaluation and criticism of the facility as well as of the surveyors, with constructive results.

FACILITY DEVELOPMENT

Varied approaches to meet the community's need for free-standing ambulatory surgical care are reflected in the personality of the new facility (Fig. 2–1). However, construction and operational trends are surfacing that suggest preferred patterns.

Construction

Few facilities have fewer than two operating rooms, and most planners consider four to be serviceable and practical. The Salt Lake Surgical Facility is believed to be the largest free-standing surgical unit, with eight operating rooms.

One functional design is shown in Figure 2–2. A holding area large enough to accommodate one patient for each operating room is suggested (Fig. 2–3); this would include a toilet and changing room. The recovery area must be sufficient to accommodate at least four patients for each operating room (Fig. 2–4), and a waiting room large enough for six adults per operating room is needed (Fig.

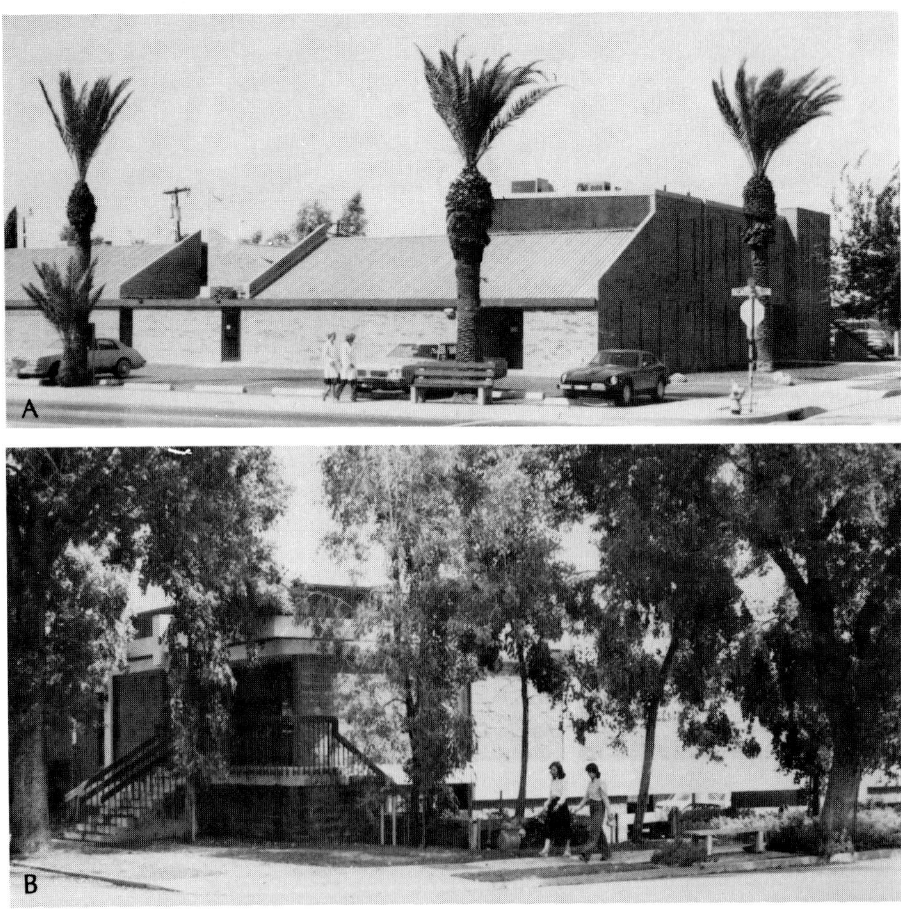

Fig. 2–1. *A*) Phoenix Surgicenter, (*B*) The Palo Alto Surgicenter.

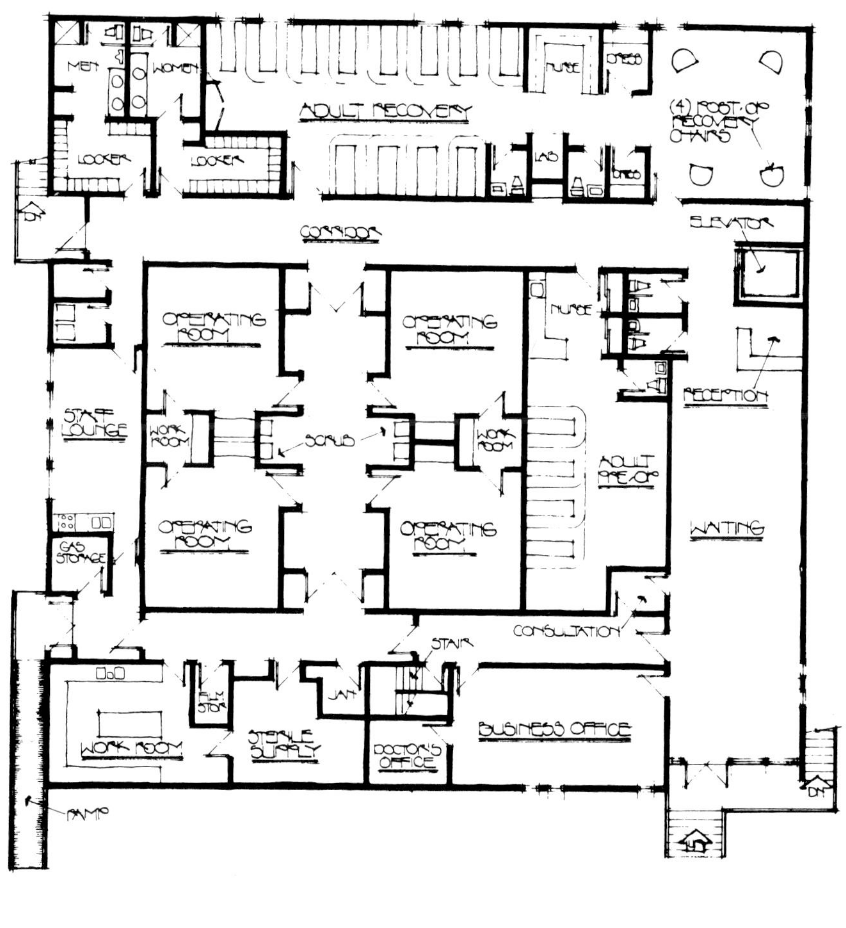

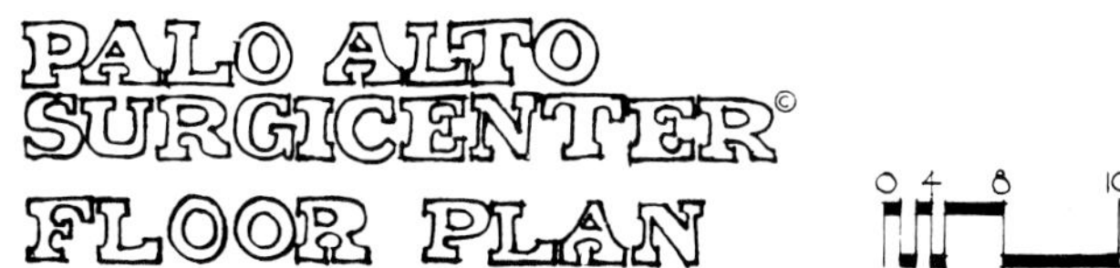

Fig. 2–2. Floor plan of the Palo Alto Surgicenter shows one effective layout.

2–5). At least ten parking spaces are necessary for each operating room to accommodate patients, family, staff, surgeons, and service staff. Storage and equipment areas are usually too small. The lounge and dressing areas for the staff should be comfortable and give each planner an opportunity to develop the personality of the facility. Bright and cheerful colors and innovative architecture make a free-standing unit strikingly different from a hospital (Fig. 2–6).

Staff

The basic staff includes a head nurse and two other nurses, with 1.25 recovery-room nurses and 0.5 orderlies for each operating room. One instrument technician is needed for every four operating rooms. Key office staff includes one reception and admitting person, one scheduling person, and three persons for business and accounting. A secretary can often assist with admitting and scheduling during heavy periods and also func-

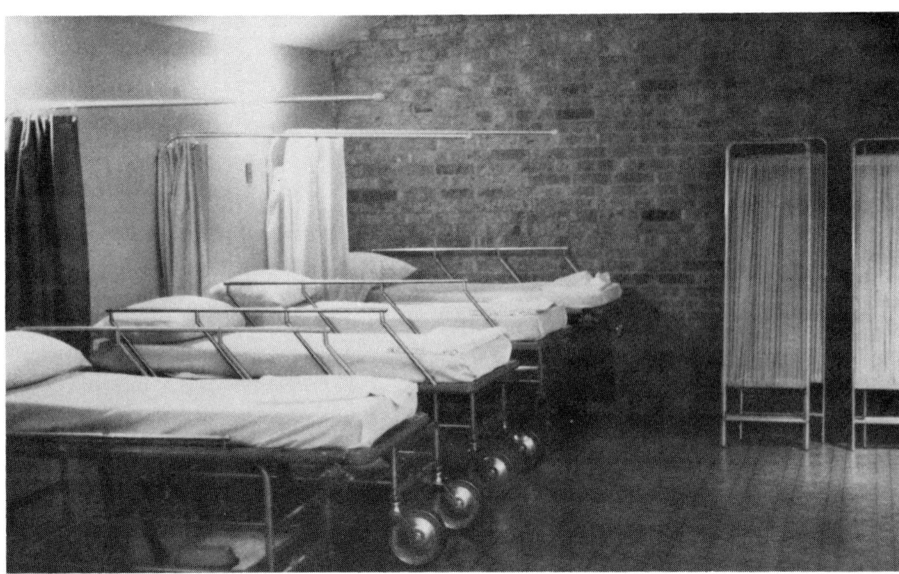

Fig. 2–3. Adult preoperative holding area.

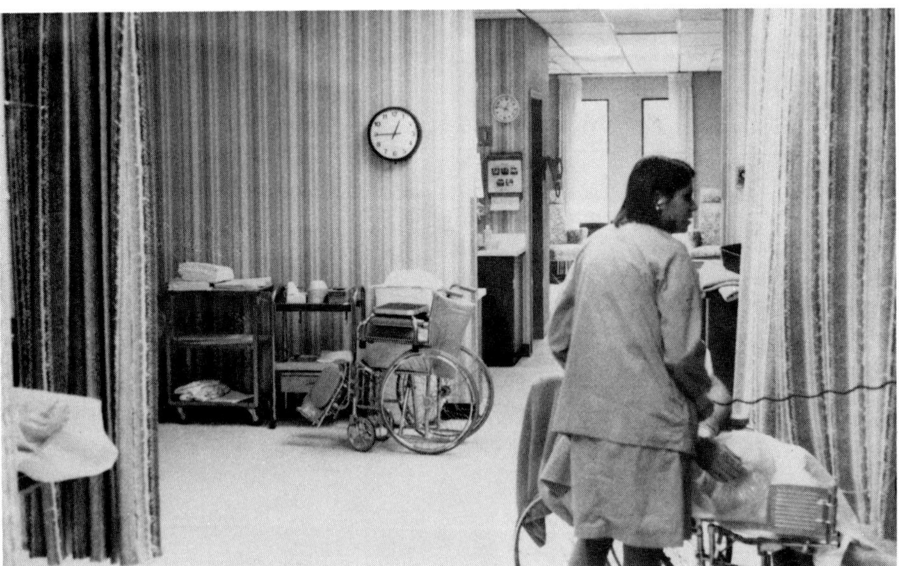

Fig. 2–4. Adult postoperative recovery area.

tion as a transcriptionist. General accounting services may be obtained from an outside source when needed. A medical director and an office manager are basic in the personnel structure. Thus, the total number of staff members is approximately 25, excluding janitorial and grounds maintenance staff.

THE FUNCTIONING FREE-STANDING AMBULATORY SURGICAL UNIT

Each activity in the daily operations of the unit is aimed at meeting all the goals previously enumerated in this chapter.

The facility and staff of a free-standing surgical unit can be scheduled in advance

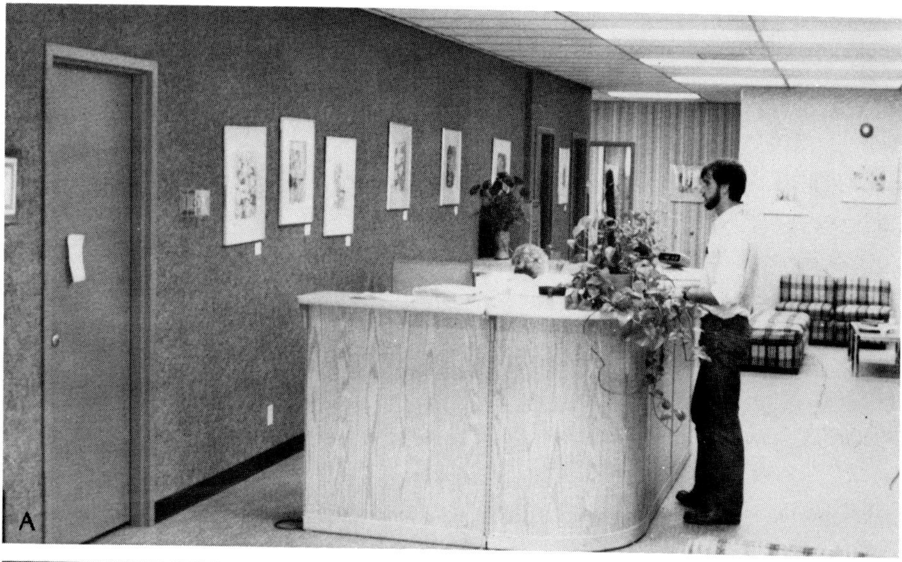

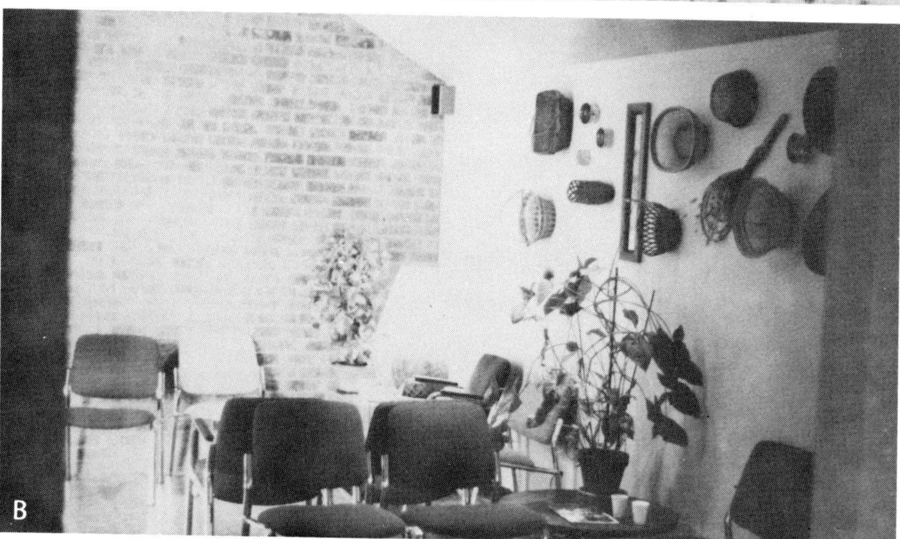

Fig. 2–5. Reception (*A*) and waiting (*B*) areas. Arrangement and decoration are strikingly different from those of hospitals.

to assure treatment of a patient for a particular length of time on a specified day. This allows efficient scheduling as well as smooth operating-room turnover. Many facilities are using a one-page record designed by Doctors Reed and Ford of the Phoenix Surgicenter, which conserves paper and time in scheduling, case development, and chart retrieval. The surgeon's efficiency is enhanced by having the evaluation history and physical examination done by the anesthesiologist, who is also responsible for the anesthetic record, discharge summary, postoperative management, and discharge. The surgeon performs the operation, dictates a descriptive note, and signs the chart.

The patient is asked to arrive at the facility no less than 45 minutes before the time scheduled for the operation. This requirement, and the assurance that the procedure will be performed as sched-

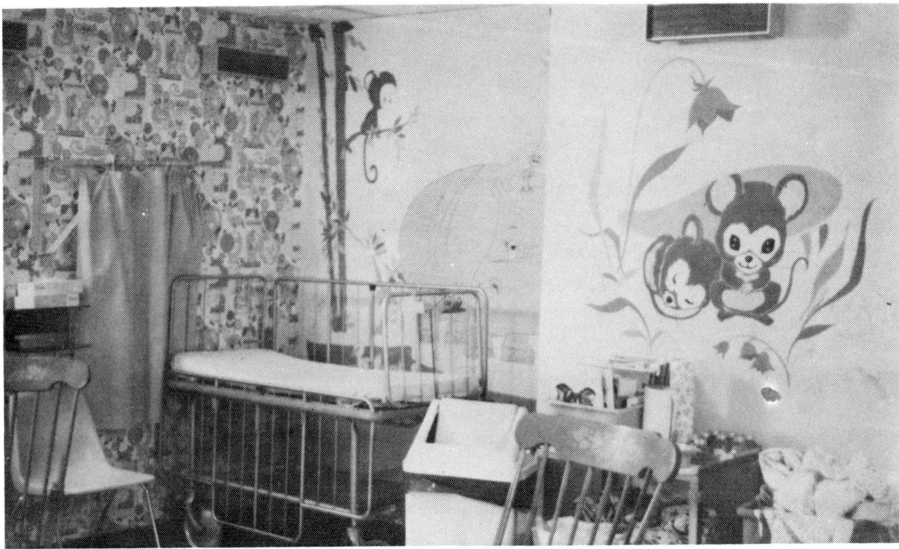

Fig. 2–6. Pediatric area. Designs and bright colors help reduce the child's fears.

uled, allows the patient's family to plan their day. This conserves home expense, a factor usually not included in determining health-care costs, but nonetheless significant.

Most facilities operated by members of FASA have adopted an all-inclusive fee schedule, which means that the entire facility charge can be known before the patient is admitted. This policy has been welcomed by insurance companies as well as patients, because it facilitates budgeting and actuarial planning.

Since the patients are basically well and their condition has already been diagnosed, a full diagnostic work-up is not indicated. The cost of unnecessary routine laboratory tests, radiologic examinations, and electrocardiograms can thus be avoided. The laboratory examinations that are usually required are dip-stick urinalysis and hemoglobin determinations, which are helpful to the anesthesiologist in making a preoperative evaluation. If needed, more extensive tests can be done through independent laboratories. Preoperative evaluation of healthy children has made it possible to eliminate hemoglobin determinations for most of them. Except for patients undergoing long procedures with local or regional anesthesia, preoperative medications are seldom needed.

Scope of Care

Procedures that do not require extensive invasion of the dura, pleura, or peritoneum generally can be performed in a free-standing facility. The limiting factors in ambulatory surgical care include the physical status of the patient and the anticipated extent of postoperative care in relation to the ability of the home to provide it. The most frequently performed procedures are diagnostic dilatation and curettage, laparoscopy, arthroscopy with or without meniscectomy, myringotomy, inguinal herniorrhaphy, and various plastic surgical procedures. Ophthalmologic procedures have increased, with cataract extraction and retinal detachment repair being performed more frequently. The early return of elderly patients to a known home environment has usually proved to be advantageous.

Physician Involvement

The involvement of qualified anesthesiologists is vital to the successful day-today operation of an outpatient surgical facility. Also, surgeons are recognizing the importance of becoming involved with the development of these facilities in their communities. It is interesting that most free-standing ambulatory surgical facilities have been developed as for-profit organizations yet have lowered the surgical charges in their communities.

CONCLUSIONS

The development of the free-standing ambulatory surgical concept has brought a new dimension to the health-care delivery system. Improved care for "well" surgical patients and the reduction of costs have been notable achievements. Physicians are beginning to realize that their involvement in the facility aspects of surgical care will preserve freedom for their patients and themselves, and that such freedom will continue to improve the quality of health care. The satisfaction of direct involvement in the delivery of health care is real. The facilities are small, and the staff works closely and develops a good rapport. The bureaucratic maze of larger hospitals is avoided. Direct physician involvement in the development of free-standing facilities, and the continued dedication to high-quality care and cost containment, will assure the expansion of the free-standing outpatient surgical concept.

REFERENCES

1. Nichole, J.H.: The surgery of infancy. Br. Med. J., *2*:753, 1909.
2. Thurm, R.H.: Doctor Benjamin Waterhouse and the Boston Marine Hospital. Ann. Intern. Med., *76*:801, 1972.
3. Waters, R.M.: The down-town anesthesia clinic. Am. J. Surg., *33*:71, 1919.
4. Cohen, D.D., and Dillon, J.B.: Anesthesia for outpatient surgery. J. Am. Med. Assoc., *196*:1114, 1966.
5. Levy, M.L., and Coakley, C.S.: Survey of in and out surgery—first year. Report by the Department of Anesthesiology of George Washington University Hospital, 1967.
6. Reed, W.A.: The Surgicenter experience. Contemp. Surg., *20*:66, 1982.
7. The Orkand Corporation: Comparative Evaluation of Costs, Quality, and System Effects of Ambulatory Surgery Performed in Alternative Settings. Executive Summary, December, 1977.

3

Office-Based Outpatient Surgical Units

HAROLD P. McDONALD, JR., M.D.

Endoscopic procedures have been part of office surgery since the early days of urology, when cocaine was used to anesthetize the urethra. Currently, lidocaine and similar drugs are used. Unfortunately, too many cystoscopic examinations have been done under such local anesthesia and have resulted in undue suffering.

As increased financial resources became available to even the poorest patients, cystoscopic procedures were increasingly performed in hospitals or outpatient surgery clinics under general or spinal anesthesia. Unfortunately, this approach has several disadvantages, namely increased expense, uneconomical use of the urologist's time, and increased anesthetic hazard.

DISADVANTAGES OF IN-HOSPITAL UROLOGIC PROCEDURES

Expense

The size of hospital and anesthesia charges is not appreciated by the public or even by physicians, because such charges are usually paid by third-party insurance or government plans. In 1982, the cost of the hospital or outpatient surgical unit and anesthesia ranged from 800 to 1,200 dollars at our hospital for cystoscopy or short surgical procedures. The urologist's charge may be less than 20% of such a sum. Although most third-party carriers will pay the surgeon's fee no matter where the procedure is performed, the facility fee for a physician's office is not reimbursable at present; consequently, the patient's out-of-pocket costs may well be higher for a cystoscopy in the physician's office than in the hospital.

Urologist's Time

The total effort required for a cystoscopy and many other urologic operations in a hospital is much greater than the surgical procedure itself and is an uneconomical and inefficient use of the physician's time. The writing of the medical history, results of the physical examination, operative notes, progress notes, discharge summary and orders; the visits to the patient and family; the wait between cases; the wait for anesthesia to begin and end; the traveling from the office to the hospital; the hospital committee activity—all create a significant burden to the surgeon and add unnecessary time and effort to the short time actually needed to perform the surgical procedure. In contrast, the same procedure done in a urology office can be integrated with other activities, so that the physician's time is maximally utilized. For an office-based surgical procedure, the patient's chart has already been developed, the patient and family are already in the office so the physician can easily visit with them, and the time wasted at the hospital in waiting between cases, waiting for anesthesia induction, and synchronizing one's actions with the hospital's timetable is conserved.

Hazards of Anesthesia

The risks of general or spinal anesthesia are often greater than the risks of the urologic surgery or endoscopy; hence the need for preoperative and postoperative visits by the anesthesiologist, electrocardiograms and chest radiographs, and the frequent requirement for a battery of blood tests. Also, the morbidity of endotracheal intubation, "spinal" headaches, and occasional phlebitis in the veins used for infusions are often more significant than the morbidity of the urologic procedure.

OFFICE SURGERY

Since the introduction of safe, rapid-acting, and effective medications to relieve pain and anxiety, many urologic procedures can be performed best in an office surgery setting. We have performed more than 3,000 urologic procedures in our office in the past ten years and found that the analgesia, sedation, and local anesthesia to be described are safe and effective. Office surgery patients acquire postoperative infections less commonly than hospitalized patients. Patients prefer to have their urologic operation in the office without general or spinal anesthesia if possible.

Despite these desirable features, there are limitations. For example, patients must be able to follow instructions and have a satisfactory home environment, preferably with someone there with them at least for the rest of the postoperative day. Patients who have serious medical problems that significantly increase the risk of surgery, as well as those who require other in-hospital evaluations or operations, should have their urologic operation done in the hospital. As experience with office surgery broadens, however, the number of medical problems that restrict the patient to in-hospital investigations is decreasing.

ANALGESIA AND ANESTHESIA FOR OFFICE SURGERY

With the continued evolution of analgesic and anesthetic drugs suitable for office use, patient comfort and satisfaction with office surgery continues to improve. We have found two combinations of drugs to be most useful.

Fentanyl and Diazepam

For all adults and older children, we use a combination of fentanyl (Sublimase) and diazepam (Valium) intravenously plus lidocaine (Xylocaine) in the urethra (for cystoscopic procedures) or operative site.

Technique. A butterfly needle with attached tubing is secured in a vein in the patient's arm. Usually, 2 ml (0.1 mg) of fentanyl is injected through it; but for procedures that may cause considerable pain, such as ureteral basketing, transurethral resections of bladder tumors, transurethral incisions or resections of the prostate, or fulguration of the area around the bladder neck or urethra, 4 ml (0.2 mg) may be given initially. After the fentanyl injection, diazepam is injected slowly by the surgeon until the patient shows one of several signs that the drug is taking effect: a relaxed facial expression, some slurring of speech, forgetfulness of family birthdays, or a glassy look to the eyes. Usually, the amount needed is $\leq$ 10 mg, although for patients who take tranquilizers or drink alcohol regularly, the amount needed may be as much as 40 or 50 mg. After the procedure is under way, small additional amounts of diazepam may be given if the patient becomes very talkative or otherwise appears to be emerging from sedation.

The patient's blood pressure, pulse, and breathing are monitored throughout the procedure. A semiautomatic blood pressure cuff (Fig. 3–1) is used, and a pulse monitor with an audible beep is attached to the patient's finger (Fig. 3–2).

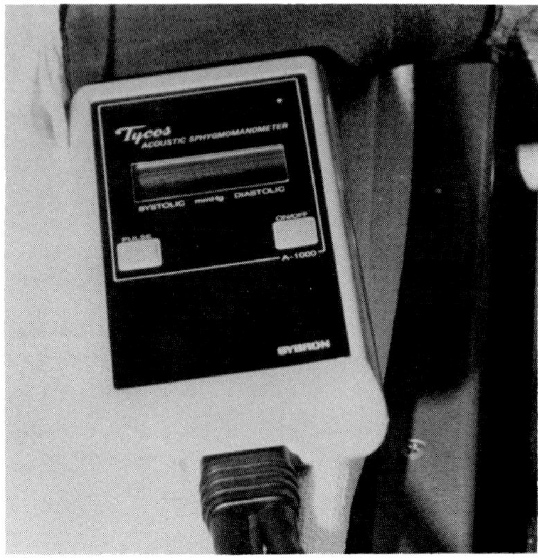

Fig. 3–1. Semiautomatic blood pressure and pulse monitor (Tycos Acoustic Sphygmomanometer; Sybron Corp., PO Box 23077, Rochester, N.Y. 14692).

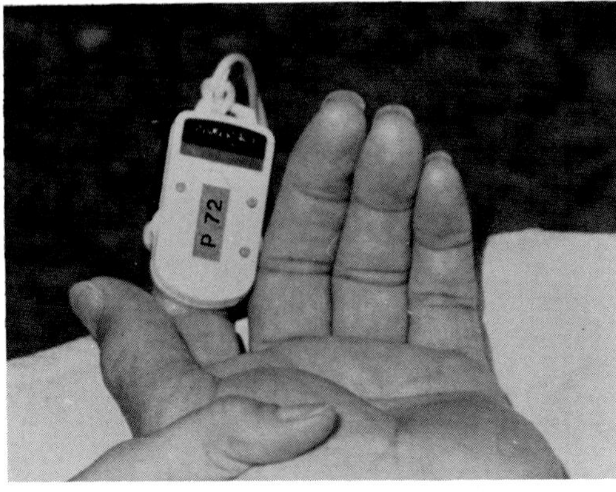

Fig. 3–2. Audible and readout pulse-rate monitor (Pulse Tach; Prime Microelectronic Instruments, Inc., 2319 Foothill Drive, Salt Lake City, Utah 84109).

During the procedure, the patient usually listens to peaceful music through small earphones. After the operation, the patient is usually ready to get dressed within 30 minutes or less.

Advantages. The advantages of using a combination of fentanyl and diazepam are its rapid onset and short duration of action, its safety, and its amnesic effect. Patients do not suffer nausea, vomiting, or diarrhea, and pulse and blood-pressure changes are rare. Not only are patients relieved of their anxiety during the procedure, but afterward they generally do not remember its discomforts or even its events. Because of this amnesic effect, the immediate postoperative instructions and precautions must be given to the patient and his companion both orally and in writing.

Antidotes. Both fentanyl and diazepam can cause respiratory depression. Thus, we insist that the patient breathe deeply, especially during the first 3 or 4 minutes after receiving the drugs, and take deep breaths periodically throughout the procedure. Drugs in well-identified containers, and equipment that includes oxygen, endotracheal tubes, and an electrocardiograph with immediate by-telephone interpretation, are readily available in case of an emergency. Routines have been established to deal with emergencies, and all staff members are certified in cardiopulmonary resuscitation. Arrangements for admission to a nearby hospital have been established.

Drugs that specifically reverse or counteract the effects of fentanyl and diazepam are easily found in the emergency drug kit, and can be injected through the butterfly needle that is left in the patient's arm through the immediate postoperative period. Naloxone hydrochloride, 1 ml (0.4 mg) is used to reverse fentanyl. Doxapram hydrochloride, 1–2 ml (20 mg per milliliter) can be injected to stimulate breathing; it also tends to make the patient more alert and awake.

Physostigmine salicylate, 1 ml (1 mg) can be given intravenously to counteract the effects of diazepam but may cause gastrointestinal cramping, particularly if administered too rapidly. Ringer's lactate and intravenous infusion containers of 500 and 1,000 ml are available.

Ketamine and Diazepam

For boys between the ages of 1 and 10 years who are undergoing circumcision or urethral meatotomy, we use ketamine (Ketalar), 1.5 mg/pound, subcutaneously in the buttocks while the patient's mother or father is holding him. About 10 minutes later, when the boy is sedated and somewhat disassociated from the activity in the room, he is given 1 mg of diazepam intravenously. For circumcisions, the penis is then blocked with 0.5% lidocaine; for urethral meatotomies, the lidocaine is injected directly into the operative site.

The dose of ketamine used is approximately 25% of the anesthetic dose and provides sufficient disassociation from the activity of the medical staff to allow injection of the local anesthetic without resistance by the patient. After the local anesthetic has been given, the child is peaceful throughout the short procedure. The postanesthesia nightmares sometimes generated by ketamine are attenuated by the diazepam, so instead of dreaming of dragons and snakes, the child may dream of pink flowers and elephants.

Local Anesthetics

As noted, a local anesthetic (0.5 or 1% lidocaine) is given after the analgesic and sedative drugs have been injected.

For vasectomy, varicocele ligation, and removal of skin lesions, the anesthetic is injected directly into the operative area. For penile skin biopsies and urethral meatotomies, the anesthetic is injected around and into the area.

For penile prosthesis insertion, a dorsal penile block with 1% lidocaine followed by anesthetic injection into the site of the skin incision is all that is necessary. (We use a vertical midline upper-scrotal incision beginning at the penoscrotal junction.) For the inflatable prosthesis, the spermatic cord is blocked on the side where the reservoir is to be inserted. Anesthetic is also needed in the area of the inguinal ring for placement of the reservoir in that area. We also use the dorsal penile block for circumcisions in adults.

Orchiectomies, operations on the vas deferens or epididymis, and vasovasostomies are usually done through a transverse infrapubic incision with a block of the spermatic cord after it has been exposed.

We do needle biopsies of the prostate perineally, with lidocaine injection at the skin site and along the expected path of the biopsy needle. For operations on the prostate and bladder neck, lidocaine is injected through the cystoscope under direct vision by means of a long needle.* Five milliliters of anesthetic may be injected into the prostate on either side or into the bladder neck area. In females, the urethra and vaginal area can be anesthetized by direct injection of lidocaine into the operative area or around the urethral meatus and the anterior aspect of the urethra from the meatus to the bladder neck[1] (see Chapters 14 and 32).

QUALITY CONTROL ACTIVITIES

Preoperative Information

When the appointment is scheduled, the patient is given a brochure describing our office surgery procedures and explaining what to do before and after the operation. Any special instructions, such as those regarding bathing, laxatives, or diet before the operation, are given in writing at this time, along with prescriptions for any drugs that may be needed

*Greenwald Surgical Company, Inc., 2688 DeKalb St., Lake Station, Ind. 46405.

postoperatively. The operative permission form is then signed (Fig. 3–3).

Perioperative and Intraoperative Activities

Circumcision of boys can be done in a regular treatment room, and most other urologic office surgical procedures can be done on a cystoscopic table in a cystoscopy suite. (We use large containers to collect outflow fluid during a cystoscopic procedure to avoid needing a drain in the floor.) The room is prepared, the patient is draped, and the operating room staff is scrubbed and gowned in the same way they would be if the procedure were being done in a hospital operating theater.

An intraoperative and postoperative flow record is maintained (Fig. 3–4). The monitoring and precautionary measures we use have been described. We have a registered nurse who has operating-room experience that supervises and circulates through the treatment and recovery areas.

Postoperative Management and Instructions

After the procedure, the patient rests in a quiet part of our office. With children, we have found that they may appear to have recovered as early as 30 minutes after the procedure, but find we avoid some of the problems of early ambulation if we insist that they wait for 3 hours before leaving the office.

As noted earlier, the patient, and anyone driving him home, must be given the instructions both orally and in writing (Fig. 3–5). The person who is driving the patient home is identified on the patient's records. Patients sign a form confirming that they have received the postprocedure instructions; this form is kept in the patient's records.

Patients who go home with an indwelling catheter have a leg or night drainage bag and instructions for its proper care. They are encouraged to drink sufficient fluids to maintain a good flow through the catheter.

On occasion, we have performed office surgery on patients who were then admitted to the hospital for other medical or surgical care, thus shortening their hospital stay and often lowering their costs.

Postdischarge Procedure

The office nurse calls the patient the following day to inquire about his or her condition, specifically about the amount of pain and any bleeding, difficulty in urinating, fever, or nausea. Should there appear to be a significant problem, the surgeon is notified and appropriate action taken.

REVIEW

At present, there is no professional review body for office urologic surgery. With possible changes in federal and state legislation and insurance company regulations, it is advisable that record keeping meet the highest standards, so that any questions about quality and patient safety can be answered readily. We keep thorough records of the surgical procedure in the patient's chart. (A typed or printed format can be designed for each type of operation, with blank spaces for the details of the specific case.) We also keep an operative book, which lists each surgical procedure performed, with the date, the patient's and surgeon's names, and the names and dosages of all drugs given.

Needless to say, one must maintain the highest standards in office surgery to assure the quality of care and one's professional reputation, and to avoid malpractice claims. These standards should be reassessed periodically by a formal audit.

McDONALD UROLOGY CLINIC, P.C.
98 CURRIER STREET, N.E.
ATLANTA, GEORGIA 30308
TELEPHONE
404—688-3321

PREOPERATIVE INFORMATION FORM

1. Statement of Informed Consent:

   I authorized the performance upon ______________________________
   of the following surgical procedure to be performed by Dr. ____________________
   and/or such associates as may be selected by him.

2. Suggested surgical procedure: ______________________________

3. The nature and purpose of the surgical procedure, possible alternative methods of treatment, the risks involved, and the possible complications have been explained to me by my physician. I acknowledge that no guarantee or assurance has been made as to the results that may be obtained.

4. I consent to the performance of other surgical procedures in addition to or different from those now contemplated, which the above named doctor or his associates may consider necessary in the course of the surgical procedure.

5. Fee for the surgical procedure:

   Operating Surgeon: ____________________

   Assistant: ____________________

   The above fee is the usual and customary charge of the McDonald Urology Clinic. I understand that the fee may be increased if complications develop. The fee includes the usual surgical and post surgical hospital care as well as care in the office for the first operative visit. I understand that I am responsible for the surgical fee and that insurance or Medicare may not cover all of the charges.

6. My signature below constitutes my acknowledgement:

   A. THAT I HAVE READ AND AGREED TO THE FOREGOING
   B. THAT THE PROPOSED SURGICAL PROCEDURE HAS BEEN SATISFACTORILY EXPLAINED TO ME AND THAT I HAVE ALL THE INFORMATION I DESIRE; AND
   C. I HEREBY GIVE MY AUTHORIZATION AND CONSENT.

Signed ______________________________
(patient or person authorized to consent for patient)

____
(relationship to patient)

Witness ____________________

Date ____________________

Fig. 3–3. Preoperative information and consent form.

OFFICE SURGERY RECORD

NAME: ______ DATE ______

CHART NO.: ______ PHONE NO. ______

ALLERGIES: ______

ANESTHESIA: Sublimaze: 0.1mg 0.2mg
Valium: 5mg 10mg 15mg 20mg
Xylocaine 2% ______cc

Narcan: ICC
Other: ______

OPERATIVE NOTE:
Procedure ______ ______
PHYSICIAN
Dx. ______
Drains/Implants ______
Specimens Obtained ______

Patient Assessment Flow Sheet

TIME	BP	P	R	Cir	Res	Col	Act	Pain	Nausea	Dsg	Meds - Tx - Observations

Discharge Score: 2 - 1 - 0
Discharged accompanied by ______
Comments ______
Instructions given ______

Post OP Phone Call:

PAIN	BLEEDING	DIFF URINATION	FEVER	NAUSEA

Other ______

Comments ______

______

______
Signed

Fig. 3–4. Office surgery record.

THE MCDONALD UROLOGY CLINIC, P. C.
98 CURRIER STREET, N. E.
ATLANTA, GEORGIA 30308
TELEPHONE
404-688-3321

HAROLD P. MCDONALD, SR., M. D.
HAROLD P. MCDONALD, JR., M. D.
STEVEN L. MORGANSTERN, M. D.

WILBORN E. UPCHURCH, M. D.
LAWRENCE P. MCDONALD, M. D.

DISCHARGE INSTRUCTIONS FOR OFFICE SURGICAL PROCEDURES

Patient's Name:______________________ Date:__________________

1. Do not drive or operate hazardous machinery or power tools for 12 hrs.

2. Do not drink alchoholic beverages for 12 hours.

3. You may eat your regular diet.

4. Activity:
    ____May resume normal activities
    ____Limit your activities the rest of the day today
    ____Do not engage in sports, heavy work or lifting until your doctor gives you permission
    ____Do not have sexual intercourse for ________days

5. Do not make important personal or business decisions or sign legal documents today.

6. Incision care:
    Change dressing: ____yes ____no when?______________
    May get dressing/incision wet? ____yes ____no

7. May shower? ____yes ____no
   May take tub bath? ____yes ____no
   If no, when?__________________

8. Take medications as instructed on bottle.

9. Call your doctor at 688-3321 in case of large amount of swelling or redness of incision, fever, excessive bleeding, unusual odor or difficulty with urination.

10. Your next office visit is______________________________.

11. Additional Instructions:

I HEREBY ACCEPT, UNDERSTAND, AND CAN VERBALIZE THESE INSTRUCTIONS.

______________________ ______________________
WITNESS PATIENT OR GUARDIAN

Fig. 3–5. Postoperative instruction form. This is printed on NCR paper, and the copy is kept after the patient or guardian has signed it.

FINANCIAL AND LEGISLATIVE CONSIDERATIONS

Government and Insurance Reimbursement

At present, the facility fee for office surgery is rarely paid by the government or insurance companies. However, freestanding ambulatory surgical units delivered high-quality medical care for several years before they began to receive reimbursement from third-party carriers, and it seems only a matter of time before the safety and cost-effectiveness of office surgery persuades third-party carriers to support it.

There are already some signs that this is happening. For example, the Medicare Law, as amended in 1980, provides that a facility fee be paid for surgical procedures done in a physician's office,[2] although the necessary regulations have not yet been implemented.

The surgeon's fee is usually paid by third-party carriers, regardless of where the operation is performed. Under some insurance plans, physicians are given slightly larger payments for procedures performed in the office, in order to encourage out-of-the-hospital surgical procedures. This practice of paying the surgeon but not covering the facility fee, however, fails to take into account the expenses of maintaining a high-quality office-surgery unit and thus discourages the establishment of such units. We believe that except for biopsies and other simple operations, the surgeon's charge should be separate from the facility charge.

Determining Facility Fees

Various mechanisms can be used to establish a facility fee for an office ambulatory surgery unit:

(1) The charges of other ambulatory surgical facilities for similar procedures;
(2) A flat fee for each type of procedure;
(3) The length of the procedure and recovery-room stay; and
(4) A variable fee for each procedure based on the time, equipment, and supplies required.

The easiest system is the second alternative: a flat fee for each type of procedure based on the staff, equipment, supplies, and time usually needed. In locations where third-party reimbursement is available for supplies but not the other components of the fee, an itemized supply list can be provided separate from the other charges. Whatever the mechanism chosen for determining the fee, one should seek the help of an accountant knowledgeable in this field.

Coding of Facility Fees

There is no satisfactory Current Procedure Terminology (CPT-4) code for the facility charge for office surgical procedures. The number 99070 can be used for supplies but is not sufficiently broad to encompass a complete facility fee. Therefore, we give each office facility fee our own code number; and for the third-party listing, we use the CPT code of the surgical procedure.

As office surgery is recognized by third-party carriers, a satisfactory coding system will surely be developed. One satisfactory scheme would be to add a suffix to the present CPT code to indicate the facility charge. For example, 55535 is the CPT-4 code for a varicocele repair; 55535-FF could be used to indicate the facility fee for that operation.

CONCLUSIONS

Office-based ambulatory surgery enables urologists to make maximum use of their time, and keeping patients out of the hospital reduces the frequency of postoperative infections as well as the cost. With the available antianxiety, analgesic, and anesthetic drugs, many types of procedures can be done safely and to the patient's satisfaction in an office. Unfortunately, third-party payers rarely cover facility fees for office procedures, and this must change if use of this safe and cost-effective form of urologic care is to be maximized.

REFERENCES

1. Orandi, A.: Local anesthetic proves painless urethrotomy paradox. Wellcome Trends in Urology, *1*(7):3, 1979.
2. Omnibus Reconciliation Act of 1980, PL 96-499.

4

Outpatient Urologic Surgery—Past, Present, and Future

ELWIN E. FRALEY, M.D.

Outpatient surgery has been done on a regular basis for a long time. Historically, "outpatient" was usually equated with "minor," so the facilities were often primitive. Of course part of this attitude was a response to the medical equipment of the times: without real time imaging methods and flexible optical instruments, there were narrow limits to what could be done without major surgery. Finally, there were no financial incentives for the physician and patient to avoid hospitalization. Indeed, as earlier chapters in this book have made clear, the opposite was true: medical insurance seldom covered even the most simple outpatient operations.

TODAY

It scarely needs saying that much has changed in the past decade. Extraordinary developments in surgical, anesthetic, and imaging techniques and equipment, as well as in the several areas of perioperative care,[1] have made it possible to do many things faster and more efficiently and to get patients out of the hospital sooner. At the same time, the public has become, not only willing, but insistent on taking more responsibility for its own health care, thus reducing the demand for hospitalization. The growth of home hemodialysis is but one example of this trend. Finally, the high cost of new equipment (the CAT scanner comes immediately to mind), combined with several years of soaring inflation, has turned health care into what other authors have aptly called the "Green-Backed Dollar Gobbler."[2]

A public need for financial relief brought a sudden change in the way reimbursement costs are calculated. The Tax Equity and Fiscal Responsibility Act of 1982 (TEFRA) established 467 diagnosis-related groups (DRG) and directed that the average cost of care for patients in each group be determined. That average has become the standard rate for reimbursement through Medicare. In similar fashion, the Health Care Financing Administration recently made several rule changes designed to encourage home dialysis and set maximum rates at which it would reimburse outpatient clinics and hospitals for the care of patients on chronic dialysis. Both of these measures are designed to make health care facilities acutely cost conscious; to make "medicine put on a business suit."[3] A significant sign of the changing times comes from the University of Alabama–Birmingham, which recently received a 64,000 dollar grant from the

W. K. Kellogg Foundation to continue instructing its third-year medical students and resident physicians in the reduction of health care costs while maintaining the quality of health care.

The burgeoning cost of health care has contributed significantly to the growth of outpatient surgery, including urologic surgery. As the cost of insurance claims escalated, insurance companies took a new and more approving look at the outpatient surgery unit and decided to stop paying for some procedures, such as hydrocelectomies, if they were done on inpatients. Increasingly, third-party payers are willing to consider approving the adaptation of other procedures to the outpatient clinic or office.

The impact of these changes in instrumentation, health care sophistication, and financial pressure are dramatically visible in Table 4.1.

TOMORROW

What is likely to happen in the next decade? An answer to this question requires some speculation about the future of hospitals.

It is my opinion that the hospital of today, with its centralized administration and financial management, will largely disappear. The hospital of the future will consist of integrated units—each of which has its own cost accounting, profit structure, and mission—around a core consisting of beds for intermediate and long-term care, operating rooms for major procedures that would be shared by the several surgical specialties, an intensive care unit, and the requisite support facilities such as dietetics. Such a system will permit identification of the true costs of various procedures and thus lower the hospital bill by ensuring that the patient pays only for what he or she actually uses. (This approach will also facilitate identification of physicians whose methods increase costs inordinately.) Accompanying this change will be an increase in home-care services and community outreach activities, which already are significant growth areas in health care delivery. In my view, it is only through such a radical restructuring that the hospital-based outpatient surgery unit is likely to be financially competitive with a free-standing one.

If this is indeed the hospital of the future, the need for the present large, terribly expensive inpatient care facilities

TABLE 4.1. Procedures Performed on Outpatient Basis or with One-day Admission

10 Years Ago	Additional Procedures Now Being Done	Procedures Likely to Be Added in Future
Vasectomy	Hydrocelectomy	Transurethral resection of prostate
Circumcision	Transurethral incision of urethral strictures	Transurethral resection of bladder tumors
Cystoscopy	Varicocelectomy	Ureteral reimplantation
	Implantation of penile prosthesis	Transluminal angioplasty
	Implantation of testicular prosthesis	Simple nephrostolithotomy
	Embolization of varicoceles	Needle suspension of the bladder
	Vasovasostomy	
	Repair of undescended testes	
	Herniorrhaphy	
	Meatoplasty	
	Angioaccess	
	Urodynamic tests	
	Percutaneous nephrostomy	
	Cyst puncture	
	Renal, prostatic, and nodal biopsy	
	Suprapubic cystostomy	

may well be diminished to the point where most of those that survive will be regional facilities confined to large urban areas. Of course, this would be a reversal of the trend of previous generations, when, under various government programs, elaborate hospitals were built even in rural communities. A forewarning of the present difficulties soon appeared, in the form of excess maternity beds that typically were a loss center for all or most of a regional group of community hospitals. These problems have since spread throughout the hospitals with the general decline in the utilization of beds, to the point where, if the experience in Minnesota is representative, many community hospitals are no longer financially viable, relying on tax levies, community donations, and fund-raising to preserve the town's or culture's own hospital, and in some cases, such as at one of the smaller hospitals in Minneapolis, luring patients with specialties such as gourmet meals that also are available, for a price, to nonpatients with reservations.

IMPLICATIONS

The picture I have sketched certainly has implications for the practice of urology and urologic surgery, a fact that has not escaped present practitioners. In a survey recently conducted by a large supplier of urologic products, most respondents predicted a tremendous increase in the percentage of urologic surgery performed in outpatient units. This shift will involve both the increasing movement of procedures such as cystoscopy, that can now be done on an outpatient basis, out of the hospital, and the transfer of other inpatient procedures to the outpatient setting (Table 4.1).

The new situation is going to demand several things from urologists. First, they will need to become knowledgeable about the spectrum of facilities available in their communities. As Doctor Crouch has explained in Chapter 2, it may be necessary for physicians to create the necessary facilities. Second, they will need to learn the business aspects of outpatient surgery (see Chapter 6). Third, they will need to master new operative techniques, such as those of endourology (see Chapters 16 and 17); make new alliances, such as those with the rapidly rising field of interventional radiology (see Chapters 18–21); and learn which techniques previously thought to be inpatient procedures, can be safely transferred to the outpatient unit (see Chapters 12–15). These changes may be particularly difficult for older urologists but are essential if the individual is to remain competitive. Finally, urologists will have to stimulate and educate their colleagues so they can develop a provider group for outpatient urologic surgery.

CONCLUSIONS

It will be obvious even to the casual reader that this textbook details precisely those requisite skills outlined in the foregoing paragraphs. For this reason, I see it as a significant contribution to urologic practice. Through it, urologists can prepare themselves for the radically different structure of medicine in the 1980s and 1990s and take the lead in reducing the cost of health care while improving its quality.

REFERENCES

1. Sheldon, C. (ed.): Urologic perioperative care. Urol. Clin. North Am. *10*:1, 1983.
2. Brindley, G.V., Jr., and Williston, C.L.: Of miracles, ethics, and the green-backed dollar gobbler. Tex. Med., *79*:69, 1983.
3. Anonymous: The upheaval in health care. Business Week, 25 July 1983, p. 44; Fisher, A.B.: Washington reins in the dialysis business. Fortune, *108*:66, 1983.

5

Outpatient Anesthesia, Recovery, and Discharge

JOHN W. PENDER, M.D., and JOHN H. REDPATH, M.D.

Each outpatient surgical unit is unique. In this chapter, we present the practices, procedures, and philosophies that have served to promote the objectives selected for our unit. Other outpatient units will need to select and alter these practices to attain their own objectives in view of the geographic arrangement of their units, the surgical procedures performed, the experience and ability of their surgeons and anesthesiologists, and many other factors.

SELECTION OF PATIENTS

As in all medical practices, the patient makes the final decision about what surgical procedures will be performed and where, but he usually follows the surgeon's advice about whether a proposed procedure is to be done in an outpatient or inpatient setting. Many factors influence this decision; the most important is the surgeon's prediction of the nature and progress of the patient's recovery from the operation. The technical requirements of almost any operation can be met in an outpatient setting; it is the need for observation or treatment postoperatively that makes some procedures less adaptable than others. Most outpatient units, however, find that after several years of experience they are doing many procedures that were not selected originally. When a new procedure is being considered for the unit, the proposal should be reviewed by a professional outpatient committee that will recommend a protocol incorporating precautions needed to preserve high-quality care.

Most outpatient units admit only patients of physical status I or II; that is, patients who have no or only slight systemic disease. However, good arguments can be advanced for sparing certain patients in physical status III, and possibly in status IV, from the dangers of the pathogenic bacteria so prevalent in many acute-care hospitals;[1] and strict rules are difficult to formulate and justly supervise. For example, we admit insulin-dependent diabetic patients but only after careful evaluation of the stability and degree of control of the disease, the past ability of the patient to regulate his diet and medication, and the supervision available in the home to which the patient will return after discharge.

The surgeon also must be considered in the choice of the location. Our unit puts no limit on the length of the procedure that can be performed, but some outpatient units do so. Certainly, recovery of a patient takes longer after a long procedure than a short one, especially if general anesthesia is used. Also, the same procedure that is done by one surgeon in an average of 20 minutes may take 2 hours when done by another. The experience of the anesthesiologist in the outpatient setting is also important; the anesthesiologist who seldom works in an outpatient unit tends to use the same long-acting drugs that are administered to inpatients. Use of these agents and techniques, however, may conflict with the objective of having the outpatient able to move about soon after the surgical procedure. Thus, outpatient anesthesia is becoming a subspecialty within anesthesiology.

Another consideration in selecting patients is the difficulty in obtaining reliable information about the home environment in which recovery will take place. Only with such information in hand can an intelligent decision be made about whether a patient with special postoperative disabilities will be safe at home. One rule is that very young and very old patients require more experienced care than most young or middle-aged patients.

Admission to our facility is not dependent on age. Patients from a few days to more than 90 years of age have been safely afforded the advantages of outpatient surgery. In a published study of more than 5,000 outpatient surgical procedures, approximately 30% of which were genitourinary procedures, the criteria for selection were more strict for older patients, especially in regard to postoperative care.[2] If an elderly patient is to be discharged with a recently inserted indwelling urinary catheter, arrangements must be made for supervision of the emptying of the collecting receptacle and for monitoring the catheter for obstruction.

Which patients, after *what* procedures should then be allowed to spend their first 24 hours after discharge in an area where the operating surgeon is not available to treat possible complications? Some surgeons have admitted patients for outpatient surgery who plan to board an airplane immediately after discharge to travel long distances. Somewhere, a line must be drawn restricting such practices. Patients referred from considerable distances are usually told to spend at least the first postoperative night at a hospital, extended-care facility, or even a nearby motel where they can be seen by the operating surgeon should the need arise.

PREPARATION OF PATIENTS

The most important aspect of patient preparation for an outpatient procedure is maintenance of adequate lines of communication. In the inpatient setting, such lines between the patient, surgeon, anesthesiologist, and hospital staff are well established, whereas in the outpatient setting, care must be taken to ensure that each member of the outpatient care team remains informed about the procedure and the part for which each is to be responsible. The scheduling person is a good hub for this communication. The surgeon calls the scheduling person and arranges for a clearly defined procedure on a certain day at a precise hour.

Written Instructions

The patient must then be provided with written preparation instructions, and if these are not available in the surgeon's office, the scheduling person mails a copy to the patient. Our instructions include:

(1) A warning about not eating or drinking before the procedure, regardless of the type of anesthesia being planned;
(2) A map showing the location of the facility;
(3) When to report for admission;
(4) The type of clothing suggested for convenience;
(5) Bringing a urine specimen;
(6) A list of the insurance data that will

be required at the time of admission.

It is emphasized that a responsible adult must accompany every patient to his home, regardless of the type of anesthesia administered. (Unfortunately, even written instructions about preparation for outpatient operations are often ignored.[3]) Also included are some indications about the postoperative course to be expected. Our instructions say that postoperative care and medication will be provided by the surgeon, that dizziness and sleepiness may persist for several hours, and that the patient's judgment may be impaired until the day after the operation. At the end of the pamphlet is a checklist for patients to use before arriving:

> Have you had anything to eat or drink?
> Urine specimen will be needed.
> Insurance form/card will be needed.
> Valuables left at home?
> Ride home arranged for?
> Plan to arrive on time?

The scheduling person tries to telephone every patient the day before the operation to make sure that the information is understood.

Medical Evaluation

Various methods have been used to screen patients before operations in an ambulatory setting. Almost all patients are screened in the surgeon's office before the operation is scheduled, but additional medical screening is usually considered advantageous. For example, some outpatient units insist that each patient be examined by an internist or a primary-care physician shortly before the operation and that the patient bring the internist's findings and recommendations at the time of admission. Other units require that patients come to the unit the day before the operation to meet and be examined by the anesthesiologist who will be responsible for their care, although many patients object to the inconvenience of this additional preoperative visit to see a physician other than their surgeon. Certainly, ambulatory surgery units are concerned primarily with treatment, not diagnosis, and each unit must decide what it considers essential. We have found it sufficient to evaluate the patient at the time of admission; however, surgeons are encouraged to discuss any medical problems of an individual patient with the anesthesiologist before admission, so that adequate preparations for special laboratory tests can be made. Facilities for a 16-lead electrocardiogram are available in our unit.

ADMISSION AND PREOPERATIVE PROCEDURES

On arrival at our facility, the patient or guardian provides the patient's name, address, telephone number, and any insurance affiliation. This is typed onto the single sheet that serves to record all the data generated at the facility. On the back is the consent form for the operation, which the patient or guardian signs.

In the preparation room, a specially trained nurse records the answers to questions concerning the medical history, recent ingestion of drugs, any drug intolerances, and previous surgical procedures. The patient's height, weight, temperature, blood pressure, and pulse rate are determined and recorded, as are the presence of dental or ocular prostheses. The urine is tested with Ames N-Multistix Reagent® Strips, and the hemoglobin concentration is measured by a calibrated extinction technique. The patient is then asked to remove all clothing and to don a paper gown, cap, and boots. The patient's personal possessions are placed in a plastic basket that is kept under the gurney on which the patient lies.

In the privacy of a curtained area, an

anesthesiologist visits with the patient and reviews his medical history, especially of any previous operations and anesthesia. In female patients, pregnancy is ruled out by the menstrual history and, if necessary, by a pregnancy test. A physical examination is performed as indicated, stressing examination of heart and lungs. The proposed operation and anesthesia are discussed with the patient and any relatives, including a prediction of the probability of complications during or after the procedure. If all agree that the procedure is desirable, the patient is taken into the operating room.

If some new or previously unrecognized problem is discovered by the anesthesiologist, it is discussed with the surgeon, then with the patient; however, the final decision about cancellation of the operation is the responsibility of the anesthesiologist. To justify cancellation, a problem must reduce the safety of the patient or the likelihood of success of the scheduled procedure. The most common reason is recent ingestion of food by the patient despite the repeated warnings.

CARE OF PATIENTS IN THE OPERATING ROOM

Anesthesia Equipment

Operating rooms used for outpatients should contain the same anesthesia and emergency equipment available for inpatient operating rooms. Although outpatients are generally healthier and their surgical procedures shorter, high-quality, well-maintained equipment should be available. Equipment maintenance schedules are essential for the provision of safe anesthesia and should not be neglected. Although extensive monitoring equipment is not required for simple operations, the entire range of resuscitation equipment, including a defibrillator and emergency drugs, must be available and properly maintained. A mobile "crash cart," with a cardiac defibrillator, electrocardiograph, equipment for endotracheal intubation, and various drugs, is readily available for use in any section of our facility. Readily available protocols outline the orderly steps to be taken in the treatment of emergency complications such as cardiac arrest and malignant hyperthermia. To treat the latter, a supply of dantrolene is kept.

Each operating room has a multidrawered chest for sorted equipment readily available to the anesthesiologist. An efficient scavenging device removes excess anesthetic gases and vapors from the operating rooms.

Monitoring Equipment

Standards for monitoring vary regionally, but we require that certain monitoring equipment be available during outpatient surgery. An electrocardiograph, a finger pulse monitor, and precordial stethoscope provide methods of continuous monitoring for patients receiving general anesthesia. Blood-pressure determinations, either manual or automatic, are required for all patients. Anesthesia machines are equipped with oxygen analyzers to ensure proper oxygen concentrations. Temperature monitoring is available for selected cases but is not routine. Plastic strip thermometers are not accurate enough to be acceptable for this purpose.[4] Peripheral nerve stimulators and dipsticks (Dextrostix) for blood glucose determination are also available.

Staff

In addition to the anesthesiologist's expertise, nursing and ancillary staff must be knowledgeable about the anesthesiologist's equipment and tasks. Nurses must be efficient and adaptable to the requirements of the anesthesiologist, especially when dealing with children or emergencies. An inept operating-room staff is a major crippler of the safety and efficiency of an outpatient facility.

Intravenous Fluids

Virtually all patients who require general anesthesia, extensive regional anesthesia, or local anesthesia with large doses of drugs are started with an intravenous drip of balanced salt solution before the operation. This is used for administration of anesthetic or sedative drugs and to provide a route for the administration of emergency drugs should a toxic or hypotensive complication occur. Our experience suggests that adult patients are better able to walk around after general anesthesia if they have received 500–1000 ml of intravenous fluid. An intravenous drip maintained during early ambulation allows for rapid fluid infusion should syncope occur, and if necessary, vasopressors can be administered rapidly by this route. Exceptions to our use of intravenous fluids include patients receiving only minor local anesthesia and children, for whom inhalation induction is used and fluid requirements are inconsequential.

A protocol for obtaining blood for transfusion from a nearby bank should be established in advance of actual need.

Efficiency

Maintenance of an attitude of efficiency by the anesthesiologist helps set the tone for the rest of the operating-room team. Patient anxiety is minimized and staff morale is encouraged when every effort is exerted to facilitate a smooth operating schedule. Minimization of turnover time between operations is a team effort that the anesthesiologist can encourage. Although the challenge of complex cases is lacking in an outpatient facility, there is a definite feeling of a job well done when a full schedule is smoothly managed by the operating-room team.

CHOICE OF ANESTHETIC TECHNIQUE

Site of Operation

Most urologic surgery is confined to the abdominal and pelvic regions, but the precise site of the operation must be considered in selecting the type of anesthesia. Low subarachnoid anesthesia, for example, would not be adequate for a renal biopsy, and topical urethral anesthesia would be unsuitable for fulguration of a bladder tumor. This subject is reviewed in Part II. Regional anesthesia of the arm is useful for vascular shunts for renal dialysis.

Surgeons' Requirements

Some surgeons are adept with local anesthesia they administer themselves, whereas others function poorly unless adequate regional or general anesthesia is established. Consideration of the surgeon's requirements is mandatory.

The Patient's Preference

As long as the patient's wishes can be met safely within the confines of the surgical requirements, the anesthesiologist would do well to try to accommodate them. In general, patients arrive in the operating room with less anxiety, have a smoother anesthetic course, and recover faster with fewer complaints when their wishes have been considered.

Speed of Recovery

Since the objective of outpatient surgery is to have the patient return home soon after the operation, the length of time needed to recover from the proposed anesthesia must be considered. As a rule, our patients recover to street fitness faster after general anesthesia than after major regional anesthesia with long-acting anesthetic agents and heavy sedation. Every effort should be made to reduce the recovery time, and a well-conducted subarachnoid anesthesia that requires a long recovery period has few advantages over a similarly well-conducted general anesthesia. Also, because most outpatient facilities close in the late afternoon, a long recovery can lead to problems that can be avoided with proper planning.

Minimization of Complications

Even minor complications of general and regional anesthesia decrease the patient's satisfaction and interfere with the smooth functioning of an outpatient unit.[5,6] Headache is common after general anesthesia but is rarely severe enough to require hospitalization. On the other hand, the postspinal headache encountered in the outpatient setting may be severe enough to require hospital admission or outpatient blood-patch therapy, which turns a smooth anesthetic procedure into a complex problem (see Chapter 8). Similarly, a sore throat may follow any well-conducted general anesthesia, but it is more common when endotracheal intubation has been performed. Since some of our patients have complained that the sore throat was the worst part of their surgical experience, it is likely that reduction of unnecessary intubations will lead to a greater percentage of satisfied patients.

Postoperative muscle pains from succinylcholine use can be severe, especially in patients who are mobilized immediately after the operation. Pretreatment with a small dose of a nondepolarizing relaxant can significantly reduce this complication. Postoperative vomiting can prolong the recovery, but an adequate medical history helps prevent nausea by revealing drug sensitivities. Intravenous administration of antinauseant drugs may help reduce the incidence, and we have used 0.5–1.0 mg of perphenazine intravenously to decrease postoperative nausea and vomiting without prolonging the recovery time. Droperidol or other antinauseants may be used in small doses in similar fashion.

LOCAL ANESTHESIA

Agents

Local anesthetic agents used most frequently include 0.5 to 2% lidocaine, 0.25 to 0.5% bupivacaine, 2% chlorprocaine, and 1 to 2% mepivicaine. Epinephrine may be added in concentrations of 1:200,000 to 1:400,000 to prolong the anesthetic action and reduce bleeding at the operative site. Bupivacaine is especially useful for long-term (3 to 8 hours) anesthesia, whereas chlorprocaine provides anesthesia of shorter duration (45 to 90 minutes). The characteristics and safe doses of these drugs are reviewed in Chapter 8.

Method of Administration

Local Infiltration. Vasectomies and excision of skin lesions can be performed satisfactorily with local infiltration of anesthetic around the involved areas.

Urethral Instillations. Outpatients undergoing endoscopic examination of the urethra and bladder do well with urethral instillation of a topical anesthetic agent. Lidocaine gel (2%) is available for this purpose (see Chapter 13).

Block of the Penis. This local block is useful for patients requiring circumcision (see Chapter 8).[7] Infiltrating with local anesthetic as the needle is advanced increases the patient's comfort. Because the penile arteries are end arteries, some authors suggest that epinephrine not be used in the anesthetic solution for fear that tissue necrosis may result.[8]

Inguinal Area Blocks. This block is useful for outpatient repair of inguinal hernias and for hydrocelectomy.[7] The surgeon should be prepared to supplement it by injecting local anesthetic into sensitive areas that become apparent during the operation.

Sedation

Anxious adult patients presenting for procedures in which local anesthesia will be used may be given 5–10 mg of diazepam orally with a sip of water 1 to 2 hours preoperatively. Alternatively, they may be given intravenous diazepam 2.5–5.0 mg and fentanyl up to 100 μg or 12.5–25 mg of meperidine at the time of the procedure. Overdoses may be avoided if sedation is produced with small doses given intravenously every 3 to 5 minutes until the desired effect is attained. Special care should be used with elderly patients, who may become heavily sedated with small doses of drugs. Airway equipment should be available should apnea occur. If the patient experiences severe anxiety or is at high risk because of concomitant medical problems, an anesthesiologist may be asked to stand by to administer the sedative medication and monitor the patient.

Complications

Because local anesthesia is usually administered by the operating surgeon, it is important for him to have a thorough knowledge of the agent being used. The person administering drugs to a patient should know what doses are safe and have a clear plan of action should toxicity occur. In general, the inclusion of epinephrine delays systemic absorption and allows larger doses of the local anesthetic to be used.

Inadvertent intravascular injection of local anesthetics may cause immediate toxic symptoms. Therefore, equipment and drugs for the management of convulsions, apnea, and cardiovascular collapse should be readily available when local anesthetics are used in the outpatient setting.

REGIONAL ANESTHESIA

Subarachnoid Anesthesia

This method of anesthesia has traditionally been useful in urologic surgery (see Chapter 10). The duration of action of the agent must be appropriate for the anticipated duration of the surgical procedure, yet not so long that the patient will require hospital admission when the outpatient unit closes for the day. An average of 3 to 4 hours from injection to ambulation should be allowed for tetracaine, whereas after lidocaine, 1 to 2 hours is usually sufficient. When long-acting anesthetic agents are to be used, the operation should be scheduled early in the day.

Epidural Lumbar Anesthesia

This method of anesthesia, which involves injecting local anesthetic into the peridural spaces, is useful in many of the same situations in which subarachnoid anesthesia is used. Advantages include a reduction in the incidence of postspinal headache, since the subarachnoid space is not entered and, therefore, spinal fluid will not leak. The block can be performed either by a single injection or by repeated instillations through a catheter as the operation proceeds; the former is better for most outpatient procedures. Chloroprocaine has been useful for short-term anesthesia by this method, but there have been recent reports of neurologic injury after inadvertent subarachnoid injection.[9] Thus, the status of this drug is controversial, and the anesthetist is encouraged to review the evidence before using it. Lidocaine solutions generally are used at our facility. Recent studies indicate that the incidence of nausea and vomiting is reduced when epidural anesthesia is used in comparison with general anesthesia.[10]

Epidural Sacral (Caudal) Anesthesia

This method involves the peridural injection of local anesthetic solution into the caudal canal. The anesthetic can be administered as a single injection or as intermittent injections through a catheter. It may be difficult to locate the sacral hiatus, especially if the operator is not experienced. Caudal anesthesia can be used for procedures in the lower urinary tract and for circumcision.

Brachial Plexus Blocks

An axillary nerve block is most commonly used by urologists for the installation of vascular hemodialysis shunts and is successful in most cases. Supraclavicular approaches may be less desirable because of the possibility of causing pneumothorax or bleeding that cannot be controlled by local pressure. Local anesthetic supplementation may be advantageous when sensitive spots are discovered during the operation.

Sedation

The anesthesiologist will frequently use methods of sedation similar to those used with local anesthesia. Care must be taken that heavy sedation does not prolong the recovery period.

GENERAL ANESTHESIA

Premedication

Except in unusually anxious patients, premedication is generally omitted. If atropine or an antinausea drug is used, it is generally given intravenously at the time of induction.

Induction

Thiopental or another short-acting barbiturate is used unless contraindicated. If intubation is planned, a small dose of a nondepolarizing agent is given beforehand. Succinylcholine is used to facilitate endotracheal intubation.

Maintenance

Anesthesia is maintained with nitrous oxide and oxygen supplemented by nonflammable inhalation agents such as halothane, enflurane, or isoflurane, or by narcotics such as fentanyl or meperidine. In general, it is desirable to keep narcotic doses small to avoid postoperative respiratory depression; larger doses given intraoperatively may require naloxone administration at the end of the procedure, and this increases the incidence of nausea and vomiting. Succinylcholine 0.1% is given by continuous intravenous infusion when muscle relaxation is required in order to avoid the difficulties that often result when polarizing muscle relaxants must be reversed soon after their administration.

Endotracheal Intubation

The need for intubation of outpatients is continually being reassessed, since it is a source of many patient complaints about sore throats. We try to restrict its use to those situations where it is necessary for the safe conduction of anesthesia. If an endotracheal tube is used, it is removed before the patient is returned to the postanesthesia recovery room.

Postoperative Analgesia

When it is believed that there will be more than mild postoperative pain, surgeons are encouraged to infiltrate 0.5% bupivacaine into the operative site to reduce the postoperative need for narcotics.[11] If this is not possible, small doses of meperidine or fentanyl are given intravenously before anesthesia is over for comfort in the early recovery period.

SPECIAL CONSIDERATIONS

Pediatric Patients

When dealing with children, it is important that waiting times be minimized. Children become anxious and noisy when smooth anesthetic routines are interrupted. Premedication is generally omitted, but heavy sedation can be induced by the anesthesiologist with 25 mg/kg of methohexital administered rectally.[12] This has been restricted to children younger than 3 years of age and produces heavy sedation or sleep in 5 to 10 minutes without prolonging the recovery time.

This method requires the constant attention of the anesthesiologist, who must have at his disposal suitable means for ensuring adequate ventilation should apnea ensue. Parents can be with the child until he becomes sleepy.

Ketamine induction is not used because it causes postoperative psychic disturbances in some patients. Rather, anesthesia for children younger than 3 years is generally induced with a mask using halothane or enflurane with nitrous oxide and oxygen. Older children may have an intravenous or mask induction, depending on the anesthesiologist's assessment. Intubation is used as required, and atropine is given intramuscularly or intravenously as required. Older children may have the dorsal nerve of the penis blocked after circumcision using 0.5% bupivacaine (total dose of 0.5 mg/kg) to relieve postoperative discomfort.[13]

Temperature monitoring is used for infants, and alterations in body temperature are reduced by the use of warm (72° to 75° F) operating rooms plus heating lamps and water mattresses if necessary.

Elderly Patients

Frequently, the patient presenting for urologic surgery is elderly and may have concurrent diseases that complicate anesthetic management. Careful evaluation is required to select those patients who will tolerate outpatient anesthesia and surgery. Care in the administration of anesthetic drugs will reduce the long recovery periods sometimes experienced by these patients. The action of sedatives such as diazepam may be prolonged in the elderly and make walking difficult.

RECOVERY

After the operation, monitoring of the patient becomes the primary consideration. Most outpatients are well adjusted to their environment before the operation, but the treatment and required anesthesia may inhibit their protective reflexes temporarily so that support is needed. The type of monitoring and support will vary widely, and rigid rules cannot be applied.

Transit from operating to recovery room is supervised by the anesthesiologist and an operating-room nurse. Until discharge, immediate care and monitoring become the primary responsibility of the recovery-room nurses, with supervision by a surgeon and an anesthesiologist. Until the patient has been discharged from the surgical unit, a nurse and a physician are always available.

Such responsibility requires that the nurses be trained in postanesthesia recovery rooms or intensive-care units. One nurse is required for every two or three disabled patients. Bleeding, inadequate breathing, and deficient circulation become the greatest threats to the patient's safety, and all must be monitored. Equipment for treatment of emergencies, including suction apparatus and equipment for tracheal intubation and artificial respiration with oxygen, is immediately available, as is the "crash" cart described earlier.

Medication is kept to a minimum to reduce undesirable or prolonged effects. Outpatients generally expect and receive less analgesic medication during the postoperative period than do inpatients. Bupivacaine infiltration into the operative site often reduces postoperative pain to the point that no narcotics are required. From the time the operation is scheduled, both physical and psychologic preparation is made for the patient to be able to walk out of the facility. Success comes with experience.

Nausea and vomiting was the most frequent postoperative complication (15%) of 7,015 of our outpatients. Usually this is brief, and patients are encouraged to drink clear liquids even when nauseated unless this is otherwise contraindicated. Only 2% of our patients required postoperative antiemetic drugs, and none had to be admitted to a hospital because of protracted nausea.

The second most common complication is dizziness, which usually occurs as the patient gradually resumes an upright position, but this is soon dissipated. If it persists, the patient can be put back into the supine position for a while and then encouraged slowly to resume the erect position. Rarely, a small intravenous dose of ephedrine will be needed for hypotension or an intravenous dose of atropine for bradycardia.

Urinary retention has not been a problem. More than 800 inguinal hernias have been repaired using general anesthesia and local infiltration without catheterization of the bladder being necessary. This result is attributed to early ambulation and limited use of narcotic medication.

Of all the areas in an outpatient surgical unit, the recovery area has the greatest potential for generating good public relations. It is here that the patient feels the greatest insecurity, which needs to be allayed by "tender loving care" sprinkled with genuine sympathy. A little urging is necessary to get postoperative patients to move around, but it must be done gently and diplomatically. The most frequent criticism by our patients is that they felt as if they were being rushed out of the unit. This criticism has been almost eliminated since we provided a sitting area for ambulatory postoperative patients. They are allowed to remain in this area under the surveillance of the recovery-room nurses until discharge.

DISCHARGE

Many objective methods have been recommended for evaluating the patient's readiness for discharge.[14–17] Most are time consuming and do not take into account all the variables applicable to an individual patient. By necessity, the final decision is almost always a subjective one on the part of both the attending nurse and the responsible physician. It is their estimation of the degree to which the patient's protective reflexes have returned to normal that determines when it is safe for that particular patient to leave.

It is essential that written instructions about continuation of care and monitoring be given to the patient at the time of discharge. Both the patient and the guardian must understand the instructions, especially what is to be done if a complication is suspected. The patient is given a self-addressed, stamped postcard questionnaire for return two weeks after the operation. This method permits recording of long-term postoperative complications.

One of the criticisms leveled at ambulatory surgery is that, after the operation and discharge from the outpatient unit, patients are abandoned to their own devices. This is an unjust accusation. At the time of discharge, a telephone number is recorded in the patient's chart where he can be contacted the following day, and a record of the condition of the patient 24 hours postoperatively is kept. A determined effort is necessary if adequate communication is to be maintained with the outpatient and those responsible for care, in spite of language barriers, distance, or irresponsibility on the part of the patient.

CONCLUSIONS

No outpatient ambulatory unit can function safely without the backup of an acute-care hospital. A written protocol for transfer of a patient from the outpatient unit to a hospital must be prepared in advance so that the transfer can be made with a minimum of delay and confusion. An unscheduled hospital admission was deemed desirable after only 0.4% of 7,015 operations in our unit. The transfers made directly from the outpatient unit to the hospital usually resulted from an operation being more extensive than was anticipated. Only one patient of the

7,015 was admitted to a hospital after discharge from the outpatient unit, and this was for the reinsertion of a nasal pack after nasal polypectomy.

REFERENCES

1. Othersen, H.B., and Clatworthy, H.W.: Outpatient herniorrhaphy for infants. Am. J. Dis. Child., *116*:78, 1968.
2. Cloud, D.T.: Outpatient pediatric surgery. Int. Anesthesiol. Clin., *20*:99, 1982.
3. Mallins, A.F.: Do they do as they are instructed? a review of outpatient anaesthesia. Anaesthesia, 33:832, 1978.
4. Lewit, E.M., Marshall, C.L., and Salzer, J.E.: An evaluation of a plastic strip thermometer. JAMA, *247*:321, 1982.
5. Riding, J.E.: Minor complications of general anesthesia. Br. J. Anaesth., *47*:91, 1975.
6. Brindle, F.G., and Soliman, M.G.: Anaesthetic complications in surgical out-patients. Can. Anaesth. Soc. J., *22*:613, 1975.
7. Moore, D.C.: Regional Block. 4th Ed. Springfield, Charles C Thomas, 1973.
8. Murphy, T.M.: Nerve blocks. *In* Anesthesia. Vol. I. Edited by R.D. Miller. New York, Churchill Livingstone, 1981.
9. Kane, R.E.: Neurologic deficits following epidural or spinal anesthesia. Anesth. Analg., *60*:150, 1981.
10. Bridenbaugh, L.D.: Regional anesthesia for outpatient surgery. Can. Anaesth. Soc. J., *30*:548, 1983.
11. Shandling, B., and Steward, D.J.: Regional analgesia for postoperative pain in pediatric outpatient surgery. J. Pediatr. Surg., *15*:477, 1980.
12. Goresky, G.V., and Steward, D.J.: Rectal methohexitone for induction of anaesthesia in children. Can. Anaesth. Soc. J., *26*:213, 1979.
13. Steward, D.J.: Manual of Pediatric Anaesthesia. New York, Churchill Livingstone, 1979.
14. Steward, D.J.: A simplified post-anaesthetic recovery scoring system. Can. Anaesth. Soc. J., *22*:111, 1975.
15. Newman, M.G., Trieger, N., and Miller, J.C.: Measuring recovery from anesthesia: a simple test. Anesth. Analg., *48*:136, 1969.
16. Steward, D.J., and Volgyesi, G.: Stabilometry: a new tool for the measurement of recovery following general anaesthesia for outpatients. Can. Anaesth. Soc. J., *25*:4, 1978.
17. Asbury, A.J.: Measuring immediate recovery from general anesthesia using a scoring system. Can. Anaesth. Soc. J., *28*:567, 1981.

6

Financial Considerations

GEORGE L. FRALEY

Ambulatory surgery units offer many benefits for both patient and surgeon. For the patient, these units offer personalized care and friendly surroundings, thus reducing anxiety and the time spent away from home and work. The unit meets the needs of the surgeon by eliminating unnecessary tests and "bumping" of scheduled procedures, minimizing paperwork, and delegating admission and discharge procedures to the unit's staff.

Of course safety and convenience are not the only appealing features of outpatient surgery: the monetary savings for patients and third-party carriers, most of whom now pay for outpatient procedures done in accredited facilities, are considerable. It is the financial aspects of ambulatory surgery that are the focus of this chapter.

SOURCES OF SAVINGS

Accommodations are the most obvious area of savings in the ambulatory surgery unit. There is no need to construct and maintain dozens of rooms with beds, or provide a food service* with the many specialized diets and staff of nutritionists required by a hospital. Also, the few laboratory tests the facility must perform are simple and do not require sophisticated equipment, so there is no need to maintain expensive inventories of reagents and machines. Radiographic studies are also simple, so there is no need for a staff of radiologists or expensive equipment such as a computed tomography scanner. Finally, rehabilitation and pharmaceutical services are not needed.

As a result of these factors, the staffing requirements of an ambulatory surgery unit are small, with an average staff to patient ratio of 1:1 rather than 3 or 4:1, which is common in hospitals. Additional savings can be effected by using disposable gowns, basins, etc., and by restricting the anesthetics used to nonexplosive agents.

It is evident, however, that these considerations do not apply equally to all types of ambulatory surgery units. In particular, hospital-based units usually work with the laboratory, radiology, and central supply facilities of the hospital; and this contributes to the generally higher cost of maintaining hospital-based units compared to free-standing ones. Thus, the charges in free-standing units are 41 to 83% of those of a hospital-based unit and 13 to 43% of those for the same procedure performed on an inpatient basis (Table 6–1).[2]

DETERMINING FEES

There are several ways to determine the facility charge for a procedure per-

*Perhaps this is not entirely true. On the list of operating expenses for the Phoenix Surgicenter in 1977 is an entry of 246 dollars for Coca-Cola![1]

TABLE 6–1. Comparison of Facility Fees for Urological Procedures in Ambulatory Surgery Units and Inpatient Settings*

Procedure	Free-Standing Unit ($)	Hospital	
		Outpatient ($)	Inpatient ($)
Cystoscopy, pediatric (1977)[1]	142	301	456
Cystoscopy, adult (1977)[1]	142	406	605
Hydrocele repair (1982)†	—	250	966
Vasovasostomy (1982)†	—	657	1,668

*Surgeon's fee not included.
†University of Minnesota Ambulatory Surgery Unit.

formed in an ambulatory surgery unit. Most of the free-standing units in the United States charge a single fee representing the average cost of supplies, staff time, and other resources needed for a particular procedure. The surgeon and anesthesiologist usually submit a separate bill. Provided the standard fee has been based on adequate research, this approach has many advantages, including simplified bookkeeping and encouragement for the expeditious and efficient use of resources.

The surgeons and anesthesiologists can determine their charges in one of two ways, both of which are based in part on the difficulty of the procedure. One method takes into account the actual time required in a particular case; the other considers only the average time required for that procedure. The former approach can create difficulties, because insurance carriers have set standard fees for procedures, and if more time than usual is required, they may not cover the extra costs. The latter approach encourages efficiency, simplifies billing, and is reassuring to the patient, because the full cost will be known before the operation.

THE FINANCIAL TRANSACTION

With so much emphasis being placed on the financial aspects of medicine, I think it is important for ambulatory surgery units to establish guidelines to aid the business office and relieve surgeons of the daily involvement in this aspect of medical care. One policy that aids in the management of accounts receivable is to require patients who have no insurance, or who are undergoing a noncovered procedure such as vasovasostomy, to pay the estimated bill in full before the operation is performed. The same rule is advisable for patients in health maintenance organizations who have not been referred to the unit. (Such a policy provides another reason for establishing a standard fee for a given procedure.) Patients with insurance other than Medicare should be required to deposit 20% of the estimated bill for a covered procedure, as most third-party carriers pay 80% of the cost of required surgery. Medicare patients should make a deposit of 40% of the estimated bill, as Medicare typically covers 67 to 80% of allowed charges. In all cases in which part of the cost is paid by insurance, the business office should make it clear to the patient whether he is responsible for submitting the bill to the carrier.

Another valuable policy is to provide a statement, prepared by the unit's attorneys, that must be signed by the patient or guardian whenever the bill will not be paid in full before the procedure. It should state that if the account must be turned over to another party for collection, the costs of this action will be borne by the patient. If the unit is willing to allow payment of the bill in installments, this should also be stated, with the interest charges specified and a statement included in which the patient agrees to pay these interest charges.

The business office also requires a simple system for ensuring that everyone who undergoes a procedure that is not paid for beforehand receives a bill. One such system is based on the sign-in sheet, on which patients provide their names, addresses, and telephone numbers when they enter the unit. The receptionist records the number of the charge ticket beside the name on the sign-in sheet. At the end of the day this sheet is given to the bookkeeper, who checks to see that all the charge tickets have been turned in. Ideally, charge tickets will have numbers printed on them in sequence, and any gaps will be accounted for at the end of each day.

Patients carry their charge tickets, which bear their names and addresses, the name and address of the responsible party, and insurance and employer information, with them. When the procedure has been completed and the operative note dictated, the charge ticket and the patient's chart are given to the business office for processing.

OFFICE MANAGEMENT

For many ambulatory surgery units, a computer is a cost-effective tool and a wise investment. Not only does it simplify record keeping, but it enables the unit to keep patients' account records up to date, which greatly reduces the frequency of annoying bills sent to patients who have already paid. It also enables the unit to closely monitor its cash flow. The great reduction of computer costs in recent years, and the ease with which most business systems can be operated by people who know little about computers, are added incentives.

Several introductory-level books on computers are available,[3–5] and the would-be user should read one or more in order to be able to converse intelligently with the vendors.

Essentially, a computer system has four parts: hardware, software, documentation, and a storage medium. The hardware is the computer: a video display terminal (VDT; also called a cathode ray tube or CRT) with a keyboard and printer. The software is the program; that is, the instructions that tell the computer what to do. The documentation is the user's manual: the instructions that tell the user how to tell the software to tell the computer what to do. The storage medium is exactly what its name implies and is most often either a floppy disk, which looks like a rusty 45 rpm record in a jacket, or a hard (Winchester) disk, which is larger and often silver in color. Of these parts, the choice of hardware is least important: the wise computer buyer will select software that can do the jobs that need to be done and then select hardware that will run that software.

The first step in selecting a computer is deciding exactly what functions it should perform.[6]* This decision should be made in consultation with those who will be using the system, such as the bookkeepers, laboratory technician, appointment secretary, and typist, not only because these are the people best able to describe in detail what needs to be done, but because if the staff is involved in the computerization of the unit, their resistance to the conversion will be reduced. These people should also examine a system's documentation before a purchase is made, to be certain it is clear and easy to follow. If the system is to be used for word processing, such as in the typing of operative reports, the ergonomics of the terminal become a consideration, be-

---

*Many computer consulting firms are available. If there is one in your area knowledgeable in medical business procedures, it may be worthwhile to hire them to analyze your needs. Although such services are expensive (≥ $250/day), a few days of their help can save many thousands of dollars by preventing the purchase of an inappropriate system. Before selecting a consulting firm, however, talk to some of their previous clients.

cause the operator must spend many hours at the machine. Some designs are more likely than others to produce eye strain and fatigue; this subject has been reviewed by Makower.[7]

One final point about the computerized office: it is imperative that a complete duplicate set of the medical and financial records be created, with the disks being stored somewhere other than the surgery unit and updated at regularly scheduled intervals. This will prevent loss of the records in case of accident or sabotage.

ESTABLISHING AN AMBULATORY SURGERY CENTER

Readers of this book may wish to establish an ambulatory surgery unit themselves. Such a project will require competent professional, financial, and legal advice that will take into account local laws and regulations and one's own financial position. In many cases, an S corporation is advantageous. With this arrangement, the partners borrow the money to capitalize the surgery center, with each partner having a sufficient basis in the corporation to obtain tax advantages. When the center begins to make a profit, it can then be reorganized as a regular corporation. Before a form of financing is chosen, however, a long-term cash budget should be generated in order to choose the method that will produce the best tax situation. In determining the construction costs, the special needs of a medical facility must, of course, be included. We have estimated that the construction costs of an ambulatory surgery unit in Minneapolis in 1982 would have been 100 to 120 dollars per square foot.

CONCLUSIONS

If an ambulatory surgery unit is to flourish, it must do more than provide good health care. It must be run efficiently, and it must be suited to its market. A center may wish to consider offering incentives such as a discount to elderly persons with Medicare coverage. Certainly, if the center is to succeed, those who manage the business side of it must be as competent and professional as the physicians and nurses who staff it.

REFERENCES

1. Reed, W.A., and Williams, R.C.: Unique financial considerations. *In* Outpatient Surgery. Edited by R. Schultz. Philadelphia, Lea & Febiger, 1979, p. 435.
2. Orkand Corp.: Selected Use of Competition by Health Systems Agencies: Final Report Summary and Findings. Submitted to the Bureau of Health Planning and Resources Development, Department of Health, Education and Welfare (Contract No. ITEW-HRA 230:75-0071), 1976, pp. iv, 42-46.
3. Shrum, C.: How to Buy a Personal Computer. Sherman Oaks, Alfred Publishing Co., 1982.
4. McWilliams, P.A.: The Personal Computer Book. Los Angeles, Prelude Press, 1982.
5. Kember, N.F.: An Introduction to Computer Applications in Medicine. London, Edward Arnold, 1982.
6. Linn, N.A., and Pugliese, D.F.: Trends in ambulatory care information systems. Computers Health Care 4(1), Jan. 1983.
7. Makower, J.: Office Hazards. Washington, D.C., Tilden Press, 1981, p. 85.

7

Legal Aspects

RODNEY J. REPKO, Esq.

"The life of the law has not been logic: It has been experience."

Oliver Wendell Holmes, Jr.
The Common Law

As the payment and delivery of health-care services evolve, so too will the legal standards of care by which physicians, practicing in both the inpatient and outpatient settings, are measured. With the implementation of the Tax Equity and Fiscal Responsibility Act of 1982 (TEFRA), as well as the enactment of Medicare prospective payment in the 1983 amendments to the Social Security Act, the system of incentives whereby inpatient services are delivered has undergone radical change. As a result, a new impetus will be added to the development of less costly outpatient delivery systems; and, as in other endeavors, increased activity will carry an increased risk of liability at law. This is no doubt the case with the development of ambulatory surgical centers.

Serving as backdrop to the emerging legal issues facing ambulatory surgical centers and practitioners is the ever-increasing frequency and size of medical malpractice claims. The *American Bar Association Journal* has noted an increase in the average size of malpractice verdicts against physicians from nearly 95,000 dollars at the height of the "malpractice crisis" in 1975 to more than 244,000 dollars in 1981, along with a steady annual increase in the rate of malpractice filings over recent years. This problem is compounded by the fact that the courts have not yet clearly formulated the standards of care to be applied to developing methods of delivering health-care services, leaving physicians and institutional providers to voyage warily into new and unknown waters.

The current is nonetheless running toward the development of alternative methods of delivery, and if we are to reasonably anticipate the legal perils that lie ahead, some effort must be made to apply established principles of law to the developing ambulatory surgical setting. With Mr. Holmes' observation in mind, such will be the objective of this chapter.

THE SCOPE OF THE LAW

A discussion of the law of professional liability is essentially a discussion of the law of negligence as applied to physicians and other health-care providers. Although in many jurisdictions theories of contract law may still be asserted in professional liability actions, the prevailing practice finds plaintiff's counsel framing issues of liability in terms of negligence. While developments in the rules of civil procedure in most jurisdictions generally make it easier to join allegations of negligence (referred to as actions "in trespass") and breach of contract (referred to as actions "in assumpsit") in one action, it is also the case that some jurisdictions have erected other barriers against asserting a contract theory in medical malpractice cases. By way of illustration, the Pennsylvania Health-Care Services Malpractice Act contains a provision raising a presumption against the validity of any "contract" between physician and patient not actually set forth in writing: "In the absence of a special contract in writing, a health-care provider is neither a warrantor nor a guarantor of a cure" (40 P.S. § 1301.606). Likewise, the Georgia courts have affirmed the Georgia Voluntary Sterilization Act prohibition against malpractice actions based in contract, permitting liability only when a physician was negligent in performing the sterilization procedure, Shessel v. Gay, 228 S.E.2d, 361 [1976]. As many contract-based malpractice actions involve contentions that a guaranteed result was not achieved, such statutory provisions serve to inhibit the assertion of such theories in all but exceptional circumstances.

NEGLIGENCE

The law of negligence is only one component of the broader Common Law, the doctrines and principles of which have been developed and refined over the centuries by courts in both Great Britain and the United States. More precisely for our purposes, the Common Law, as distinguished from statutory or codified law, refers to those principles assumed from English law at the time of our independence and subsequently interpreted and applied by the American judiciary. The law of Torts, in turn, refers to that body of Common Law setting forth the principles whereby an individual injured by a wrongful act (a tort) of another may be compensated, with the law of negligence comprising but one category among a number of torts (others include assault, battery, libel, and a variety of other actions for which a civil remedy will lie).

Negligence law proceeds from the principle that in the course of everyday human interaction, a duty to act in an ordinary, prudent, and reasonable fashion with respect to others should be imposed on individuals under certain circumstances. In general, a plaintiff in a negligence action must establish four separate elements of negligence in order to prevail, those elements being (1) a *duty*, or obligation recognized by the courts, requiring an actor to conform to a certain standard of conduct, for the protection of others against unreasonable risks; (2) a *breach*, or failure on his part to conform to the standard required; (3) *causation*, or a reasonably close causal connection between the conduct and the injury; and (4) an *injury*, or some actual loss or damage resulting to the person to whom the duty is owed. That is, in an action against a physician, an individual would first have to establish the existence and nature of the duty owed by the physician to the patient, that the duty was in fact breached, and that the breach caused the injury of which the plaintiff is complaining and for which he is asking money damages.

Duty and Breach

The first two elements of a negligence action when applied to medical malpractice become interlocked in the concept of the standard of care. In general, the standard of care owed by a physician to his patient requires that he act with respect to that patient as would any ordinary, prudent, and reasonable physician in treating the same patient for the same condition under the same or similar circumstances. As in all negligence actions, the standard is imposed in order to prevent the occurrence of a reasonably foreseeable injury to the patient. The standard is an objective one, turning on the legal fiction of the "reasonable physician," who is deemed to possess and exercise the same degree of knowledge and skill as other members of his profession in good standing in the medical community. It should only be noted that although physicians have historically been held to the standard of practice in existence in the same or similar locality, the development of mandatory continuing medical education, national boards for the certification of specialty and subspecialty practice, widespread circulation of scholarly articles and medical publications, and the general transient nature of the medical profession have often served as the basis for the abrogation of the "locality rule" in favor of a broader national standard of practice.

In addition, as would no doubt be the case for a physician performing outpatient urologic surgery, in the event a practitioner possesses or attests to possess superior knowledge or skill in a given area, the law will hold him to the higher standard of care of other practitioners with the same degree of knowledge, training, and expertise. A board-certified urologist would, therefore, be held to a higher standard in treating a urologic condition than would a family practitioner or general surgeon; he might also be held liable for untoward results where his colleagues would not.

In determining the precise nature of the standard of care owed by a physician to a patient under any given circumstances, the law generally requires the introduction of expert testimony into the trial in order to inform and educate the judge and jury of information outside the ordinary scope of their knowledge. Likewise, the plaintiff in a malpractice action is in most cases required to produce expert testimony to the effect that the duty of care thus established has been breached by the physician. In most jurisdictions, failure to produce such testimony on either count will prevent the case from being submitted to a jury and will result in the dismissal of the case in favor of the defendant.

Causation and Injury

Having established the first two elements of negligence, the medical malpractice plaintiff must then establish some causal relationship between the physician's breach of duty and injuries suffered as a result. In many cases, as for example in the postoperative development of a fistula in a patient's bladder where before there was none, the argument for a causal relationship may be compelling and require little further proof. There may, however, be circumstances where the causal relationship between a physician's breach and a given injury is seriously in question and will require extensive expert testimony in order to be established. Thus, in the case of the patient who postoperatively suffers a stroke, but who previously suffered from medical conditions independently capable of causing a stroke (for example, arteriosclerosis), the plaintiff would bear the difficult burden of proving that the surgery rather than the pre-existing condition occasioned the injury.

The realization of some reasonably foreseeable injury is the final factor in the negligence equation. It is also often the most demonstrable in a malpractice action and the one least often subject to dispute. In addition to presenting a deceased or visibly debilitated plaintiff, injury may be proved by showing the medical expenses of the procedure in question and any additional costs incurred for the repair of an alleged injury. Plaintiffs may also receive compensation for such items as lost wages and pain and suffering. One should not suppose, however, that the injury is a given in this equation. Recent cases have illustrated how a plaintiff's damages, which are essentially a measure of the injuries incurred, may be subject to legal dispute.

Among the most hotly debated issues in malpractice litigation over recent years has been the question of recovery for the "wrongful birth" of a child following a surgical attempt at sterilization. At the center of the controversy has been the public policy question of whether, and to what extent, the courts should provide a legal remedy for the birth of an otherwise healthy child notwithstanding the failure of the procedure in question to achieve its desired result. In the case of Mason v. Western Pennsylvania Hospital, 453 A.2d, 974 [1982], the Pennsylvania Supreme Court, following other jurisdictions, held that the plaintiff in such an action would be unable to recover the costs of rearing such a child, reasoning that the costs of raising a child to the age of majority are more than offset by the love, affection, and society enjoyed by the parents of that child over the years. Although a given physician may have acted without due diligence in performing such a procedure, the courts in Pennsylvania and similar jurisdictions may limit or prohibit recovery of damages in such cases as being against public policy.

Without proving some injury, no matter how egregious a physician's conduct, the malpractice plaintiff will be barred from recovering any compensatory damages previously noted. As noted by Dean Prosser, "negligent conduct in itself is not such an interference with the interests of the world at large that there is any right to complain of it, or to be free from it, except in the case of some individual whose interests have suffered."

Negligence and Informed Consent

Whereas the doctrine of informed consent originally derived from the tort theories of assault and battery, the prevailing practice among American courts recently has been to frame consent cases in terms of negligence. Although the court and commentators have often been (and often remain) confused as to the proper tort category in which to place the doctrine, few would argue that the underlying principle of all consent cases was best expressed by Justice Cardozo in the seminal case of Schloendorff v. Society of New York Hospital, 105 N.E. 92 [1914]:

> Every human being of adult years and sound mind has a right to determine what shall be done with his own body, and a surgeon who performs an operation without his patient's consent . . . is liable in damages.

While the doctrine and its ancillary principles have evolved through case law, and have been codified through legislative enactment, the original principle remains sound. Thus physicians and institutional providers have been obliged to continuously reassess consent practices and procedures in order to avoid claims predicated on the doctrine of informed consent.

The standard against which physicians will be measured in adjudicating consent cases will be determined by the particular jurisdiction in which either the physician resides or the action is filed. Generally, however, the courts have chosen between two competing tests in assessing whether the plaintiff has met his burden of proving lack of informed consent. The majority of jurisdictions have adopted the professional disclosure or "reasonable physician" standard exemplified in Karp v. Cooley, 493 F.2d, 408, 419 [5th Circuit, 1974]. This standard judges a given disclosure according to what the reasonably prudent medical practitioner would disclose to the patient under the same or similar circumstances. As elsewhere, such a standard necessarily requires the introduction of expert testimony.

The second test, adopted by a minority of jurisdictions, involves the "materiality rule." As expressed by the California Supreme Court in Cobbs v. Grant, 502 P.2d, 1 [1972]:

The scope of the physician's communication to the patient, then, must be measured by the patient's need, and that need is whatever information is *material* to the decision. Thus the test for determining whether a potential peril must be divulged is its *materiality* to the patient's decision. (Cobbs v. Grant 502 P.2d, at 15 [emphasis added]).

Unaddressed by the *Cobbs* v. *Grant* court, yet problematic for physicians practicing under the "materiality rule," is the question of how one determines what is and is not "material." Although courts and legislators have both gone to the extreme of defining materiality in terms of a statistical likelihood that a risk will be realized, such an approach was itself rejected by the Pennsylvania Superior Court in Cooper v. Roberts, 286 A.2d, 647 [1971]. Rejecting the lower court's verdict against a physician for failing to disclose a 0.04% risk to the patient, the Pennsylvania appellate court wrote:

A more equitable formulation would be: Whether the physician disclosed all those facts, risks and alternatives that a reasonable man in the situation which the physician knew or should have known to be the plaintiff's would deem significant in making a decision to undergo the recommended treatment. This gives maximum effect to the patient's right to be the arbitor of the medical treatment he will undergo without either requiring a physician to be a mindreader into the patient's most subjective thoughts or requiring that he disclose every risk lest he be liable for battery. (Cooper v. Roberts, 220 Pa.Super., at 267).

Thus the Pennsylvania court rejected the stricter materiality rule for a "reasonable man" standard which may be less obtrusive to the practice of medicine than its rigid alternative. A "material risk," as expressed by the court in the leading case of Canterbury v. Spence, 464 F.2d, 772 [1972], may be deemed as that which a reasonable person "would be likely to attach significance to . . . in deciding whether or not to forego the proposed treatment" (Canterbury v. Spence, 464 F.2d, at 787).

Proving the necessary elements of causation and injury in an informed consent case likewise calls into play competing judicial standards. The majority view accepts the formulation of the standard adopted by the *Canterbury* v. *Spence* court and expressed by the California Supreme Court in *Cobbs* v. *Grant*. Focusing on the question of whether the patient/plaintiff would have rejected the treatment were the risks disclosed, and whether he may so testify, the *Cobbs* v. *Grant* court wrote:

The patient/plaintiff may testify on this subject, but the issue extends beyond his credibility. Since at the time of trial the uncommunicated hazard has materialized, it will be surprising if the patient/plaintiff did not claim that had he been informed of the dangers he would have declined treatment. Subjectively he may believe so, with the 20/20 vision of hindsight, but we doubt that justice will be served by placing the physician in jeopardy of the patient's bitterness and disillusionment. Thus an objective test is preferable: i.e., What would a prudent person in the patient's position have decided if adequately informed of all significant perils. (Cobbs v. Grant, 502 P.2d, at 11).

Thus in proving causation under the above formulation, the plaintiff must show that the reasonable person would have foregone treatment if informed of the previously undisclosed risks. Unlike the "reasonable physician" standard applied to the issues of duty and breach above, the application of this test lies well within the abilities of a lay jury and should not require the production of expert testimony.

Notwithstanding the reasoning set forth in the *Cobbs* v. *Grant* case, a minority of courts have adopted a subjective test to determine the issue of causation for the purposes of informed consent. In the case of Wilkinson v. Vesey, 295 A.2d, 676 [1972], the Rhode Island court held that the testimony of the patient/plaintiff himself may be conclusive proof that the failure to disclose "caused" him to undergo the procedure and, therefore, suffer the injuries associated with it (medical expenses, pain and suffering, lost wages, and so on). In this regard, it should be noted that here, as in all consent cases, the plaintiff need not prove that the procedure was negligently performed; rather, the measure of the plaintiff's injuries may be solely based on those damages normally associated with the procedure itself.

There is no single rule or precept capable of lending certainty to a physician's determination of what should be disclosed. Such a determination must, in the final analysis, rest on a physician's judgment, his experience with the procedure in question, his knowledge and understanding of the particular patient, and his assessment of the patient's ability to comprehend the risks disclosed. No preconceived consent form is capable of accurately reflecting the substance of a communication which by its nature will be unique to the physician and patient in question. While consent forms may be a necessary administrative burden, or while a signed consent may in some jurisdictions be required by statute, the executed consent form will serve in most states only as prima facie evidence that the duty to inform has been met.

AMBULATORY SURGERY

The most significant question with respect to negligence and ambulatory surgery may be stated thus: When and to what extent does the performance of a given procedure on an outpatient basis constitute a deviation from the standard of care owed by the physician to the patient? In addition, the physician performing ambulatory surgery in a free-standing facility, as opposed to a hospital-based outpatient surgery department, may incur personal liability from other, more indirect sources. That is, issues of liability may arise from attending questions concerning the nature and size of the facility itself, the credentialing of its staff, the sophistication and adequacy of its equipment in meeting unanticipated situations, and the training and qualifications of its employed support staff.

In determining whether the performance of a particular procedure on a given patient on an outpatient basis will constitute a breach of the standard of care, the courts will look first to the testimony of physicians introduced as experts. As knowledge and experience in this field continues to grow, the courts will no doubt look to scholarly articles and treatises, medical textbooks, and other authoritative sources on outpatient surgery as compelling evidence of the applicable standard of care. The practitioner, therefore, would do well to document knowledge of and compliance with established practice and protocols in this area and should be prepared to demonstrate continued efforts to keep abreast of developments in his field. In this context, written policies should be regularly reviewed and revised as appropriate.

Some of the legal perils unique to the performance of outpatient surgery derive from the lack of control over the patient's activities in the preoperative and postoperative periods. For example, the failure of a patient to respect dietary restrictions before presenting for surgery or to follow his postoperative instructions may, in the event of an injury, expose the physician to a malpractice claim. Considerable care, therefore, should be taken to document the patient's receipt and knowledge of any instructions given either prior or subsequent to surgery. In the event of a malpractice claim, the ability to demonstrate the communication of necessary information to the patient, as well as the patient's failure to comply with instructions, will be of obvious advantage.

The 1974 Florida case of Pierce v. Smith, 301 So.2d, 805, may illustrate the hazards of releasing a patient into an uncontrolled environment after outpatient surgery. In the *Pierce* v. *Smith* case, the patient underwent a vasectomy in his physician's office and successfully alleged that he was prematurely released from the facility while still bleeding, and that the ultimate loss of his testicle was therefore due to a failure to adequately render appropriate postoperative care. In instructing the patient in the course of his postsurgical care, a physician may guard against such liability in one of two ways. First, the patient may be informed of the normal anticipated course of recovery and instructed to return to the clinic or to the nearest emergency facility in the event of a sudden or unanticipated turn of events. Otherwise, the physician may provide the patient with the names of colleagues with whom coverage arrangements have been made in the event of an emergency. Furthermore, state licensing laws for such facilities may require a written agreement with a nearby hospital, or the nearest hospital at which the physician has privileges, for the emergency admission of postsurgical patients who require hospital inpatient care. To the extent that such licensing requirements are violated, or the physician otherwise fails to adequately treat or make provisions for appropriate postsurgical treatment he may, as in the *Pierce* v. *Smith* case, be held liable at law.

CORPORATE OR INSTITUTIONAL LIABILITY

Like individuals, corporations may also be held liable for negligence. The oldest and most frequent source for such liability is the Common Law doctrine of "Respondeat Superior," whereby a person may be held liable for the negligent acts or omissions of his agents (employees, officers, and directors). Inasmuch as corporations are deemed "persons" for most purposes under the law, the doctrine has been applied to create liability in corporate entities. Thus the New York State courts, in the case of Connell v. Hayden, 83 AD.2d, 30, 443 NYS2d, 383 [1981], held that a professional corporation, like any other business corporation, may be vicariously liable for the torts of their agents committed within the scope of the corporate business.

The leading case on the corporate liability of health-care providers remains that of Darling v. Charleston Community Memorial Hospital, 211 N.E.2d, 253 [1974]. Notable for our purposes in the *Darling* v. *Charleston Community Memorial Hospital* case was the court's holding that state licensing requirements, standards set forth by voluntary accreditation agencies (JCAH), and the institution's own rules, regulations, policies, and procedures may be introduced into evidence as to the standard of care owed to its patients. The lesson of *Darling* v. *Charleston Community Memorial Hospital* is, therefore, that should a facility voluntarily assume a higher standard of care or more exacting policies and procedures with respect to outpatient surgery than is generally practiced by the medical community at large, it may be held liable in the event its failure to meet those standards results in an injury to one of its patients. Again, care should be taken to regularly review and, where appropriate, revise any written policies, procedures, or protocols that may be in effect at the ambulatory surgical facility.

Since ambulatory surgical facilities may be organized as a partnership rather than a corporation, some note should be made of the differences between the two for the purposes of liability. While the shareholders or members of a corporation are generally shielded from personal liability for the acts or omissions of corporate employees, a professional partnership is governed by the same legal principles relating to business partnerships in general. Thus, the individual physicians in such a partnership may be held jointly and severally liable for each others' acts of malpractice. The otherwise important, and in some states obligatory, credentialing and peer review functions in an ambulatory surgical facility may therefore be of heightened significance when the facility is organized along the line of a partnership, as each of the practitioners may have a peculiar interest in the qualifications of his partners.

Although professional liability claims may come to many of those engaged in the practice of ambulatory surgery, approaches can be taken to minimize exposure to liability. Some of those that have been discussed in this chapter, including sound documentation and adherence to an ongoing review of published protocols, may at times seem burdensome or unnecessary to a physician in his daily practice. By devoting attention to such considerations in advance, however, and by taking steps to control information important to litigation while it is still within the physician's power to do so, a practitioner may in time enjoy more of the benefits and suffer fewer of the hazards involved in heeding the national call for lower health-care costs and participating in safe, cost-effective alternatives of delivery.

CONCLUSIONS

The law governing outpatient surgery units is in flux. One crucial question requiring an answer is, when does performance of a given operation on an outpatient basis constitute a violation of the usual standard of care? The surgeon wishing to do outpatient operations must keep abreast of developments in the field and document his knowledge of and compliance with established outpatient practice. Also, because the preoperative and postoperative control of the patient is minimal, special care is needed in documenting preoperative and postoperative instructions. Finally, urologists considering affiliation with an outpatient surgery unit must carefully consider the adequacy of its facilities and the qualifications of its staff.

Section II

Special Anesthetic and Investigative Techniques

8
Anesthetic Blocks

JOSEPHINE N. LO, M.D.

The use of regional and nerve blocks in outpatient surgery is gaining popularity because it is safe, simple, cost-effective, and spares the patient the nausea and drowsiness that may follow general anesthesia. This chapter introduces anesthetic-block techniques that are simple and suitable for relatively healthy patients undergoing outpatient urologic diagnostic or therapeutic procedures.

Although serious toxic reactions to local anesthetics are rare, personnel and equipment must always be immediately available to treat them. The basic equipment includes a respiratory resuscitation kit, an oxygen source, and suction apparatus. Cardiovascular resuscitation drugs must always be on hand: atropine, epinephrine, phenylephrine or other vasopressors, and anticonvulsants such as diazepam.

Proper choice of patients is essential for success. For example, small children and very anxious patients are not suitable candidates for regional anesthesia. Also, the physician who performs the block should be skilled, preferably as a result of experience with hospitalized patients. Finally, knowledge of the pharmacology of local anesthetics is essential for both safety and selection of the optimal amount of anesthetic.

LOCAL ANESTHETIC DRUGS

The local anesthetics are either esters or amides. Esters are hydrolyzed in the plasma, whereas amides are metabolized by the liver. The most commonly used amides are lidocaine and bupivacaine. Procaine and tetracaine, both esters, are seldom used for nerve blocks.

Lidocaine (Xylocaine)

Lidocaine hydrochloride is a water-soluble salt with excellent penetrative capabilities that make it the agent of choice when rapid onset of action is required.

Topical Anesthesia. A 4% solution provides sufficient topical anesthesia for mucous membranes; the urethra can be anesthetized effectively with a 2% jelly. Analgesia begins in 5 minutes and lasts 30 minutes.

Infiltration Anesthesia. With this approach, the onset of action is immediate. The 0.5% solution provides anesthesia for approximately 75 minutes and the 1% solution for approximately 120 minutes.

Peripheral Nerve Block. Both the 0.5% and the 1% solutions may be used for peripheral nerve blocks. The onset of action is in approximately 5 minutes; anesthesia lasts approximately 60 minutes if epinephrine is not used and 120 minutes if it is used.

Spinal Anesthesia. The most commonly used solution is 5% lidocaine in 7.5% dextrose. The onset of action is immediate, and the duration is approximately 60 minutes without and 90 minutes with epinephrine.

Safe Dosage. The toxic threshold is a plasma concentration of 5 μg/ml.[1] The maximum safe dose depends on the weight of the patient, ranging from 200–400 mg without epinephrine; toxic symptoms usually appear at doses > 6 mg/kg of body weight. Addition of epinephrine decreases capillary absorption of the drug, lowering the plasma concentration and increasing the safe dose to 500 mg.

Elimination. Lidocaine is rapidly extracted and metabolized by the liver. Elimination through the urine is negligible.

Bupivacaine (Marcaine)

Bupivacaine hydrochloride is a water-soluble salt. It is four times as potent as lidocaine but proportionally more toxic. Preparations are not available for topical anesthesia, and the drug is not approved for spinal anesthesia.

Infiltration Anesthesia. A 0.125% or 0.25% solution may be used with or without epinephrine. The action is almost immediate and lasts 200 to 300 minutes. Bupivacaine is, therefore, indicated for procedures in which postoperative analgesia is sought.

Peripheral Nerve Block. Solutions of 0.25% to 0.5% are usually used. The onset is slow (10 to 20 minutes), but analgesia lasts approximately 400 minutes and occasionally as long as 24 hours. Epinephrine prolongs its effect only marginally.[2]

Safe Dosage. The maximum safe dose is 150 mg for preparations without and 200 mg for those with epinephrine.

Elimination. Bupivacaine may be eliminated both by liver metabolism and by renal excretion;[3] its metabolic pathway has not been established.

Procaine (Novocain)

Procaine's poor spreading capacity limits its popularity for infiltration and nerve block. The effective doses are similar to those of lidocaine; but the onset of action is slower, and its duration is shorter. However, procaine has little toxicity; the maximum safe dose is as large as 750 mg. Procaine is metabolized rapidly by plasma cholinesterase.

Tetracaine (Pontocaine)

Tetracaine hydrochloride is a water-soluble salt. The solution may be degraded during repeat autoclaving,[4] and many clinicians prefer the heat-stable crystalline form. Tetracaine is six times as potent as lidocaine but is ten times as toxic.

Topical Anesthesia. A 1% solution is effective and has a long duration of action: approximately 60 minutes.

Infiltration and Peripheral Nerve Block. Infiltration and peripheral nerve block are performed with a 0.1% or 0.2% solution. Onset of the blockade is slow (15 to 30 minutes); the duration of action is 4 to 6 hours.

Spinal Anesthesia. A 1% solution is mixed with 10% dextrose. Anesthesia begins in 5 to 10 minutes and lasts approximately 90 minutes if epinephrine is not used and 120 to 180 minutes if it is used.

Safe Dosage. The maximum safe dose is 100 mg without and 150 mg with epinephrine.

Elimination. Tetracaine is metabolized slowly in the plasma.

TOXIC REACTIONS TO LOCAL ANESTHETICS

Intoxication with local anesthetics affects the central nervous system primarily, with the most hazardous effect being a generalized seizure. Premonitory signs such as sleepiness, irritability, and shivering mandate stopping the injection of anesthetic and administering oxygen by mask. Diazepam, 10 mg intravenously, raises the convulsive threshold.[5,6]

If a convulsion does occur, the first steps in management are maintenance of the airway and protection of the patient from hypoxia and self-injury. Controlled or assisted ventilation with 100% oxygen is essential. Frequently, there are depressive effects on the cardiovascular system, and it may be necessary to maintain the blood pressure by raising the patient's legs or administering a vasopressor. Although barbiturates remain the most effective drug for terminating a seizure caused by a local anesthetic, their use should be restricted to settings in which immediate endotracheal intubation can be ensured.

ALLERGY TO LOCAL ANESTHETICS

True allergy to local anesthetics is rare and may be manifested as dermatitis, urticaria, or anaphylaxis. Virtually all reports of allergy involve the ester group of drugs rather than the amides, and nearly all reported allergies to amides were subsequently found to be sensitivity to the preservative methylparaben.[7] Hence, amide-type local anesthetics without preservatives are the best agents for avoiding allergic reactions.

Mild urticaria and itchiness can be treated effectively by an antihistamine. Diphenhydramine (Benadryl), 30–50 mg, is given intravenously every four hours until the symptoms abate. If a bronchospasm occurs, 0.01–0.02 mg of isoproterenol is given intravenously.

In the extremely rare case of anaphylaxis, 0.1–0.5 mg of epinephrine and 100 mg of hydrocortisone should be given intravenously. Cardiopulmonary resuscitation, ventilation, and fluid support should be instituted immediately.

PREMEDICATION FOR ANESTHETIC BLOCKS

Early discharge of the patient precludes heavy sedative premedication. A thorough explanation of the procedure reassures the patient and often replaces sedative drugs. However, some sedation is indicated in children and anxious patients. Diazepam, 0.15 mg/kg intravenously, is often the drug of choice; it is considered specific for the relief of anxiety and does not cause vomiting or significant cardiorespiratory depression. Elderly patients are sensitive to the central depressant effects of diazepam, so the dose should be reduced by half.

SPINAL ANESTHESIA

The subarachnoid block is a simple procedure that provides profound, predictable, controllable anesthesia with a small dose of drug. The onset of action is virtually immediate, and its duration can be varied between 45 minutes and 3 hours. The occurrence of postoperative spinal headache may make some outpatient units reluctant to use spinal anesthesia; however, headache can be prevented by using small-bore needles.[8] Spinal block is not a contraindication to early ambulation.

In an ambulatory surgical center, the following conditions should be observed to minimize complications from spinal anesthesia.

(1) Personnel and equipment for general anesthesia must be immediately available in case there is a complication such as a high-level blockade or failure of spinal anesthesia.
(2) The person giving the anesthetic must be experienced and knowledgeable in the physiology of spinal anesthesia.
(3) Short-acting anesthetics, such as procaine or lidocaine, should be used. The patient should be discharged only after both sensory and sympathetic blockades have disappeared.
(4) The patient should be in good general condition and free of cardiovascular disease. As with any anesthesia, the patient should not eat or drink anything for at least 6 hours before the block is given.

Indications

All outpatient surgical procedures below the level of T-10 (umbilicus) may be done with spinal anesthesia. Sensations aroused by bladder distension are mediated by the afferent sympathetic nerves terminating in the T-9–L-2 segments of the spinal cord. Nerves to the testes are derived from the T-10 segment of the spinal cord. Therefore, in operations involving bladder distension or the testes, a T-10 level is required. Cystoscopy, perineorrhaphy, transurethral resection, and vasectomy require an anesthetic level to the inguinal ligament (L-1).

Drugs

The drugs available provide spinal anesthesia lasting 30 to 180 minutes (Table 8–1). Lidocaine, 5% in 7.5% dextrose, a hyperbaric solution, is recommended. The precise dose needed for each vertebral level depends on the height of the patient.

Technique

The spinal puncture is performed with a 25-gauge, 3½-inch spinal Lok-needle at the L-3 or L-4 interspace with the patient in the sitting or lateral decubitus position. The syringe containing the 5% lidocaine solution is connected to the needle, and 0.5 ml of spinal fluid is aspirated, making a total volume in the syringe of 1.5–2 ml. The contents of the syringe are discharged into the subarachnoid space over 5 seconds. To assure the proper position of the needle at the completion of injection, 0.2 ml of spinal fluid is withdrawn into the syringe and reinjected. The needle is withdrawn, and the patient is immediately placed in the supine position with the head and shoulders elevated on a pillow. The table should remain level, and no positional change should be made for at least 10 minutes. Blood pressure must be monitored closely during the first 10 minutes after the subarachnoid block.

Complications

Hypotension. Hypotension is the most common complication, especially in elderly patients who are unable to compensate for the vasodilation resulting from the sympathetic blockade. A sensory block of the T-10 dermatome causes peripheral pooling of approximately 500 ml of blood, and a block of the T-4 dermatome blocks the sympathetic nerves to all the abdominal viscera, in which another 500 ml of blood is pooled. Hypovolemia must be treated before spinal anesthesia is given, and in elderly patients, extra fluid should be given to compensate for the vasodilation.

Hypotension is most effectively treated by rapidly infusing fluids and giving oxygen by mask. If it persists, a vasoconstrictive drug may be given intravenously; 10–15 mg of ephedrine sulfate is recommended because of its inotropic effect in addition to its α-stimulating action. Accompanying respiratory arrest is rare and is probably caused by reduced perfusion of the brain stem rather than by a

TABLE 8–1. Drugs for Spinal Anesthesia at T-10

			Duration (min)	
Drug	Dose (mg)	Onset (min)	Without Epinephrine	With Epinephrine*
Procaine 5%	100–150	5–10	30–45	60– 75
Lidocaine 5%	50– 75	2– 4	45–60	60– 90
Tetracaine 0.5%	8– 10	4– 6	60–90	120–180

*1:200,000

motor block at the C-4–C-5 level. It should be treated immediately with artificial ventilation by bag and mask. As soon as the blood pressure is restored, spontaneous breathing usually resumes.

Headache. Spinal headache occurs in 1 to 9% of patients, usually 24 to 48 hours after the lumbar puncture. The most plausible explanation concerns the diameter of the needle (Table 8–2). Use of a 26-gauge needle resulted in a negligible incidence of headache. In the past, patients were kept flat in bed after spinal anesthesia to prevent headache, but there is no evidence that this practice is effective. Leakage of cerebrospinal fluid (CSF) probably occurs even if the patient is recumbent.

More than 70% of spinal headaches resolve within a week, and in most cases, hydration and analgesics should be sufficient treatment. If the headache persists or is incapacitating, especially if it is associated with nausea, vomiting, or diplopia,[9] an epidural "blood patch"[10] should be considered. Approximately 10 ml of the patient's venous blood is collected aseptically and injected into the epidural space at the leakage site; the clot thus formed stems the escape of CSF. Although the success rate for this technique is better than 90%,[11] it is not without its own complications, such as fever, root pain, and ataxia;[12] and thus it should be reserved for cases of severe or persistent headache.

EPIDURAL BLOCK

The principal advantage of epidural block over subarachnoid block is that headache from CSF leakage does not occur unless the dura is inadvertently punctured. The precautions, indications, and complications of epidural block are similar to those of spinal anesthesia. However, because a much larger dose of drug is used for epidural block, the potential for toxic reactions is greater.

The epidural space lies between the dura on the one side and the ligament and periosteum lining the vertebral canal on the other side (Fig. 8–1). It extends from the foramen magnum to the sacrococcygeal membrane. The space, filled with loose areolar tissue, blood vessels, and lymphatics, has a negative pressure in the normal person.

Drugs and Dosage

The rapid onset and consistent results of lidocaine make it the agent of choice for outpatient epidural block. Bupivacaine epidural block lasts 4 to 12 hours and thus is not recommended. Lidocaine, 1.5% with or without epinephrine provides operating analgesia of 75 to 120 minutes. The dosage correlates closely with age and only weakly with weight or height. A dose of 2–2.5 ml of 1.5% lidocaine per segment can be used in patients between the ages of 20 and 40; that is, 25–30 ml to achieve a T-10 level anesthesia. A 30% dose reduction is recommended for pregnant women and a 50% reduction for elderly patients and those with severe arteriosclerosis.

Technique

The "loss of resistance" technique is popular because of its ease and reliability,

TABLE 8–2. Relation of Gauge of Needle Used for Lumbar Puncture to Frequency of "Spinal" Headache

Gauge	No. Cases	No. Headaches (%)
16	839	151 (18)
19	154	16 (10)
20	2698	377 (14)
22	4952	430 (9)
24	634	37 (6)

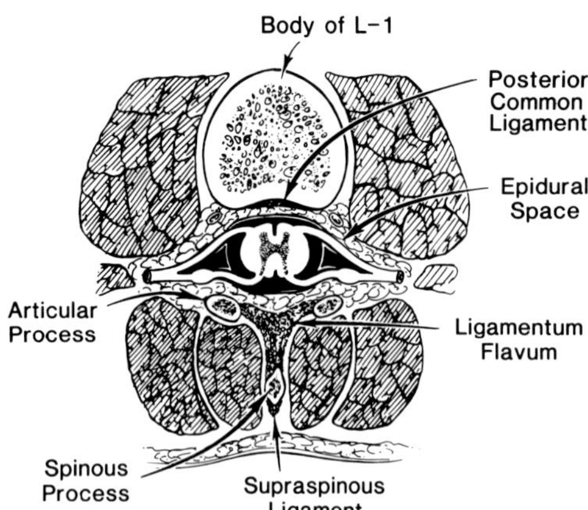

Fig. 8–1. Location of the epidural space.

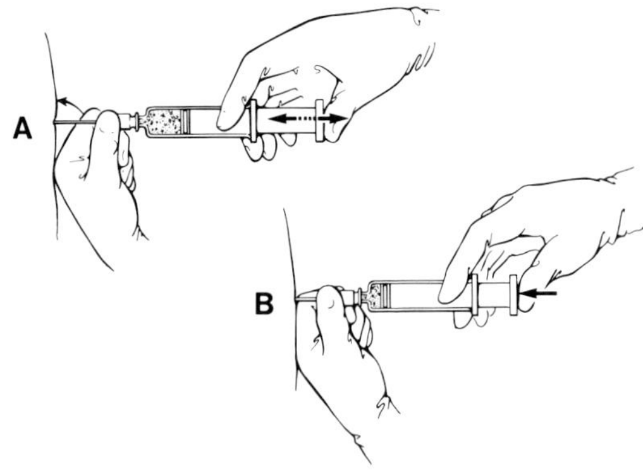

Fig. 8–2. Technique of epidural block. *(A)* Constant pressure on the plunger with the thumb allows the operator to tell when the needle has entered the epidural space. *(B)* If aspiration yields neither blood nor CSF, the anesthetic is injected.

and a single injection is preferred to the insertion of a catheter for patients undergoing brief procedures.

After the aseptic preparation, the skin and the interspinous region at the center of the L-3 or L-4 interspace is infiltrated with 1 ml of 1% lidocaine. After the drug has taken effect, the skin is punctured with an 18-gauge needle to facilitate the insertion of the epidural needle. A 20-gauge epidural Lok-needle is connected to a glass syringe containing 5 ml of saline or air. The needle is gripped and advanced with the left hand, and the syringe is held with the right hand with the thumb applying constant pressure on the plunger (Fig. 8–2); this permits immediate perception of the loss of resistance when the needle tip enters the epidural space. Gentle aspiration is carried out, and if neither CSF nor blood is produced, one third of the calculated anesthetic dose is injected at the rate of 0.5 ml per second. If the patient does not have any untoward reaction, such as numbness or hypotension, the remainder of the dose is injected.

BLOCK OF THE INGUINAL REGION (ILIAC-CREST BLOCK)

The inguinal region, which includes the inguinal canal, spermatic cord, and surrounding soft tissues is supplied by the twelfth thoracic, iliohypogastric, ilioinguinal, and genitofemoral nerves. At the level of the anterosuperior iliac spine, the ilioinguinal and iliohypogastric nerves lie between the internal and external oblique muscles. Thus, with the anterosuperior iliac spine as the landmark, an infiltration block of the inguinal region can be performed; success depends on the spread of a large volume of anesthetic solution between the muscle layers. Because of these large doses, one must watch for toxic reactions with special care.

The usual drug for iliac-crest block is lidocaine, approximately 70 ml of a 0.5% solution with or without 1:200,000 epinephrine. (Use of epinephrine is recommended, as it reduces the rate of absorption and thus the toxicity.) Anesthesia is established in 5 to 15 minutes and lasts 75 to 150 minutes.

Technique

With the patient supine, a skin wheal is made 3 cm medial and 3 cm inferior to the anterosuperior iliac spine (Fig. 8–3). A 3½-inch, 22-gauge security Lok-needle is inserted and directed almost horizon-

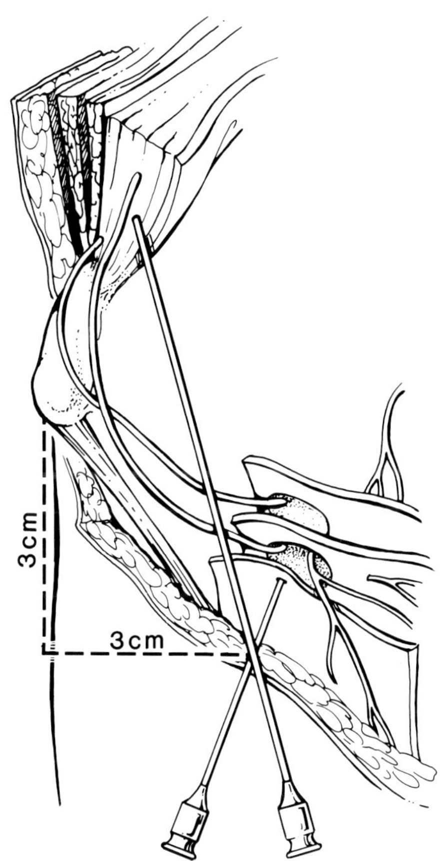

Fig. 8–3. Iliac-crest block.

tally to contact the inside shelf of the iliac bone, and 10 ml of the anesthetic is injected as the needle is slowly withdrawn. The needle is reinserted at a steeper angle to penetrate the external and internal oblique muscles and the transversalis muscle, and again 10 ml of the anesthetic is injected as the needle is slowly withdrawn. This maneuver is repeated two more times, with the needle directed slightly more medially each time.

To anesthetize the genitofemoral nerve and the peritoneal sac, another skin wheal is made 2.5 cm above the midinguinal point, and the needle is inserted to a depth of 1½ to 2 inches with 20 ml of local anesthetic being injected during insertion and withdrawal of the needle. Another 10 ml of anesthetic is injected subcutaneously along the line of incision.

PENILE BLOCK

The penis is innervated by left and right dorsal nerves that enter from beneath the symphysis pubis, run below the deep (Buck's) fascia, and divide to supply the entire surface of the penis. The skin around the base of the penis is innervated by the ilioinguinal nerve, which is not blocked for circumcision.

Lidocaine, 1% or 0.5% bupivacaine may be used; epinephrine should not be added because of the risk of penile ischemia. Bupivacaine is preferred because it provides postoperative analgesia.

Technique

With the patient supine, the tubercles of the pubic bone are palpated and marked with X's. An "O" is marked on the median raphe of the scrotum at the base of the penis.

To block the ilioinguinal and genitofemoral nerves, intradermal and subcutaneous infiltration is carried out with a 2-inch, 25-gauge needle. With 10 ml of the anesthetic solution, a triangular ring is formed around the base of the penis, joining the two X's and the X's and the O (Fig. 8–4).

The dorsal nerves of the penis are blocked at its base. With the penis held vertically, a 2-inch needle attached to a syringe of anesthetic is inserted in succession through the X's and the O. When the needle has pierced the deep fascia, it is aspirated to be certain no blood returns; 0.5 to 3 ml of the anesthetic solution, adjusted for the patient's age, is then deposited fanwise between the corpora cavernosa and Buck's fascia (Fig. 8–5).

SPERMATIC CORD BLOCK

A regional block that has proved valuable for outpatient vasovasostomy, hydrocelectomy, spermatocelectomy, and

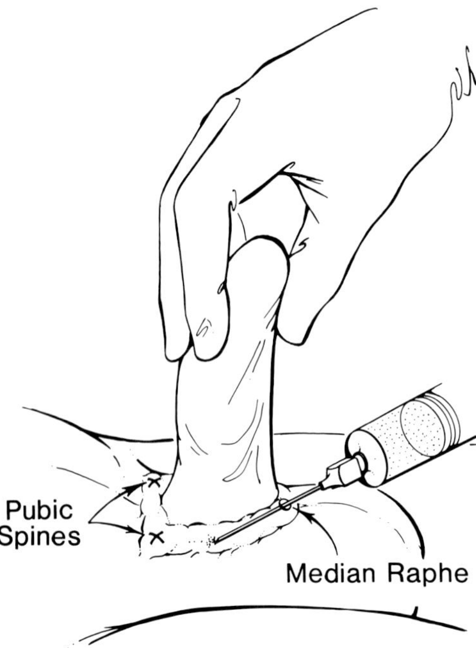

Fig. 8–4. Penile block. Anesthetic ring around base of penis to block ilioinguinal and genitofemoral branches.

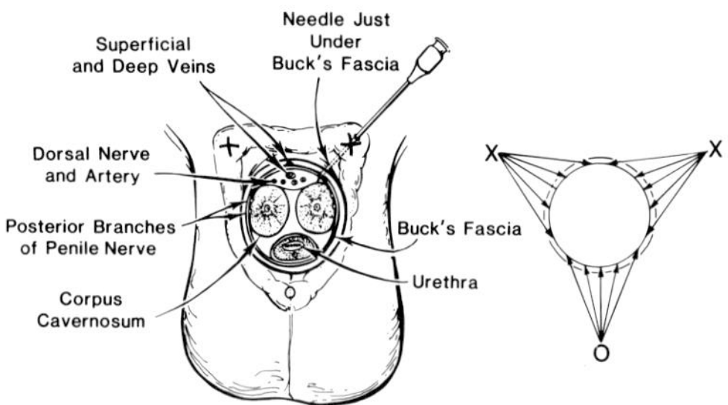

Fig. 8–5. Blockage of the dorsal penile nerves. Inset at right shows fanlike distribution of anesthetic injection sites.

orchiectomy is the spermatic-cord block.[13] It is described in Chapter 24.

DIAGNOSTIC USES OF REGIONAL BLOCKS

Transsacral Block

Sometimes the patient with a spinal cord injury cannot void, although the cystometric readings show good bladder tone. A block of the second, or more often, the third sacral nerve bilaterally may relieve the sphincter spasms and help the patient void (see Chapter 9).[14] The procedure is usually performed for diagnosis, and the preferred drug is 0.5% bupivacaine because of its long action.

The patient lies prone with a large pillow under the iliac bones to elevate the sacrum approximately 40° from the horizontal; this makes the sacral foramen easier to palpate. The sacral cornua are located, and the median sacral crest and the posterosuperior iliac spine is palpated. The second sacral foramen lies ½ inch caudad and ½ inch medial to the posterosuperior iliac spine (Fig. 8–6). The third foramen is 1 inch below the second and 1 inch lateral to the median sacral crest. A 22-gauge, 3-inch Lok-needle is placed in each foramen until there are paresthesias in the leg, penis or vagina, or buttock. Radiography may be used to verify correct needle placement. After aspiration fails to yield blood or CSF, 5 ml of the anesthetic solution is deposited in each foramen.

After the block is established, the cystometrogram is repeated and compared with previous readings. The amounts of urine voided and retained after each micturition indicate whether surgical intervention is appropriate.

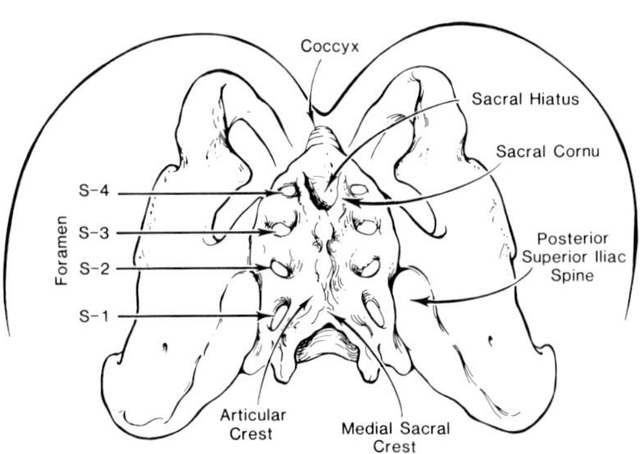

Fig. 8–6. Landmarks for transsacral block.

Orchalgia and Saddle Block

A saddle block is defined as anesthesia in the area of the perineum that would touch the saddle when riding a horse.

After the subarachnoid block has been administered, the patient remains sitting for 3 to 5 minutes. Only the sacral nerves are anesthetized, and the patient will be ready for cystoscopy or perineal surgery. The penis and scrotum are partly supplied by the ilioinguinal nerves derived from L-1 and thus are not entirely anesthetized by this procedure (see Chapter 10.) A saddle block may be used to differentiate referred pain from prostatitis and orchalgia; prostatic pain is relieved by a saddle block, whereas pain in the testes is not relieved until a T-10 block is achieved.

Incisional Pain

Pain at the site of a healed incision is often caused by nerve entrapment. Local anesthetic blocks are performed principally for diagnostic purposes. Lidocaine, 3–5 ml of a 1% solution, is injected either subcutaneously, proximal to and around the incision, or at the intercostal nerves of the involved dermatomes. The effectiveness of the block differentiates nerve-entrapment pain from referred pain of visceral origin. Nerve-entrapment pain is best treated either by surgical lysis or by infiltration of local anesthetic solutions containing steroids.

CONCLUSIONS

Outpatient surgery has tremendous benefits for the patient and is rapidly gaining popularity. It is imperative, therefore, that surgeons and anesthesiologists become proficient in all the useful local anesthetic block techniques.

REFERENCES

1. Foldes, F.F., et al.: Comparison of toxicity in intravenously given local anesthetics in man. J. Am. Med. Assoc., *172*:1493, 1960.
2. Telivuo, L., Svinhufrud, U., and Nuuttila, K.: An infrared thermography study on duration of intercostal nerve blocks using bupivacaine with or without Adrenaline. Acta Anesthesiol. Scand., *15*:131, 1971.
3. Reynolds, F.: Metabolism and excretion of bupivacaine in man: a comparison with mepivacaine. Br. J. Anaesth., *43*:33, 1971.
4. Chalaresanthervatee, P., and Thomas, R.G.: The stability of solutions of amethocaine hydrochloride. Aust. J. Pharm., *42*:800, 1961.
5. Ausinsch, B., Malagodi, M.H., and Munson, E.S.: Diazepam in the prophylaxis of lidocaine seizures. Br. J. Anaesth., *48*:390, 1976.
6. Moore, D.C., and Bridenbaugh, L.D.: Oxygen: the antidote for systemic toxic reactions from local anesthetic drugs. J. Am. Med. Assoc., *174*:842, 1960.
7. Nagel, J.E., Fuscaldo, J.T., and Fireman, P.: Paraben allergy. JAMA, *237*:1594, 1977.
8. Tarrow, A.B.: Solution to spinal headache. Int. Anesthesiol. Clin., *1*:877, 1963.
9. Bryce-Smith, R.M., and Macintosh, R.R.: Sixth-nerve palsy after lumbar puncture and spinal analgesia. Br. Med. J., *1*:275, 1974.
10. DiGiovanni, A.J., and Dunbar, B.S.: Epidural injections of autologous blood for post-lumbar puncture headache. Anesth. Analg., *49*:268, 1970.
11. Abouleish, E., et al.: Long-term follow up of epidural blood patch. Anesth. Analg., *54*:459, 1975.
12. Cornwall, R.D., and Dolan, W.M.: Radicular back pain following lumbar epidural patch. Anesthesiology, *42*:692, 1975.
13. Kaye, K.W., Lange, P.H., and Fraley, E.E.: Spermatic cord block in urologic surgery. J. Urol., *128*:720, 1982.
14. Moore, D.C.: Regional Block. 4th Ed. Springfield, Charles C Thomas, 1978, p. 473.

9

Sacral-Nerve Blocks for Neurogenic Bladder

GAYLAN L. ROCKSWOLD, M.D., and CIRIL J. GODEC, M.D.

Normal micturition requires a balanced interplay between the forces of urinary storage and those of urinary expulsion. Coordinated function between the bladder and urethra depends on intact innervation from the peripheral nerves, spinal micturition center, brain stem, basal ganglia, and cerebral cortex.[1] Any disturbance along these nerve pathways can cause clinical voiding dysfunction. Bladder inhibition is derived principally from the brainstem and is, phylogenetically, the "youngest" achievement in the development of micturition control. It is also the most vulnerable. Parasympathetic innervation originating from the spinal cord via the sacral nerves, predominantly S-3 and S-4, is responsible for bladder contraction.[2]

A hyperreflexic bladder is probably the micturition dysfunction the urologist most often sees. Detrusor hyperreflexia is defined as detrusor contractions during bladder filling that cannot be inhibited voluntarily and which increase intravesical pressure > 15 cm H_2O.[3] When detrusor hyperreflexia is neurologic, it is usually caused by a lesion above the parasympathetic outflow to the bladder. A hyperreflexic bladder can also be associated with nonneurogenic lesions, most frequently in males with outflow obstruction. Surgical removal of the obstruction is the best treatment for this second type of hyperreflexic bladder. Lesions above the sacral micturition center (spinal cord injury or tumors, multiple sclerosis, etc.) producing a hyperreflexic bladder can also cause a lack of coordinated reflex activity between the bladder and the external urinary sphincter.[4]

A thorough micturition history, coupled with a neurourologic and urodynamic examination, usually reveals the cause of a hyperreflexic detrusor dysfunction. The urodynamic evaluation should include cystometry, urethral profilometry, electromyography of the urogenital diaphragm normally and under provocation, evoked responses, and urinary flow rates.[2] The single most important diagnostic test in unmasking a hyperreflexic bladder is cystometry, which should be performed with the patient in the supine and standing positions. If a hyperreflexic bladder is diagnosed, the urologist should try to convert detrusor overactivity to normal bladder functioning in the urodynamic laboratory. Initially, conversion can be attempted with an anticholinergic drug such as pro-banthine or with electrical stimulation or anal dilatation. If this test is successful, conversion to normal bladder functioning should be possible with temporary or permanent sacral-nerve block.

TECHNIQUE

Sacral-nerve blocks are performed as a 30- to 50-minute outpatient procedure by a neurosurgeon or by a urologist trained in nerve blocking. Just before the block, prone and standing cystometrograms and sphincter electromyograms should be performed. The sacral nerves are then anesthetized with a transsacral approach with the patient prone. Initially, all blocks are unilateral, in an attempt to reduce the hyperreflexia without abolishing the detrusor responses.

The posterosuperior iliac spine and the cornua of the sacrum are identified and marked with indelible ink. The S-2 sacral foramina are usually located 1.5 cm medial and caudad from the posterosuperior iliac spine. The S-3 and S-4 sacral foramina lie approximately the same distance caudad and slightly medial to the more rostral foramen. After the landmarks have been identified, the skin is prepared with povidone–iodine solution. A skin wheal is then made unilaterally over the S-3 and S-4 foramina using 1% lidocaine and a 25-gauge needle, and anesthetic is injected into the subcutaneous tissue. A 22-gauge spinal needle is then directed perpendicular to the skin until it strikes the periosteum of the sacrum (Fig. 9–1). An attempt is made to enter the foramina of S-2 for approximately 1.5 cm, of S-3 for 1 cm, and of S-4 for 0.5 cm because of the decreasing depth of the foramen; therefore, after the needle strikes the periosteum of the posterior sacral surface, these distances are marked on the needle. The initial blocks are usually made with either lidocaine or bupivacaine, which is longer acting; 1–1.5 ml anesthetic is usually adequate. The appropriate sacral dermatome is checked before and after the block for the hypalgesia that proves that the desired sacral nerve has been anesthetized and that the effect has not spread beyond the area the operator desires to have blocked. Dermatomal hypalgesia usually begins rapidly, although occasionally it takes 5 to 10 minutes to develop. Once it has been obtained in the desired nerve roots, the cystometrogram and electromyogram can be repeated to determine the effect of the block. Sacral block can increase bladder capacity without abolishing the detrusor reflex when that capacity is reached (Fig. 9–2). In some patients, the detrusor reflex may be inhibited as well (Fig. 9–3); those patients should be watched closely, because they may suffer urinary retention.

The patient is told to chart his post-block voiding pattern, including the number of times and amount that he voids. If the results are not satisfactory, the test block can be repeated on the contralateral side. If the results are satisfactory, the procedure is repeated for the appropriate nerve root or roots using approximately 0.5 ml of absolute ethanol. Painful paresthesias are common during the injection, but they are of short duration. In a few patients, a radiofrequency lesion has been used, which has the advantage of stimulating the sacral nerve for detrusor contraction and permitting precise grading of the response.

RESULTS

Sacral nerve blocks with a local anesthetic have been used to evaluate several hundred patients with voiding problems. In a published study of 50 patients, we were able to abolish detrusor reflex activity and increase the bladder capacity in 60% of the patients and to increase bladder capacity alone in approximately 20%, leaving 20% of the patients with no effect.[5] In approximately half the patients, the detrusor reflex can be abolished with unilateral sacral blocks; these patients have various causes for their unstable bladders. As more of the sacral nerves are anesthetized, the amplitude

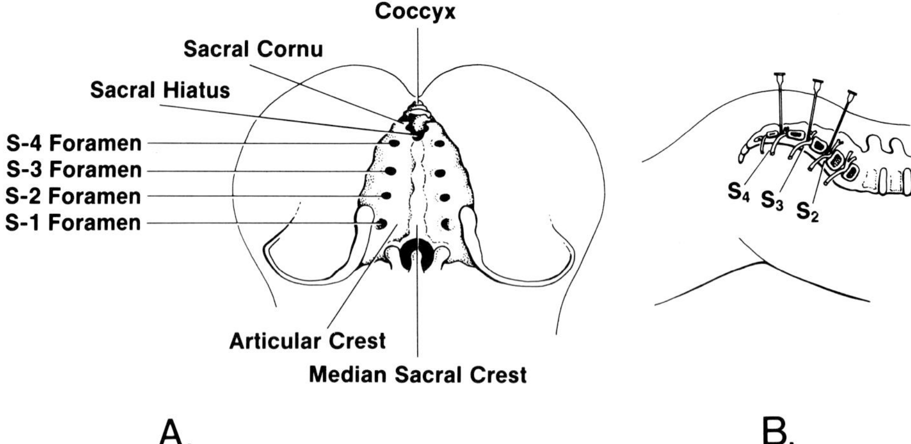

Fig. 9–1. Posterior *(A)* and lateral *(B)* views of the approach and landmarks for sacral-nerve blocks.

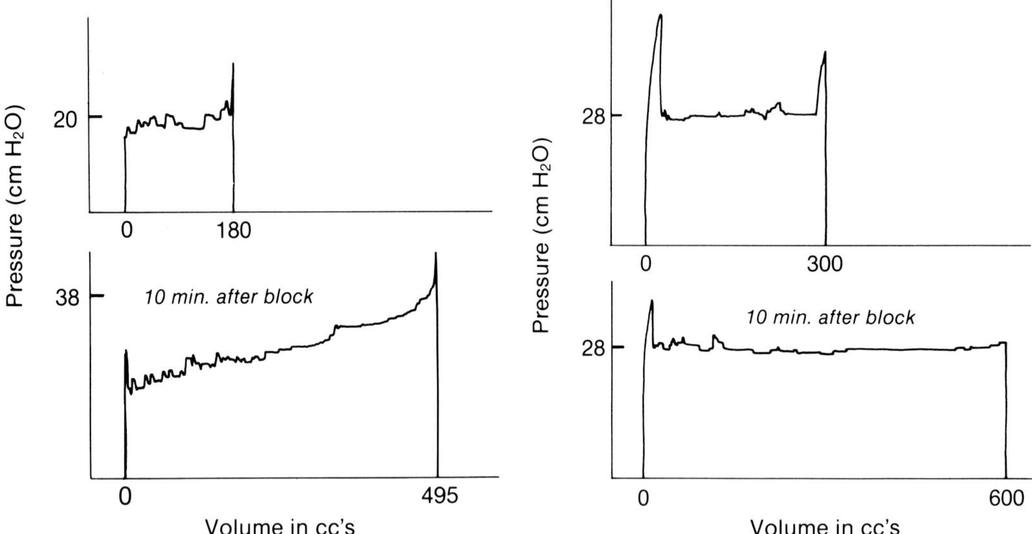

Fig. 9–2. Supine cystometrogram documents small bladder with strong detrusor reflex. Sacral block of S-3 and S-4 increases capacity and preserves detrusor reflex.

Fig. 9–3. Supine cystometrogram displaying some uninhibited contraction and strong detrusor reflex. Sacral block of S-3 and S-4 increases capacity and abolishes detrusor reflex.

and frequency of the sphincter electromyographic activity are progressively reduced.[6] When the S-2, S-3, and S-4 roots are blocked bilaterally, the sphincters become lax to palpation, and electromyographic activity ceases. Unilateral blocks, however, never abolish electromyographic activity or paralyze the external anal sphincter.

In one study, sacral-nerve blocks were used in the selection of 13 patients for differential rhizotomy.[7] When detrusor hyperreflexia could be reduced by anesthetizing one or two sacral nerves, partial rhizotomy increased bladder capacity while preserving the detrusor reflex and sphincter function and decreased frequency and urgency incontinence. However, symptoms tended to recur. More recently, we have used absolute ethanol injections of the sacral nerves or radiofrequency lesions. This procedure can be done in the outpatient department and can be repeated if symptoms recur. In our experience, two thirds of patients are relieved of symptoms for six months or longer.

DISCUSSION

The sacral-nerve block is a useful diagnostic and therapeutic tool in patients with hyperreflexic bladder dysfunction. Heimburger et al.[8] first described the use of sacral-nerve blocks in paraplegic patients with uninhibited bladder contractions. Essentially, selective sacral-nerve blocks determine which of the sacral nerves is operative in detrusor reflex activity; that is, the functional segmental innervation of the detrusor muscle is determined. The results of sacral-nerve blocks and rhizotomy indicate that the innervation of the human urinary bladder arises primarily from S-3 and S-4.[1,5,7] The effects of sacral-nerve blocks on the electromyogram of the anal and urethral sphincters indicate that the sphincter can function provided the right or the left sacral nerves to the sphincters are functioning. This protects sphincter function during rhizotomy or permanent sacral block. In addition, it has been shown in Rhesus monkeys and chimpanzees that the pudendal nerve nucleus in the sacral cord is at least one segment more rostral than the pelvic nerve nucleus;[9] the innervation of the sphincters is further protected by this anatomic arrangement.

CONCLUSIONS

In properly selected patients, a temporary or permanent sacral-nerve block will convert a hyperreflexic bladder into a normal one. This technique, which can be done on an outpatient basis in less than an hour, is also useful in diagnostic studies.

REFERENCES

1. Torrens, M.J.: The effect of selective sacral nerve blocks on vesical and urethral function. J. Urol., *112*:204, 1974.
2. Rockswold, G.L., and Chou, S.N.: Urological problems associated with central nervous system disease. *In* Neurological Surgery. Vol. II. Philadelphia, W.B. Saunders Co., 1982, p. 1031.
3. Bares, P., et al.: Standardization of terminology of lower urinary tract function. Urology, 9:237, 1977.
4. Yalla, S.V., Rossier, A.B., and Fam, B.: Dyssynergic vesicourethral responses during bladder rehabilitation in spinal cord injury patients: effects of suprapubic percussion, credé method and bethanechol chloride. J. Urol., *115*:575, 1976.
5. Rockswold, G.L., Bradley, W.E., and Chou, S.N.: Effect of sacral nerve blocks on the function of the urinary bladder in humans. J. Neurosurg., *40*:83, 1974.
6. Rockswold, G.L., and Bradley, W.E.: The use of sacral nerve blocks in the evaluation of neurologic bladder disease. J. Urol., *118*:415, 1977.
7. Rockswold, G.L., Chou, S.N., and Bradley, W.E.: Re-evaluation of differential sacral rhizotomy for neurological bladder disease. J. Neurosurg., *48*:773, 1978.
8. Heimburger, R.F., Freeman, L.W., and Wilde, N.J.: Sacral nerve innervation of the human bladder. J. Neurosurg., 5:154, 1948.
9. Rockswold, G.L., Bradley, W.E., and Chou, S.N.: Innervation of the external urethral and external anal sphincters in higher primates. J. Comp. Neurol., *193*:521, 1980.

10

Saddle Anesthesia

DAVID M. CUMES, M.D. and THOMAS A. STAMEY, M.D.

A saddle block is defined as anesthesia of that part of the body that would touch a saddle if a patient were riding a horse. There are several urologic procedures that are well handled by this selective spinal block; approximately 1,000 such anesthesias have been performed during the past 21 years in the Urology Outpatient Clinic at Stanford University Medical Center, with the anesthesia being administered by the urologist. This method has proven to be as safe and predictable as a diagnostic lumbar puncture.

There are several reasons for its inherent safety. First, a heavy solution of dibucaine hydrochloride (5 mg of dibucaine + 100 mg of dextrose per 2 ml) is used, which, because of its hyperbaricity and the patient's position, will "fix" in the lowermost sacral dermatomes of the cauda equina. Second, because of the selectivity of the block, somatic and, more especially, autonomic, hypotension are rare. Third, when a 25-gauge or, more recently, a 26-gauge spinal needle is used, the incidence of spinal headache is less than 1%.

In most outpatient surgical suites, the block will be administered by an anesthesiologist who will have the usual monitoring and anesthesiology equipment at hand, making for a virtually fail-safe form of regional anesthesia. It is so safe and effective that urologists should learn to do this technique themselves.

INDICATIONS

In the urology clinic at Stanford, saddle anesthesia has been used for the following procedures; it could well be extended to others.

(1) Endoscopic procedures in which local anesthesia alone is unlikely to be adequate, either because of the need for additional manipulation or because of the duration of urethral instrumentation. For example:

(A) Cystoscopy in a man in whom one's view is likely to be hampered by a large intravesical prostate;

(B) Ureteral catheterization studies when the cystoscope must be in the urethra for a long time, such as for bacterial localization studies, or split-function studies for renovascular hypertension (Stamey test). These patients often have mild discomfort from the ureteral manipulation, which is not blocked by the saddle anesthesia;

(C) Urethroscopy in the female when painful manipulations are necessary to search for a urethral diverticulum or ectopic orifice. Saddle anesthesia also allows painless radiologic injection studies.

(2) Perineal prostatic biopsies, especially when the nodule is small and representative biopsies would be difficult to obtain with local anesthesia alone.

COMPLICATIONS

Except for the rare headache, we have had no complications with this procedure, presumably because of the selectivity of the block and the small amount of anesthetic agent used. For example, when the heavy dibucaine solution is used and the patient is left in the sitting position for 10 minutes, sensation to pinprick is always normal over the symphysis pubis. We have become so confident about the safety of this anesthesia that we do not insert an intravenous line.

Nevertheless, with any form of spinal anesthesia, hypotension, meningitis, and neurologic deficits are possible. The incidence of hypotension is directly proportional to the extent of the autonomic block and thus has not been a problem in our patients, in whom only the lowermost sacral dermatomes are anesthetized. Meningitis is a theoretic risk if there is a breach in sterile technique. A more likely complication is meningismus from the aseptic irritating effect of the anesthetic agent. Neurologic deficits such as extra-ocular, sphincteric, and leg palsies are rare, and we have not seen these complications despite the fact that our patients sit for 10 minutes after administration of the heavy dibucaine solution to allow the agent to fix in the lower segments of the cauda equina. The manufacturers of dibucaine, however, recommend 60 seconds as the maximum permissible time for the patient to be erect; Dr. Daniel Moore has suggested that 3 minutes is sufficient and that 5 minutes is the maximum.[1] Likewise, Moore has not had a case of neurologic deficit.[2] The heavy dibucaine solution is more toxic than other drugs sometimes used for saddle anesthesia, and the lack of problems is probably a result of the small dose used.

PROCEDURE

Materials

Sterile gloves and a sterile preparation tray are required. Lidocaine (Xylocaine) 1% is used for skin anesthesia. The saddle block requires 2 ml of Dibucaine (Heavy Solution Nupercaine [0.25% dibucaine with 5% dextrose]), which is injected through a 3½-inch, 26-gauge spinal needle (Becton–Dickinson No. 5164) with a 1¼-inch, 20-gauge introducer (No. 5160). Before the patient is prepared, the drugs are withdrawn from their ampoules into syringes.

Patient Position

The patient sits with his legs over the side of the table and his feet resting on a stool. The head is flexed on the chest, and the arms are folded in front of the abdomen. The patient is steadied by an assistant (Fig. 10–1, *left*).

Landmarks

The upper edge of the iliac crest is at the level of the L-4 vertebra or the L-4–L-5 interspace. The spinal cord ends above that, at the L-1 level. The 20-gauge introducer is usually placed in line with the upper edge of the iliac crest in the L-4–L-5 interspace. In practice, however, we have placed the needle in the largest palpable interspace between L-3 and the lower sacrum (Fig. 10–1, *right*).

Method

The L-4–L-5 or other appropriate interspace is identified, and the patient's back is prepared, usually with a povidone–iodine solution, which is then wiped off with sterile 4 × 4-inch gauze sponges. A skin wheal is raised over the interspace with the lidocaine, and the interspinous ligament is infiltrated with the drug. The needle introducer is passed

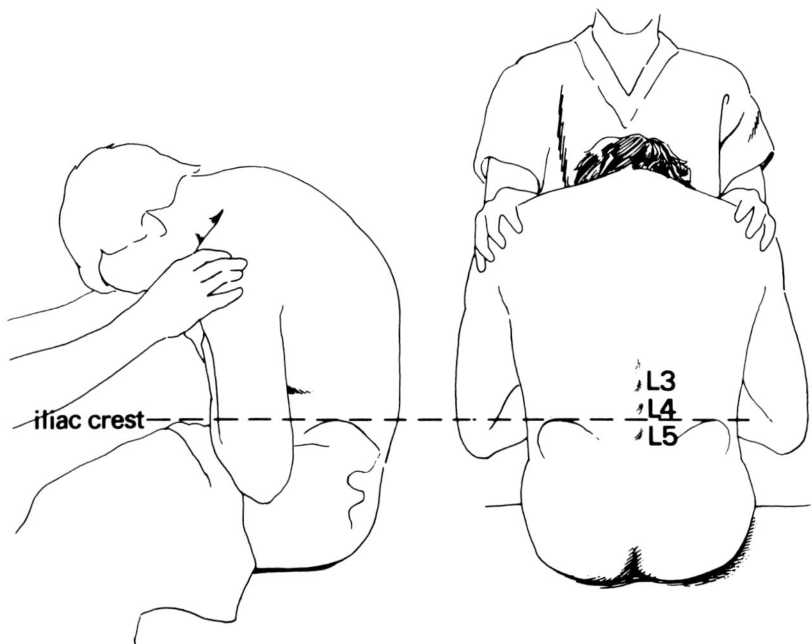

Fig. 10–1. Position of the patient and bony landmarks for saddle anesthesia.

through the wheal into the interspinous ligament and must lie in the same plane as the spinous processes and perpendicular to the transverse processes. The introducer stops short of the dura.

The spinal needle is then inserted through the introducer. If it is advanced slowly through the interspinous ligament, ligamentum flavum, and epidural space, it will encounter the dura, which it may pierce with a typical "pop" as the slight resistance is overcome. (This pop is felt much more often with the 26-gauge than with the 25-gauge needle.) The stylet is withdrawn and spinal fluid allowed to appear, which may take as long as 10 to 15 seconds with the 26-gauge needle. Alternatively, spinal fluid can be observed in the proximal part of the needle with the aid of a flashlight. When the syringe with the dibucaine is inserted into the needle, the drop of spinal fluid is forced out of the needle and easily identified as such. Spinal fluid should be withdrawn into the syringe before injecting the dibucaine and again after the injection is complete. If spinal fluid flows freely into the syringe both before and after injection, the surgeon can be assured of a perfect saddle anesthesia.

Failure to obtain spinal fluid can have a number of causes. First, the bevel of the needle may be lying against the dura or a nerve root; rotating the bevel 180° usually corrects this problem. Second, the needle may not have been advanced far enough and so may be lying in the interspinous ligament, ligamentum flavum, or epidural space. In this case, the needle should be advanced slowly while repeatedly testing for spinal fluid by withdrawing the obturator. Third, the needle may have been inserted too far and thus abuts against the vertebral body or the nucleus pulposus. In this case, it should be withdrawn a few millimeters. Fourth, there may be a small plug of tissue obstructing the bevel. This can be corrected by reinserting the stylet or injecting the needle with 0.5 ml of air. If blood is obtained and is not followed by a flow of clear spinal fluid, another attempt should be made at a higher or lower interspace.

Once the proper position of the needle is confirmed in the subarachnoid space, 1 ml of heavy dibucaine is injected slowly and the needle is withdrawn. The 1-ml dose is standard and should not be changed to accommodate differences in size and weight of the patient. Great care is taken during attachment of the syringe and injection of the solution, so as not to dislodge the needle from the subarachnoid space. A free flow of spinal fluid into the syringe at the end of the injection assures a perfect block. The patient then sits for 10 minutes before being placed in the lithotomy position for the procedure. The small dose and the 10 minutes in the sitting position ensure that the drug fixes in the lowermost segments of the cauda equina and gives a true saddle anesthesia. Operating analgesia usually appears within 5 to 15 minutes and can last 3 to 6 hours. The bladder should be emptied at the end of the procedure.

POSTPROCEDURE CARE

The patient is able to walk with assistance despite the persisting effect of the anesthesia. Although he can wait in the outpatient suite until the anesthesia has worn off, our practice is to send patients to their cars in wheelchairs and carefully instruct the accompanying family members on how to support him from the car to a sitting room at home. Some patients need to force fluids during the several hours required for the saddle block to wear off, in which case they must be instructed on how to void using the Valsalva maneuver and told that there will be no sensation of urine passing through the urethra. We instruct the patient carefully on how to walk around the sitting chair at home, holding on to the chair in order to determine when the anesthesia has worn off completely.

CONCLUSIONS

Saddle anesthesia can be performed safely and effectively by urologists, and the frequency of complications is low. Because the technique is useful for so many endoscopic procedures, as well as for perineal prostatic biopsy, urologists interested in outpatient surgery should learn how to do it themselves.

REFERENCES

1. Moore, D.C., and Thomas, C.C.: Regional Block. 4th Ed. Springfield, Charles C Thomas, 1981.
2. Moore, D.C.: Personal communication, 1982.

11

Anesthesia for Transurethral Procedures

AHMAD ORANDI, M.D., F.A.C.S.

A new device, the Resectoscope Injection Needle,* provides local anesthesia sufficient for many transurethral procedures traditionally done under regional anesthesia.

TECHNIQUE

The Resectoscope Injection Needle locks into the working element of the endoscope in the same manner as the electrode (Fig. 11–1). The Karl Storz resectoscope injection needle is inserted in the working element by threading the soft tubing through the electrode-locking aperture and advancing it until the shaft locks in place. The ACMI needle can be inserted in the cutting-loop orifice in retrograde or antegrade fashion. It is then bent at the point of the greenstick break (Fig. 11–1; *circle*), releasing the cut end, which is then advanced and fastened in the loop lock. Thus, the surgeon can maneuver the instrument and needle with one hand and inject local anesthetic anywhere in the lower urinary tract under direct vision.

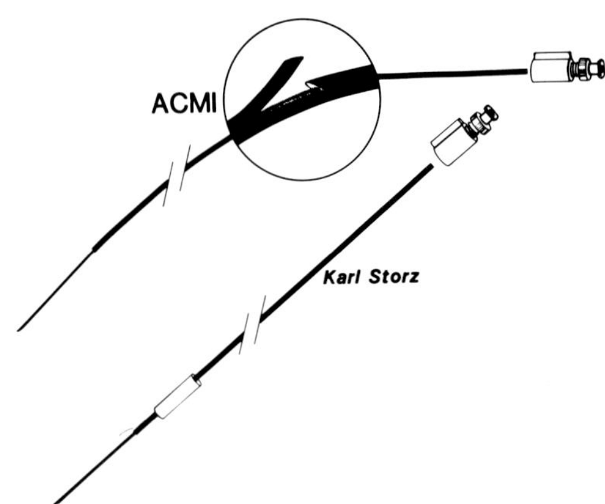

Fig. 11–1. Resectoscope Injection Needles for use with ACMI and Storz endoscopes. *In circle*: Greenstick break.

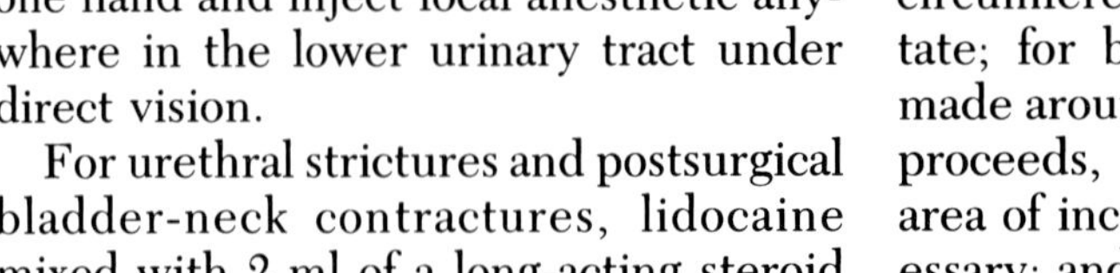

For urethral strictures and postsurgical bladder-neck contractures, lidocaine mixed with 2 ml of a long-acting steroid such as prednisolone tebutate is injected in the affected area. In prostatic surgery, the initial anesthetic injections are given circumferentially in the base of the prostate; for bladder tumors injections are made around the lesion. As the operation proceeds, subsequent injections in the area of incision or resection may be necessary; and repeated injections are made convenient by using two resectoscope working elements, one fitted with the needle and the other with the electrode.

*Patent: A. Orandi; available from Greenwald Surgical Co., Inc., Lake Station, IN 46405.

The local anesthesia thus obtained has been found adequate in selected patients for transurethral incision and resection of the prostate, resection of primary and recurrent bladder tumors, incision of the ostium and fulguration of small bladder diverticula (Chapter 14), ureteral meatotomy, and immediate postoperative pain relief when transurethral resection of the prostate is performed.

Section III

Urodynamics

12
Upper-Tract Urodynamics

ROBERT H. WHITAKER, M. CHIR., F.R.C.S.

In the late 1950s and 1960s, work was done on the general physiology and urodynamics of the upper urinary tract,[1–3] although it was not until somewhat later that the need for clinical investigation along these lines was appreciated.[4,5] During the last 15 years, there has been nothing short of a revolution in our approach to, and understanding of, the abnormal upper urinary tract. It was originally thought that any dilated system not associated with vesicoureteral reflux was obstructed, and this attitude undoubtedly led to many unnecessary operations on both the renal pelvis and the ureter.

DIAGNOSTIC ALTERNATIVES

The diagnostic task, in the presence of a wide upper urinary tract, is to distinguish between stasis alone and stasis with obstruction. Stasis alone is often harmless, and unless it is associated with a tendency to infection, there is little to be gained from operating. Obstruction implies that there is higher-than-normal pressure, often appreciated only at high urine-flow rates, and this raised pressure can damage the kidney. The combination of high pressure and infection is probably the most damaging of all.

Our approach over the last 12 years has been to measure the pressure within the renal pelvis directly during an artificially high flow rate and to deduce from this result whether the system is obstructed. Alternatives include the newer sophisticated types of renography,[6,7] which have the advantages of being noninvasive and able to measure total and differential renal function. The pressure-flow study is clearly invasive and gives no information regarding the function of the kidney, but it has the advantage of providing an immediate direct measure of the ability of the upper tract to transmit fluid. The fact that the study is independent of renal function is, at times, an asset, as one of the disadvantages of renography is that it is dependent on the ability of the kidney to handle both the isotope and the induced diuresis. In a poorly functioning kidney, this can be a considerable disadvantage, and not infrequently, it leads to a false diagnosis of obstruction.

Our policy at present is to rule out vesicoureteral reflux with micturating cystography. We then perform diuresis renography using either ^{123}I Hippuran with a gamma camera or ^{131}I Hippuran with probes. Usually within 24 hours, we perform a percutaneous pressure-flow study in the manner to be described. It has been our policy to admit the patient to the hospital for 24 to 48 hours, as we often wish to perform other studies such as renography or a creatinine clearance test, and because many of our patients must travel a considerable distance and cannot return home the same day. I will discuss the situations in which these studies could be done on outpatients.

INDICATIONS FOR PRESSURE-FLOW STUDIES

Many patients with upper-tract dilatation do not require further investigation other than a careful history and a good quality urogram to diagnose an obstruction either at the pelviureteral or ureterovesical junction. However, we seem to be seeing more and more patients with either equivocal symptoms or equivocal urographic findings who need more elaborate investigation. Particularly difficult are those patients who have had surgery or who have abnormal bladder function. In a busy practice, we estimate that one would examine some 20 to 30 patients per year in this way.

PRESSURE-FLOW PERFUSION STUDY

The principle of this study is to simulate a high diuresis and measure the pressure within the renal pelvis on the assumption that the definition of obstruction implies that increased pressure is necessary to transmit fluid through the upper urinary tract.[9] We assume that the kidney is damaged when this pressure, produced by the kidney itself, is raised above a certain level.

The main advantage of the technique that is described here over the studies that have been described previously[4,5] is that both the perfusion and the measurement of pressure are achieved by a single percutaneous cannula placed in the pelvis under x-ray control. We perfuse the system at the fast flow rate of 10 ml/min. This flow is just within the physiological range and is sufficiently fast to stress the system and show any propensity for obstruction.

Equipment

Although it is possible to perfuse the renal pelvis via an intravenous infusion set, we have found it difficult to control the flow rate precisely and thus prefer to use a syringe on a constant-perfusion pump. The pressure can be measured easily enough with a manometer tube strapped to a tape measure, but we find it more accurate and convenient to use a pressure transducer and a simple chart recorder, which produces a permanent record (Fig. 12–1). I list the basic and disposable equipment that we use but appreciate that similar suitable equipment is available from other manufacturers.

Basic Equipment

Perfusion pump (Braun acc 71104, with autoclavable 50-ml Luer-Lok syringe, acc 72465); pen recorder (Smiths Servoscribe, 1 channel, RE 501.20); and physiological pressure tranduscer (Statham, P23 Db).

Disposable Sterile Equipment

The following items are needed for each test: a four-way stopcock (Baxter, BR 62s), two three-way stopcocks (Pharmaseal, K75a), one wide-bore extension set (Avon, A60), one 200-cm manometer line (Portex, 200/490/200), two 60-cm manometer lines (Portex 200/490/060), one

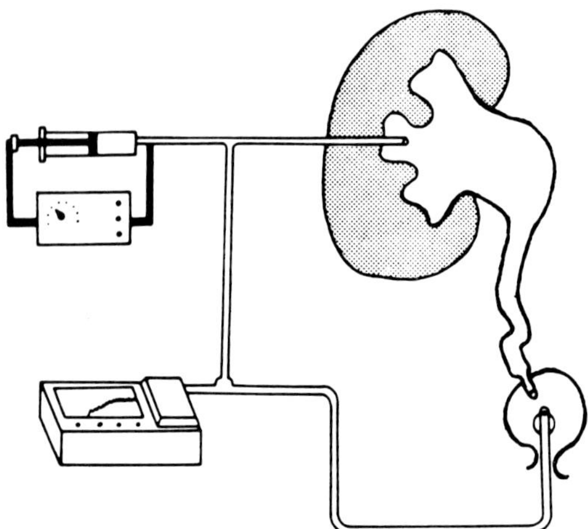

Fig. 12–1. Diagrammatic representation of the pressure-flow study (Whitaker test). (From Whitaker, R.H.: Urol. Clin. North Am., 6:529, 1979.)

double-male connector for connecting the urethral catheter and the apparatus, one bottle of saline or contrast medium (30% Urografin) for perfusion, and one Teflon cannula–Longdwel catheter, (Becton, Dickinson & Co., 18-gauge, 4- or 6-inch). The lay-up trolley with the other equipment is kept as simple as possible (Fig. 12–2).

Preparation of the Patient

We usually admit patients for these studies for logistic reasons, but many, if not most, could easily have this operation done on an outpatient basis. Only if there are problems such as hemorrhaging into the urinary system or gross extravasation of contrast medium would it be necessary to keep the patient in the hospital overnight. We do not cross-match blood, as we have not seen a worrying hemorrhage during or immediately after the procedure. Bleeding and clotting times would be determined only if there were a history suggesting that this was necessary. We always culture the urine and give appropriate antibiotics if it is infected.

We explain to the patient that this study is necessary to distinguish between stasis and obstruction and thus it helps us decide whether an operation is necessary. We also explain in some detail how the test is done, as this helps allay the patient's fears. They watch the progress on the monitor throughout and are often fascinated. Young children are often given a general anesthetic, but for older children and adults, we find this unnecessary.[10]

Technical Details

The procedure is carried out in the radiology department, where there is appropriate observation equipment. The x-ray table should be horizontal, and its height should not be changed once the procedure has begun.

With the patient supine on the table, we commence by administering an appropriate dose of an intravenous sedative such as diazepam. A plain radiograph is

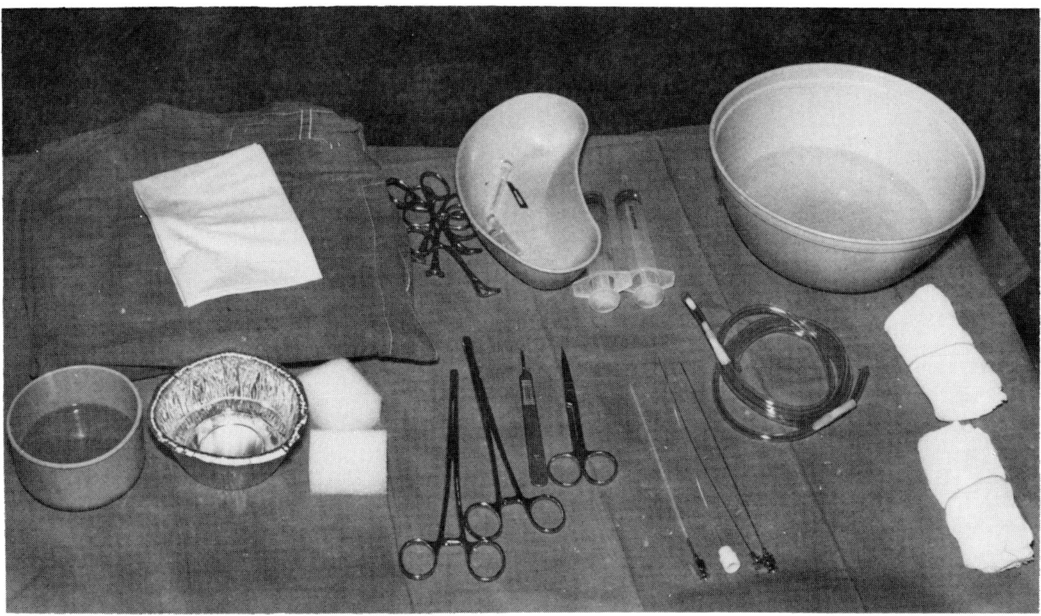

Fig. 12–2. The lay-up trolley for the percutaneous puncture is kept as simple as possible. (From Whitaker, R.H.: Urol. Clin. North Am., 6:529, 1979.)

taken of the abdomen, and an appropriate dose of contrast medium is immediately given to opacify the upper urinary tracts. A urethral catheter is then inserted; in children, we use an infant feeding tube and in adults, a 12F or 14F Foley catheter. In most cases, the bladder is emptied, although when there is outflow obstruction, we sometimes find it helpful to leave the bladder full. The bladder catheter is connected to the equipment with a 200-cm manometer line after priming with sterile water (Fig. 12–3).

The patient is then turned prone and made as comfortable as possible. We place a small foam pillow under the abdomen to displace the kidneys dorsally. By this time, the contrast medium is usually visible in the dilated collecting system; this is checked by intermittent fluoroscopy. The whole of the patient's back is then prepared with a sterile solution and the area draped (Fig. 12–4). A metal object, such as the blade of a scalpel or a needle, is placed on the skin and moved about with intermittent fluoroscopic observation to find the best spot for a vertical puncture of the collecting system. The skin is then infiltrated with local anesthetic. While the urologist is waiting for the anesthetic to numb the area, the pressure-measuring equipment is checked, and the wide-bore perfusion tubing is filled with contrast medium by activating the perfusion pump (Fig. 12–3, *Part F*). The end of this perfusion tube is held at the level of the kidney, and the baseline pressure is adjusted to zero. All further pressures are related to this level. The patency of the pressure line from the bladder is also checked at this point by asking the patient to cough. The usual resting pressure within a normal bladder is 5–8 cm H_2O.

A small incision is made in the skin with the point of a blade so that the 4- or 6-inch, 18-gauge Longdwel cannula can be advanced easily down toward the kidney. It must be kept vertical to avoid the problem of parallax. Although we have not used it ourselves, ultrasonic guidance would probably be helpful here. Patients are told to hold their breath as the needle is advanced. A point of note is that there

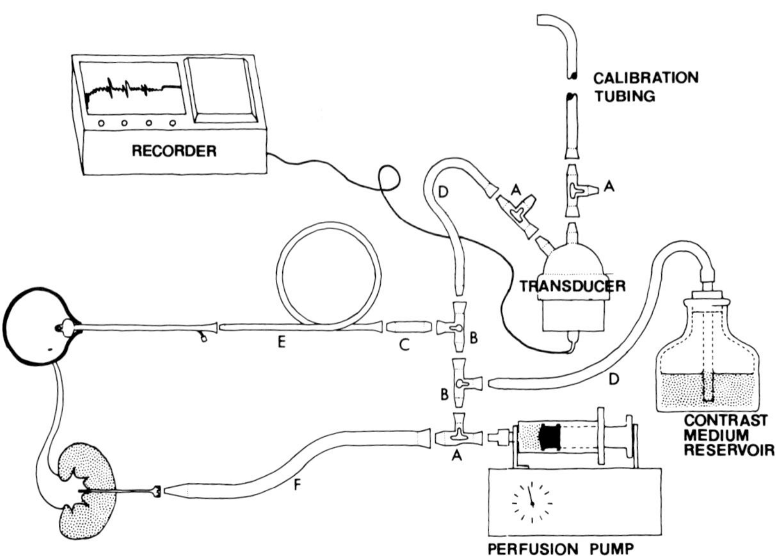

Fig. 12–3. Detailed connections of the equipment: *(A)* four-way stopcock, *(B)* three-way stopcock, *(C)* double-male connector, *(D)* 60-cm manometer tubing, *(E)* 200-cm manometer tubing, and *(F)* wide-bore extension tube. (From Whitaker, R.H.: Urol. Clin. North Am., 6:529, 1979.)

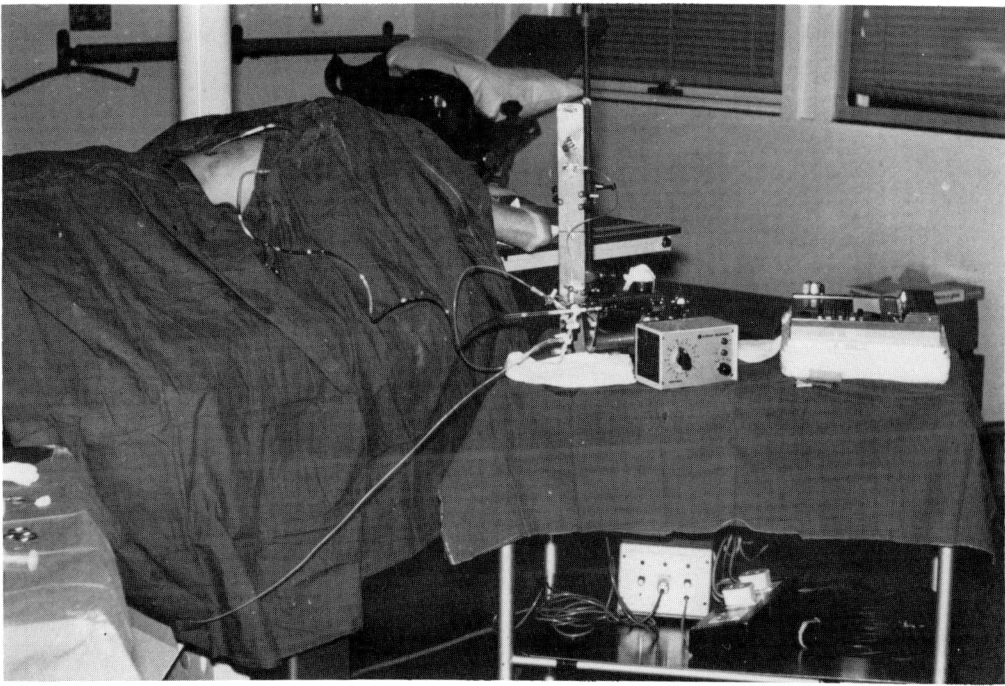

Fig. 12–4. The patient lies prone during the perfusion. The wider tube goes to the cannula, the thinner tube (under the drapes) to the bladder. (From Whitaker, R.H.: Urol. Clin. North Am., 6:529, 1979.)

is often a discrepancy between the length of the cannula and the needle, so that when urine is withdrawn from the needle, the cannula should be advanced over the needle; the needle should not simply be withdrawn.

The cannula, which is now positioned in the renal pelvis, is connected to the perfusion tubing and secured to the patient's back. We then perfuse the upper tract with 30% Urografin, commencing at the rate of 10 ml per minute. If the cannula is not lying satisfactorily within the pelvicalyceal system, this will be manifest immediately by a sudden rise in the pressure; and the cannula can be adjusted accordingly. We observe the procedure fluoroscopically during the initial stages of perfusion to make sure there is no leakage. Thereafter, intermittent screening and spot radiographs give all the information required. Thoroughout the procedure, the bladder pressure can be measured intermittently by adjusting the three-way stopcock (Fig. 12–3, *Part B*). It is imperative that perfusion continue until there is a steady flow of contrast medium in through the cannula and out through the lower end of the ureter; this may be associated with either an equilibrated pressure or, if the system is severely obstructed, a steadily rising pressure. If there is doubt as to the completeness of the filling, then the perfusion must be continued. Intermittent screening often helps to decide this point. The bladder should be allowed to fill naturally during the procedure, but if there is a rise in pelvic pressure, the bladder should be drained to see whether this allows the pressure to fall.

If the pressure within the kidney rises above 50–60 cm H_2O, it is occasionally worth seeing whether a lower flow rate, perhaps 5 or 2 ml per minute, can be tolerated. However, we seldom find that this adds much informative data. If the urinary tract is unobstructed, it will tolerate 10 ml per minute with a pressure < 12 cm H_2O.

When the pressure has risen to a high level, or has remained steady at a lower level, the procedure is terminated. It must be emphasized again that it is essential for the operator to be convinced that the system has been perfused to the point of a steady state. The residual fluid is then aspirated from the kidney, and the cannula is removed. A small dressing is applied to the wound. The cannula is reconnected to the perfusing system and perfused, away from the patient, with contrast medium so the resistance that it generates at a perfusion rate of 10 ml per minute can be measured. This information is needed to calculate the result.

After-Care

The patient is returned to the ward and kept in bed for 12 hours. The blood pressure and pulse are monitored at half-hourly intervals for 2 hours and every 4 hours thereafter. Slight hematuria can be expected, but provided this has stopped, the patient can be discharged the following day. Infection has not been a problem, and hematuria is rarely severe enough to keep the patient in the hospital for more than this limited period. Some extravasation of contrast medium probably occurs in many patients, particularly in those with an element of obstruction, but this has not been a practical problem.

If we were to change our policy and do pressure-flow studies on an outpatient basis, we would warn the patient of the possible need for hospital admission, explain the likelihood of some discomfort after the procedure, and the possibility of hematuria for a few hours. The test would be performed early in the morning, with postoperative monitoring of the pulse and blood pressure and a careful overall check of the patient's condition before discharge. Many centers now perform these studies without hospital admission; for instance, Doctor Pfister in Boston has performed hundreds of pressure-flow studies with virtually no worrying complications.

Analysis of the Results

If the pressure tracing continues to rise with no equilibration, the system is clearly obstructed and no calculations are needed. If the pressure within the renal pelvis equilibrates, it is then necessary to subtract from this level the pressure generated by perfusing the cannula alone; this provides the *absolute* pressure. If the bladder pressure is then subtracted from this figure, the result is the *relative* pressure. This relative pressure is the drop in pressure between the kidney and the bladder at the chosen flow rate. If this relative pressure is < 12 cm H_2O at a flow rate of 10 ml per minute, we can be sure that there is no obstruction in the system. If it is $> 20–22$ cm H_2O, then there is clearly some obstruction, probably to a degree that needs surgical relief. Occasionally, the levels are between 12 and 22 cm H_2O, and in this gray area, it is not yet clear whether an operation is essential.

The anatomic level of an obstruction is shown on the radiographs that are taken at the time of the study, and unless there are two or more narrowed areas, the determination of the level is not a problem. The final decision about whether an operation is necessary must be taken in the light of other factors, such as the overall renal function and the likelihood of success.

In most patients with normal bladder function, the bladder pressure remains between 8 and 12 cm H_2O throughout the study, and its actual level is needed only to calculate the relative pressure. However, if there is hypertonicity as, for instance, with a neuropathic bladder, in prostatism, or in boys with posterior urethral valves, the bladder pressure becomes critical. It is then essential to empty the bladder during the procedure to see the effect of this action on the renal pelvic pressure. If the renal pelvic pressure is 30 cm H_2O and the bladder pressure 25 cm H_2O, the relative pressure, or the pressure drop between the kidney and bladder, is within normal limits, but the absolute pressure in the renal pelvis is being maintained at too high a level because of the raised bladder pressure; and this, of course, can damage the kidney. There are other situations—for example, after reimplantation of a ureter, particularly into a neuropathic bladder—in which there may be a combination of hypertonicity of the bladder and an element of true ureterovesical obstruction. A pressure-flow study such as discussed here is the only way in which this can be determined accurately.

RESULTS

We have done more than 250 pressure-flow studies for a wide variety of clinical problems.[11,12] In 96% of the patients, the answer has been definitive as to whether there is obstruction. A small percentage of patients have shown results in the equivocal or gray area; as a rule, we have treated these patients conservatively. We also have looked at the long-term predictive value of pressure-flow studies.[13] Of 21 studies performed more than five years previously, we found there was no case that suggested that incorrect information was obtained from the initial investigation.

CONCLUSIONS

Pressure-flow studies are now a regular part of the evaluation of possible upper-tract obstruction. Although logistic considerations may necessitate overnight hospitalization, this procedure can be performed properly and safely in an outpatient unit with the necessary equipment.

REFERENCES

1. Kiil, F.: The Function of the Ureter and Renal Pelvis. Oslo, University Press, 1957.
2. Boyarsky, S., and Labay, P.: Ureteral Dynamics. Baltimore, Williams & Wilkins Co., 1972.
3. Struthers, N.W.: The role of manometry in the investigations of pelvi-ureteral function. Br. J. Urol., *41*:129, 1969.
4. Johnston, J.H.: The pathogenesis of hydronephrosis in children. Br. J. Urol., *41*:724, 1969.
5. Backlund, L., and Reuterskiold, A.G.: The abnormal ureter in children. I. Perfusion studies on the wide nonrefluxing ureter. Scand. J. Urol. Nephrol., 3:219, 1969.
6. O'Reilly, P.H., et al.: Diuresis renography in equivocal urinary tract obstruction. Br. J. Urol., *50*:76, 1978.
7. Whitfield, H.N., et al.: The distinction between obstructive uropathy and nephropathy by radioisotope transit times. Br. J. Urol., *50*:433, 1978.
8. Koff, S.A., Thrall, J.H., and Keyes, J.W., Jr.: Diuretic radionuclide urography: a non-invasive method for evaluating nephroureteral dilatation. J. Urol., *122*:451, 1979.
9. Whitaker, R.H.: Methods of assessing obstruction in dilated ureters. Br. J. Urol., *45*:15, 1973.
10. Whitaker, R.H.: The Whitaker test. Urol. Clin. North Am., *6*:529, 1979.
11. Whitaker, R.H.: Equivocal pelvi-ureteric obstruction. Br. J. Urol., *47*:771, 1975.
12. Whitaker, R.H.: An evaluation of 170 diagnostic pressure flow studies of the upper urinary tract. J. Urol., *121*:602, 1979.
13. Witherow, R.O'N., and Whitaker, R.H.: The predictive accuracy of antegrade studies in equivocal upper tract obstruction. Br. J. Urol., 53:496, 1981.

13

The Principles of Outpatient Evaluation of Lower Urinary-Tract Function and Dysfunction

RICHARD TURNER-WARWICK, B.Sc., D.M. (Oxon), M.Ch., F.R.C.P., F.R.C.S., F.A.C.S., F.A.R.A.C.S. and
JEAN PITFIELD-MARSHALL, B.Sc., M.B., Ch.B., Edin., D.M.R.D., F.R.C.R.

Many patients attend urologic clinics with symptoms arising as a direct result of detrusor or sphincter dysfunction. Unfortunately, the bladder often proves an unreliable witness even when interrogated as intelligently as possible; this problem is naturally compounded if the patient is a poor witness. The development of methods for objective urodynamic evaluation of lower urinary-tract function and their introduction into routine clinical practice have led to a fundamental revision of many functional concepts relating to symptomatology, radiographic findings, endoscopic appearances and, consequently, to treatment.

Lower-tract function can be evaluated in many ways. Some methods are invaluable, some have limited application, some have particular shortcomings, and a few are frankly inappropriate. Figure 13–1 relates some of these evaluation methods to the various aspects of urodynamic function and broadly indicates their relative value. Such a presentation is subject to widely divergent personal opinions; nevertheless, read in context with a consideration of the individual methods and the practical procedures,[1] it provides a convenient summary and basis for consideration.

MISCONCEPTIONS AND INAPPROPRIATE METHODS OF EXAMINATION

Many outdated misconceptions persist in routine urologic and gynecologic practice, even after the introduction of objective methods of evaluation more than a decade ago. This sadly reflects the amount of time it takes to effect a significant change in the practice of clinical medicine.

Symptomatology

The misleading nature of many lower urinary-tract symptoms and the importance of objective urodynamic evaluation cannot be overemphasized. The bladder is often erroneously felt to be full either as a result of hypersensitivity caused by

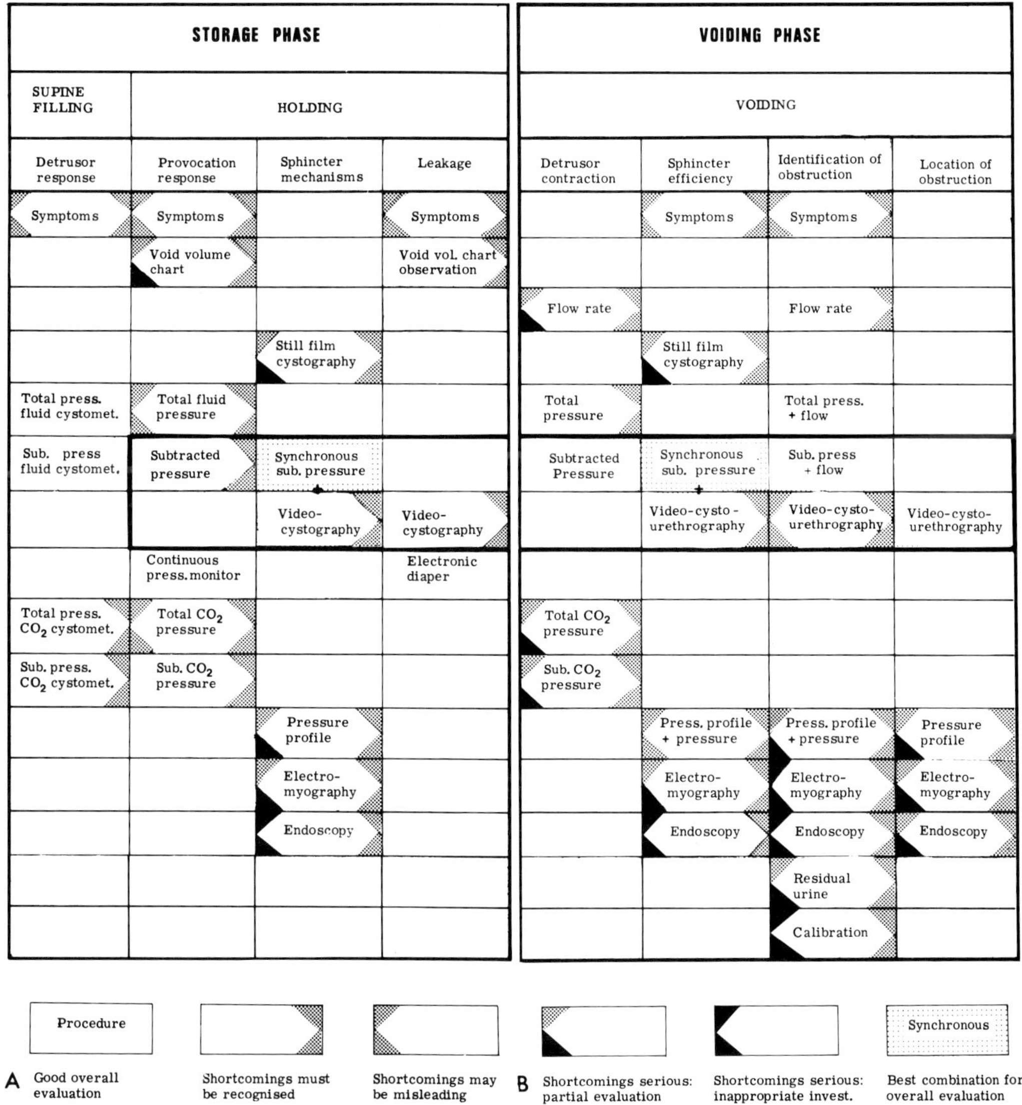

Fig. 13–1. Tests for evaluating urodynamic function.[1]

inflammation or because of a pressure rise resulting from an involuntary unstable detrusor contraction. On the other hand, under different circumstances, a full or partially evacuated bladder may feel empty.

Male patients with lifelong dyssynergic bladder-neck obstruction commonly claim that their stream is "normal" when it is, in fact, grossly impaired. Females presenting with cystitis or with retention often insist that their bladder function was previously normal, yet they subsequently prove to have been infrequent voiders who also voided inefficiently.[1] Although most females who say they leak do in fact leak, some patients who claim they do not leak can easily be shown to leak. If a female patient claims to be dry after an operation for incontinence, this can certainly be classed as a clinical success, inasmuch as the patient is satisfied;

however, the development and improvement of operative procedures requires accurate evaluation, and success may be overestimated if subjective methods of evaluation are used alone.

Clinical Examination

The size of a prostate is irrelevant to the diagnosis of bladder-outlet obstruction; large prostates do not create a proportional obstruction and sometimes create none at all. Similarly, there is a poor correlation between the extent of vaginal prolapse and urethral competence.

Endoscopy

The cystoscope and the urethroscope are virtually useless instruments for urodymanic evaluation; erroneous deductions are often made from endoscopic appearances; a diagnosis of bladder-outflow obstruction cannot be proven or excluded by these unless an impassable stricture is discovered.

Trabeculation. In the male, trabeculation is usually associated with a thick-walled bladder; this may or may not be associated with obstruction, but it is certainly not diagnostic of it. The most common correlation of hypertrophic trabeculation is with unstable detrusor dysfunction.[2,3] This is not surprising if hypertrophy is conceived as resulting from exercise, because an unstable detrusor obviously contracts against voluntarily closed sphincters much more frequently than a stable detrusor contracts against increased outlet resistance.

However, the appearance of trabeculation in females positively suggests that the bladder outlet is *not* obstructed. A trabeculated female bladder commonly proves to be thin-walled; hypotrophic trabeculation is often associated with habitually infrequent, unobstructed voiding and stable detrusor behavior.[2] A thick-walled female bladder is almost always associated with *unobstructed unstable* detrusor function, because high-resistance bladder-outlet obstruction sufficient to cause hypertrophic trabeculation, or unstable detrusor behavior secondary to it, is most unusual in females.[4]

Some aspects of the concept of hypertrophy applied to bladder muscle are open to question. The increase in the bulk of the trabeculated bladder wall or the hypertrophied bladder neck is not the result of an increase in either the number or size of the smooth muscle cells but rather of an increase in interstitial collagen; nevertheless, such detrusors commonly generate a considerably elevated contraction pressure.

Bladder-Neck Hypertrophy. The endoscopic appearance of bladder-neck hypertrophy is certainly not acceptable evidence that it is obstructing, but unfortunately it is still often erroneously conceived and treated as such. Secondary hypertrophy of a normally functioning bladder-neck mechanism resulting either from unstable detrusor dysfunction or from a distal urethral stricture in the male does not cause it to become obstructed; furthermore, many dyssynergic bladder-neck mechanisms that cause significant obstruction appear endoscopically normal in every way.[1–3]

Urethral Calibration

The concept that bladder-outlet obstruction in the female can be identified by instrumental calibration is erroneous. Meatal stenosis of a female urethra calibrating 16F–18F does not indicate that it is obstructive; if outflow obstruction coexists, it must be the result of dynamic or distortional failure of the urethra to attain its full potential caliber during voiding, because a rigid stricture does not cause a significant obstruction until it calibrates to less than 10F.[4]

Residual Urine Measurement

True postvoiding residual urine indicates inefficient voiding, and further urodynamic evaluation is required to determine whether this is the result of increased bladder-outlet resistance, an inefficient detrusor contraction, or both. However, the absence of postvoiding residual urine (often erroneously described as the bladder empties "normally" instead of "completely") by no means excludes even the severest degree of obstruction.[2,3,5] The urographic demonstration of residual urine after the patient attempts to void on command with the bladder only partially distended half an hour after the injection of contrast medium is often false.

APPROPRIATE METHODS OF URODYNAMIC EVALUATION

The proper evaluation of the function and dysfunction of the urinary tract involves the use of appropriate methods, some of which do not require special instrumentation. Some of these methods may not be included in the term "urodynamics," which, unfortunately, is used by some to denote only electronic measurements of pressures, flow, and muscle electroactivity in a urodynamics laboratory and often does not include critical radiographic studies. The diagnostic and therapeutic value of some simple outpatient tests is often overlooked.

Voided-Volume Records

The voided-volume chart is the natural cystovolumetric record.[1] A normal, stable bladder is usually not emptied until it is nearly full; however, an unstable bladder develops involuntary contractions before its full functional capacity is reached; thus, the chart characteristically shows wide variations in the volumes voided, ranging from less than 100 ml to approximately 300 ml. Thus, a simple chart kept for 48 hours may be the only urodynamic evaluation needed to confirm a clinical suspicion of detrusor instability, particularly in children. Furthermore, it is a first step in bladder inhibition training, as it provides patients with unequivocal evidence that their unstable bladders are quite untruthful when they claim to be full and convinces the patients that their urgency is caused by an intravesical pressure rise resulting from an involuntary contraction rather than by bladder-wall stretch.

Hypersensitive conditions tend to result in almost uniformly diminished voided volumes.

Uroflowmetry

A recording uroflowmeter is the essential instrument for identifying bladder-outlet obstruction. It *must* be used routinely for the evaluation of male patients, both to prevent *underdiagnosis* of clinically significant bladder-neck obstruction when the appearances of routine intravenous urography and endoscopy are normal, and also to avoid *overdiagnosis* of prostatic obstruction when the patient has a palpably enlarged prostate and symptoms of "prostatism," which may be the result of unobstructed detrusor instability.

The voiding flow patterns of some patients are greatly affected by their immediate environments. This may or may not be associated with a significant dysfunction, but it emphasizes the importance of ensuring that the uroflow records are obtained by voiding a full bladder in privacy and verifying thereafter that the patient regards the result as reasonably representative of their usual performance. The time-honored method of observing a patient's voiding stream is generally an inaccurate and impractical substitute. Indeed, even when a recording instrument is readily available, some of the patients for whom it matters most find it difficult to provide a representative uroflow record.

Procedure and Interpretation. In a busy urologic clinic, it is best to use a single-purpose uroflowmeter separate from the multichannel pressure instrument and locate it in toilet-like seclusion.

The uroflowmeter should be as simple as possible and have an automatic on–off switch because some patients find the switching too complicated and their preoccupation with this results in yards of wasted paper and sometimes in no record at all. A uroflow record can identify a grossly obstructed outlet (prolonged flow with a peak rate of less than about 10 ml per second) and an overtly normal outflow (sharp rise and termination, with a peak flow of > 20 ml per second). However, many symptomatic patients have equivocal flow patterns, with a peak rate of 10 to 20 ml per second; further information can sometimes be obtained from the shape of the flow pattern, but accurate interpretation may require measurement of the voiding detrusor pressure and determining whether this is sustained throughout micturition. Occasionally, specific symptoms in the male are related to a high-pressure, normal-flow outlet obstruction (sometimes the pressure can be very high: 100–150 cm H_2O, whereas the normal is 50 cm H_2O), or to low-pressure, low-flow states.[1–3,6]

Pressure-Flow Studies. Pressure-flow studies are required for the evaluation of equivocal flow patterns. They are best undertaken synchronously where possible, but the circumstances of the examination may cause artifactual variations of peak flow rate, so that the flow measurements obtained by voiding in privacy should be taken as the norm. The technique is described later in this chapter.

The Standard Intravenous Urogram

A review of the standard intravenous urogram (IVU) and the timing of the spot films seems overdue. It is well recognized that the yield of unexpected findings is low in many urodynamic dysfunctions such as suspected bladder-outlet obstruction in both males and females, incontinence in females, and nocturnal enuresis. Intravenous urography is, in fact, a dynamic procedure in which the natural passage of a bolus of contrast medium can be recorded as it is concentrated in the kidney and passes along the urinary tract to the point of its discharge from the urethra (Fig. 13–2); the natural process usually takes between one and four hours according to bladder behavior, so it has to be recorded adymically by spot films.

The timing of the spot films is necessarily a compromise; the standard IVU series is selected to cover the full range of clinical circumstances for which the study is generally requested. Furthermore, as the result of the longstanding urologic misconception that voiding dysfunction and inefficiency can be identified from the residual urine volume or from the endoscopic appearances of the prostate, the bladder neck, or trabeculation, the spot film series is largely focused on the upper urinary tract, and valuable evidence of lower urinary-tract function is thus lost.

The principal defect of the standard IVU series is that the postvoiding film of

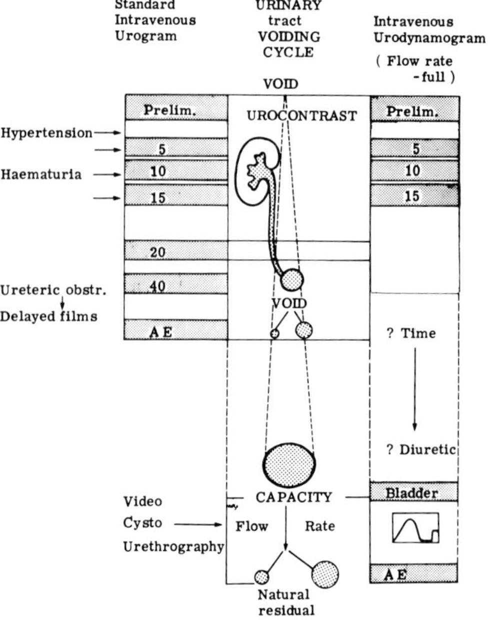

Fig. 13–2. Diagram comparing the standard I.V.U. and the intravenous urodynamogram.

the bladder is taken after the patient has voided by request 30 to 40 minutes after preinjection voiding; this may not be representative of the patient's usual voiding pattern, because many persons are unable to initiate voiding properly until their bladders feel full. Nevertheless, residual urine apparent after this unnatural voiding interval is not infrequently interpreted as evidence of voiding inefficiency, and if no residual urine is seen, this is often reported erroneously as the bladder "fills and empties normally," when in fact the snapshots justify only a report of "fills and empties completely." The absence of residual urine does not exclude even severe bladder-outflow obstruction (e.g., a flow rate of < 5 ml and a voiding detrusor pressure of > 100 cm H_2O[2,3]).

The Intravenous Urodynamogram

The basic concept of the intravenous urodynamogram (IVUD) is that, in addition to appropriate upper-tract spot films, it includes a voiding flowmetric record and a postvoiding film taken after a natural urination (see Fig. 13–2.)[7] Thus:

(1) The lower-tract films are postponed until the patient feels that the need to urinate is a matter of some urgency.

(2) Spot films are taken immediately before and after this natural voiding to outline the distended bladder and the postvoiding residual volume.

(3) Between these films, the patient voids in the privacy of an apparently conventional toilet, adjacent to the radiology facilities, which has an automatic switching device to record the flow pattern and the voided volume; this then forms an integral part of the record and the report of the examination.

Consideration should also be given to the number and the timing of the spot-film records of the upper urinary tract. Rather than adopt an extensive routine for a general all-purpose examination of the upper urinary tract, it may be economically reasonable to adopt a three-film series for the screening of many conditions and specify a "special upper-tract series," appropriately adapted, for the evaluation of specific problems such as hypertension, hematuria, and upper-tract obstruction (see Fig. 13–2, *left*).

After the initial upper-tract series has been made, the patients are free to "go walk about" and have breakfast with additional fluids to hasten bladder filling. If they are habitually infrequent voiders, it may be an acceptable expediency to give them an oral diuretic. They must understand the importance of returning to the department when they need to void; otherwise, they may void their contrast medium elsewhere.

Apart from the fact that IVUD provides a more appropriate screening evaluation of the lower urinary tract, the modified upper-tract screening series reduces not only the irradiation but also the cost; furthermore, it reduces the x-ray table time, so that more patients can be processed each hour.

In practice, an IVUD is best arranged during a morning session, partly to use overnight dehydration and partly to ensure that the examination is complete before the department closes. We find it helpful, particularly for long-distance referrals, to run a preliminary IVUD session early in the day so that we can proceed to a full urodynamic evaluation thereafter if it proves necessary.

The Intravenous Cystodynamogram

An intravenous cystodynamogram, omitting both the plain film and the upper-tract series, is sometimes an appropriate limited followup investigation to provide a true record of postoperative voiding efficiency without the artifact caused by invasive instrumentation.

The Ultrasound Cystodynamogram

The rational development of the IV cystodynamogram (IVCD) for the basic objective evaluation of the voiding efficiency is the simple noninvasive variant, the Ultrasound Cystodynamogram (USCD); the patient is required to present with a full bladder, and no other preparation is required. An ultrasound scan of the bladder is obtained before and after a full bladder uroflow record.

Voiding Cystourethrography

Simple image-intensified urographic observation of bladder-outlet and sphincter function during cystographic voiding is an important and much underutilized investigation available to every urologist; no combination of electronic pressure-flow measurements can substitute adequately for it (video = I see, non video = I do not see) (see Fig. 13–2).[1] The voiding cystourethrogram is the most accurate method of identifying the site of a bladder-outflow obstruction in both males and females after the presence of obstruction has been proved by flow or pressure-flow measurement. The technique is described later in this chapter.

EVALUATION OF SPHINCTER FUNCTION

Video studies of the sphincter mechanisms during voluntary interruption of the voiding stream—the "stop-test"—also provide detailed information about the function and dysfunction of individual sphincter mechanisms. A number of common dysfunctional varieties are discussed in detail elsewhere (Fig. 13–3).[1]

In both male and female patients, the bladder-neck sphincter and the urethral sphincter mechanism can function independently. Normally both are competent, but continence can be maintained by either one alone, and only if both are incompetent is the patient incontinent. Videocystourethrography during provocation cystometry (especially coughing in a standing position) is the most accurate procedure for determining whether a patient's continence is maintained at the bladder neck or the urethral sphincter. Minor degrees of stress leakage are incidentally detected, which is important in the critical evaluation of female incontinence when the patient claims to be cured after an operation.

Video-Audio Records

The fluoroscopic image should be videorecorded, because much urodynamic information is lost in still-film records, particularly in the assessment of vesicourethrovaginal prolapse and sphincter efficiency in incontinent women. In addition, a synchronous audio record improves the recall information on playback, especially during the evaluation of sphincter function by the voiding "stop-test." It is a simple matter to plug in a microphone.

The radiologist always observes the urodynamic behavior on the monitor screen during voiding cystourethrography; a urodynamically oriented clinician naturally insists on reviewing the audio-video record of problem cases personally before proceeding; others are satisfied with a few "comic-strip" snapshot films.

THE URODYNAMIC EVALUATION OF FREQUENCY AND URGENCY

It is often important to determine whether the symptoms of frequency, urgency, and nocturia result from unstable detrusor contractions, creating an intravesical pressure rise before the bladder is fully distended, or from abnormal bladder sensitivity. "Sensory urgency" must often be proved by ruling out un-

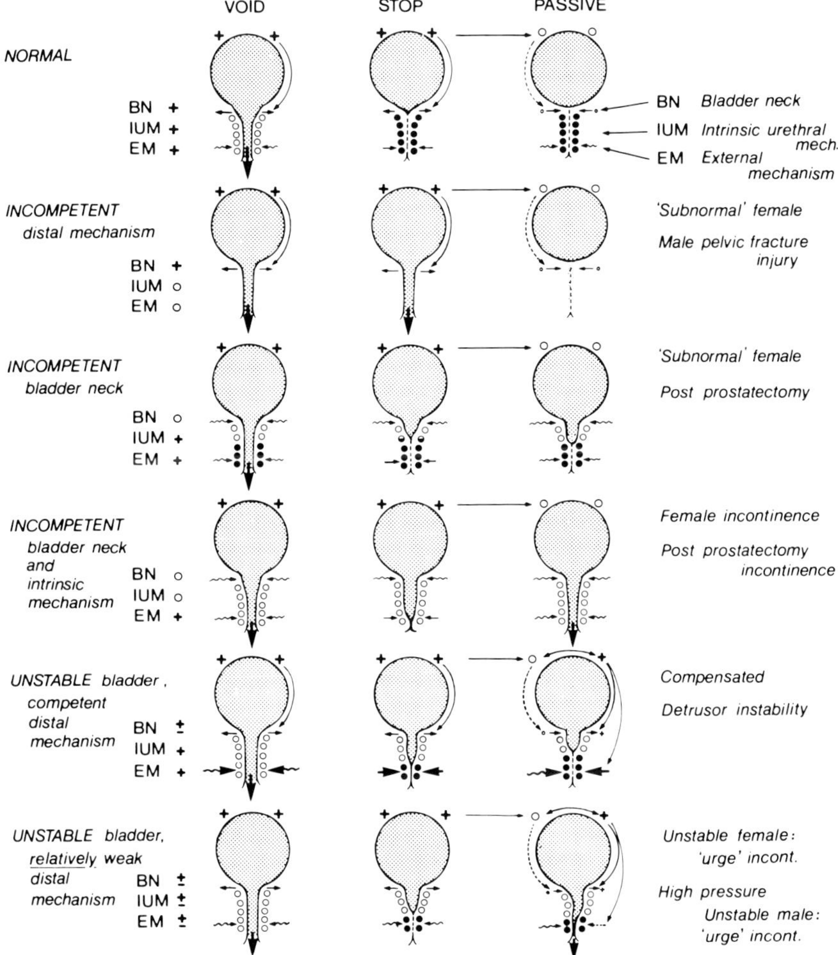

Fig. 13–3. Evaluation of sphincter function by voiding cystourethrography and the "stop-test."

stable detrusor activity by provocation cystometry.

Cystometry Under Light Anesthesia

When the voided-volume chart indicates a functional abnormality and the maximum voided volume is diminished, cystometry under light general anesthesia may be important. This technique abolishes unstable detrusor contractions, so that the small-capacity bladder distends normally and thus can be distinguished easily from a rigidly contracted undistensible bladder. The procedure is also invaluable for the evaluation of hypersensitivity dysfunction. Patients with supratrigonal hypersensitivity caused by interstitial cystitis tend to become restless and to phonate under light general (but not spinal) anesthesia when their bladders are distended by an irrigation fluid pressure of 100 cm H_2O, whereas this is not characteristic of patients with abnormally sensitive bladder bases, such as those with urethrotrigonitis.

DETRUSOR FUNCTION AND DYSFUNCTION

Many urologic problems associated with both holding and voiding are caused by disordered detrusor function and their accurate resolution depends on appropriate objective evaluation.

If a detrusor is functioning normally:

(1) It contracts only during volitional voiding.
(2) Its voiding contraction is volitionally initiated.
(3) Its voiding contraction is sustained until evacuation is complete.

Any of these elements may be abnormal, singularly or in combination; and these abnormalities may or may not be associated with a detectable neuropathy.

Description and Terminology

Itemized objective descriptions are preferred, such as "unstable detrusor with volitional but unsustained contraction" or "an acontractile bladder." It is inaccurate and unhelpful to refer to a single specific dysfunction in one phase of the storage-voiding cycle in general terms of neurological concept such as "hyper-reflexic" or "are flexic," especially when other elements are "normo-reflexic." Abnormal detrusor behavior should never be assumed to be "neurogenic" unless this is unequivocal—as in spinal cord disruption; a recently acquired incomplete neuropathy may be quite irrelevant to a lifelong idiopathic instability and, in the male, reversion to stability may occur after relief of a coincident outlet obstruction in spite of it.

When a male patient presents with frequency, nocturia, urgency, and a poor stream, it is both irrational and potentially misleading to refer to this symptom complex as "prostatism," because it is often unrelated either to the prostate or to obstruction; this symptom complex is often the result of idiopathic detrusor instability without obstruction, and a prostatic enlargement may only be a coincidence. The complaint of a "poor stream" is a natural consequence of a small voided volume, and thus uroflowmetry is essential. Furthermore, the same symptom complex resulting from unstable detrusor behavior in the female is certainly not referred to as "prostatism." However, it is important to appreciate that unstable detrusor behavior is sometimes asymptomatic.

Stability and Instability

A normally controlled detrusor does not contract during voluntary retention, and it is convenient to refer to this normally inhibited behavior as "stable," however, by definition, the term "stable" denotes that it has been proved, by provocative cystometric testing, that it is not unstable. Furthermore, it is also necessary to have objective evidence that a detrusor contracts during voiding; otherwise, one cannot be certain whether the inactivity on filling is the result of normal inhibition of its contraction potential or of an acontractile bladder, which is an abnormal state of paresis. This emphasizes:

(1) The shortcomings of supine filling cystometry and also of the use of gas for cystometry, which is quite unsuitable for measurements during voiding.
(2) The fundamental scientific inaccuracy of using the conceptual term "areflexia" to describe a flat filling cystometric pressure record so that there is no distinction between "areflexic" acontractility and "normo-reflexic" stability.

Beyond this, however, the term "unstable" has:

(1) No further implication for the extent of the abnormality; that is, whether the voiding contraction is volitional, whether it is powerful or weak, or whether it is sustained throughout voiding.
(2) No implication of aetiology; that is, whether it is idiopathic, neuropathic, or associated with bladder-outlet obstruction in the male.
(3) No implication of abnormality of the

detrusor muscle itself, just as an abnormal knee jerk does not indicate that the quadriceps muscle is abnormal. Stable behavior of the sacrovesical reflex is dependent on upper motor neuron inhibition.

The Effect of Unstable Detrusor Contractions

In addition to creating a rise in intravesical pressure, an involuntary detrusor contraction is associated with relaxation or opening of the bladder neck so that this mechanism becomes incompetent; whether this detrusor contraction pressure results in urinary leakage depends on the ability of the distal voluntary sphincter to contain the urine. In general, the distal sphincter mechanism of the male is much more powerful than that of the female.[2,3]

The Clinical Significance of the Maximum Isometric Detrusor Contraction Pressure

There is increasing evidence that the maximum detrusor contraction pressure is relevant to the management of female urinary incontinence.[8] Thus, if a female has unstable incontinence, the chances of a simple repositioning operation (which marginally improves the sphincter function) being successful are much less if there are high-pressure detrusor contractions than if the maximum detrusor pressure is low. Furthermore, a high-pressure unstable detrusor seems to respond poorly to pharmacotherapy and bladder training. An arbitrary pressure level of 35 to 40 cm H_2O is used to distinguish high and low detrusor pressures.

Supine Cystometry

The value of simple supine cystometry is strictly limited; only about 50% of unstable bladders demonstrate unstable behavior in the supine position, even on rapid filling; hence, the proper evaluation of a normally active patient requires provocation cystometry. However, slow-filling supine or sedentary cystometry is sometimes appropriate for monitoring the treatment of unstable detrusor behavior, especially in overtly neurogenic bladder dysfunction such as in patients with spinal injuries. It is unreasonable to expect pharmacotherapy to improve bladder inhibition and thus convert instability to stability; nevertheless, a striking improvement in bladder function can be obtained by a demonstrable increase in the functional capacity required to trigger the first unstable contraction.

Provocative Cystometry

Provocative cystometry, pioneered by Hodgkinson, is designed to identify unstable detrusor behavior within a short time. Although the degree of provocation is difficult to quantify, beyond a certain point a truly stable detrusor mechanism is stable, and the incidence of instability cannot be increased by greater provocation.

The usual methods of provocation testing are:

(1) Rapid (50–100 ml per minute) bladder filling with the patient supine;
(2) Changing position from supine to erect position;
(3) Bladder filling while the patient is standing;
(4) Repeated coughing;
(5) "Jouncing," in which patients gently bounce on their heels.

Provocation cystometry is sometimes objected to on the grounds that the circumstances are unphysiologic; however, some normal daily activities are very provoking. Furthermore, many unphysiologic tests are clinically useful; for instance, it is unphysiologic to hit a tendon with a hammer, but the reflex response to this assault may be diagnostically significant. Indeed, although continuous monitoring of detrusor behavior during consecutive natural filling and voiding cycles approximate to the normal physiologic conditions is particularly useful for the evaluation of certain clinical problems, this is time consuming; and for most purposes, provocation cystometry identifies clinically significant abnormalities of detrusor behavior during filling with acceptable accuracy and reproducibility.

Although high-pressure unstable detrusor contractions can be identified on the total bladder pressure record, subtracted pressures are required to identify significant unstable contractions of a low-pressure detrusor in the standing position, as they are otherwise masked by the considerable postural increase in the total pressure.

The Identification of High-Pressure Unstable Detrusor Behavior

The finding of an unstable detrusor contraction pressure peak > 45 cm H_2O on the filling pressure record is immediate proof of high-pressure unstable detrusor behavior. Unstable contractions, however, do not always produce the maximum detrusor pressure. When the voiding flow rate is less than about 10 ml per second, the detrusor contraction shortens sufficiently quickly to exert its near-maximum force, and thus the subtracted detrusor voiding pressure approximates the maximum. However, when the flow rate exceeds 15 to 20 ml per second, the apparent voiding detrusor pressure may be much lower than the isometric detrusor contraction. Thus, when the flow rate is normal or high, an isometric contraction pressure must be obtained by interrupting a detrusor contraction voiding; normally, this can be done by the stop-test.[1] However, the voluntary sphincter mechanism of many patients with stress incontinence is so weak that the stream must be interrupted either by digital occlusion of the external meatus or by occluding a large-bore indwelling catheter inserted for the test.

Although both identification of unstable detrusor voiding and measurement of the maximum detrusor contraction are important for the critical evaluation and comparison of female incontinence procedures, it may be that the identification and exclusion of high detrusor contraction pressures may prove to be the more important measurement in routine clinical practice. In our series, the results of treating low-pressure unstable incontinence by the vagino-obturator-shelf repositioning procedure are better than those of conservative treatment, although they are considerably inferior to the results of that procedure done for stable incontinence.[8]

PRESSURE-FLOW AND VIDEO PRESSURE-FLOW STUDIES

For most clinical purposes, filling and voiding cystometry and voiding cystourethrography can be performed separately. In a urodynamic referral center, however, there are advantages in performing the investigations synchronously: the provocation cystometry record can be obtained while the bladder is being filled with contrast medium, and the pressure-flow measurements can be obtained during voiding cystourethrography.[9] Our procedure for these synchronous video pressure-flow studies is outlined; the procedure for simple filling pressure-flow studies is similar but omits the valuable video element.

We take a full urologic history, the details of which are noted on a computerized pro forma to facilitate their entry into our urodynamic data base (Fig. 13–4). The six-channel recorder, radiography equipment, and videotape recorder are crosschecked and adjusted to the base line.

The terminal eyes of the 14F–16F plastic rectal pressure catheter are protected by tying a rubber finger stall over them,

NAME:
ADDRESS:
REFERRING CONSULTANT:
PRESENTING COMPLAINT:

AGE: 53. [ ][ ]
1. VIDEO NO. [ ][ ][ ][ ][ ]
HOSPITAL NO. 6. [ ][ ][ ][ ][ ][ ]
13. [ ] Male 1 Female 2
14. [ ] 1. Middlesex 2. Middx. Group 3. Elsewhere 4. Private
DATE: [ ][ ][ ][ ][ ][ ]
G.P.:

15. Frequency [ ] State No. of times or No. hours. [ ]
16. Nocturia [ ] State No. of times [ ]
17. Hesitancy [ ] 0=Never 2=Occasional 1=Usually
18. Stream [ ] 1=Normal 2=Decreased 3=Decreased + Interrupted 4=Catheter in Situ
19. Terminal Dribble [ ]
20. Post Micturition Dribble [ ]
21. Bladder Emptying [ ] 0=Normal 1=Incomplete
22. Loss of Normal Sensation [ ]
23. Straining [ ] 24. Manual Compression [ ]
25. History of Infection [ ]
26. Dysuria in absence of infection [ ]
27 Haematuria [ ]
28. Pain [ ] 1. Loin 2. Bladder 3. Urethral 4. Perineal
29. Urethral/Vaginal Discharge [ ]
30. Urgency [ ] 1.= Because of pain 2.= For fear of leaking 3.= 1 + 2
31. Incontinence [ ] 0=None 1=Stress 2=Urge 3=1 + 2 4=Continuous
32. Enuresis [ ] 1=Now 2=Childhood 3=FH
33. Impotence [ ]

34. Failure of Ejaculation [ ]
35. Dyspareunia [ ] 0=Absent 1=Superficial 2=Deep
36. Neurological Symptoms [ ] 0=None 1=Yes

State
37. Parity [ ]
38. Assisted Delivery [ ] 0=NO 1=Yes
39. Post Menopausal [ ]
40. Diabetes [ ]
41. Obesity [ ]
42. Drugs. State [ ]
43. Vaginal Examination [ ] 1. Normal 2. Atrophic 3. Cystocele 4. Rectocele 5. 3 + 4
44. Prostate Size [ ] 1. Small 2. Large
45. 1. Benign 2. Malignant [ ]

Past History of Previous Urological Surgery
46. 48. 50.
1. Bladder Neck Incision
2. Cystoscopy
3. Otis/UD
4. T.U.R.(P)
5. R.P.P.
6. Cystoplasty
7. Urethroplasty
8. Denervation
9. Vag. Repair
10. Pelvic repair
11. Hysterect. Vag.
12. Hysterect. Abdo.
13. Other Surgery

Other Diagnoses

52. Symptomatic Diagnosis.
1. Normal
2. Unstable
3. Obstructed
4. Obstructed/Unstable
5. Stress Incontinence
6. Acontractile
7. Neuropathic
8. Other

Unless Otherwise Stated
0=No or absent 1=Yes

Fig. 13–4. Data-collection form for urodynamic evaluation and data base.

URODYNAMIC INVESTIGATIONS VIDEO NO. 1. [| | | |]

6. Initial Flow Rate ml/sec [|]

8. Initial Vol Voided ml. [| |]

11. Initial Residual ml [| |]

14. C.M.G. [ ] 15. [ ]

1. Normal
2. Steep
3. Systolic-phasic
4. Systolic Non-phasic
5. Borderline.

1. Cough Instability
2. Postural Instability
3. Catheter Trigger
4. 1 + 2

16. Capacity ml. [| | |]

20. Volume at 1st unstable contraction (ml) [| |]

Volume at 1st sensation of filling (ml) [| |]

23. Pressure Rise Supine (Tick if filled [| |]

26. Erect erect) [| |]

[ ]

29. Limitation of Capacity [ ]

0=None 1=Pain 2=Instability 3= 1+2

30. Hypersensitive Urethra [ ] 0=Absent 1=Mild 2=Severe

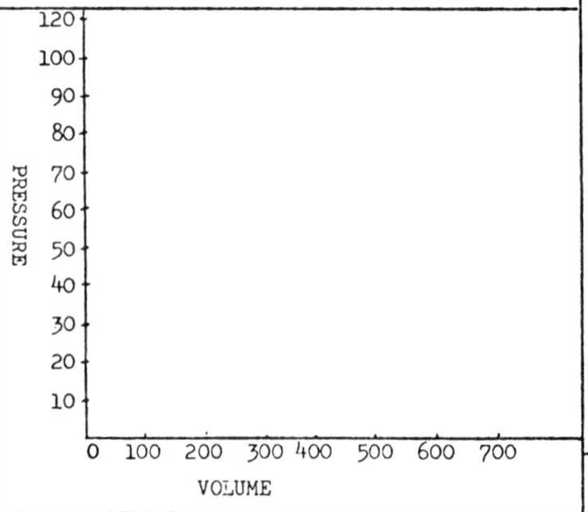
PRESSURE
120
100
90
80
70
60
50
40
30
20
10
0 100 200 300 400 500 600 700
VOLUME

Urethral Pressure Profile

31. Mamimum Urethral Pressure [| |]

34. Prostatic Plateau [| |]

37. Prostatic Length [|]

Sphincter E.M.G. 0=Not done 1=Normal 2=Abnormal

77. [ ]

Micturating Cystourethrogram

Micturition Pressure Maximum Flow

39. [| |] S 46. [|] S

42. [| |] C 49. [|] C

PISO Volume Voided

51. [| |] S [| |] S

54. [| |] C [| |] C

57. Total Volume Voided [| | |]

61. Residual Urine [| |]

(s=standing, c=commode)

64. Cystography Bladder Outline [ ] 1=Normal 2=Trabec. 3=Divertic. 4=2 + 3

65. Reflux [ ] 0=None 2=Right 1=Left 3=1 + 2

66. Bladder Neck [ ]

1=Normal
2=Open at rest stable
3=Open at rest unstable
4=Open on Cough stable
5=Open on cough + leak stable
6=Open on cough unstable

Proximal Urethra
67. [ ]

1. Tight spincter
2. B.N.O.
3. P.O
4. B.N. + P.O.
5. B.N.O. + tight sphincter

68. Bladder Base Descent [ ]

69. Distal Urethra [ ] 1=Normal 2=Tight 3=Stricture

70. Milk Back [ ] 1=Complete 2=Incomplete 3=+ve Whiteside(trapping)

71. Stop Test [ ] 1=Good 2=Poor

0=Not seen or performed.

Urodynamic Diagnosis

72. [ ]
73. [ ]
74. [ ]
75. [|]

1. Normal
2. Unstable
3. Hypersensitive ureth
4. Stress Incont. 1.2
5. Stable Obstructed
6. Unstable Obstructed
7. Neurogenic
8. Failing Detrusor
9. Detrusor Sphinct/dys
10. Acontrac/Hypot. Det
11. Others.

and the catheter is inserted. Two urethral catheters are inserted: a straight plastic filling catheter (14F for men and 12F for women) and a 2-mm plastic pressure catheter with one terminal and several side holes. Its fenestrated end is inserted into a side hole of the filling catheter and, thus piggybacked, they are passed together into the bladder. The pressure catheter is then disengaged by withdrawing it slightly to release it from the side hole. Both rectal and bladder pressure catheters are connected to water-filled pressure transducers and flushed with saline. The function of the detrusor-pressure substraction system is checked by asking the patient to cough and verifying that both show a synchronous pressure rise while the detrusor pressure remains at zero.

The filling catheter is connected to a container of contrast medium; 500 ml is sufficient for most patients. The initial filling is achieved at a rate of up to 100 ml per minute with the patient supine, and the volumes that have been instilled when the patient first notes the sensation of fullness and at the first sign of an abnormal rise (> 15 cm H_2O) in the detrusor pressure are noted. The x-ray table is then tilted into the erect position, and the bladder-transducer level is rechecked. If the detrusor pressure is borderline (15–20 cm H_2O) during supine bladder filling, or if there is no rise in the detrusor pressure even though the patient's history suggests instability (urgency, nocturia, and incontinence), the bladder is emptied and refilled with the patient in the erect position, which is more provocative. Any rise in detrusor pressure during the postural and catheter manipulations is noted. The filling catheter is then removed, and the radiographic image of the full bladder is recorded on videotape with synchronous oral comment on any abnormal findings. The patient is instructed to cough to see whether this provokes an unstable contraction; and the competence of the bladder-neck and urethral sphincter mechanisms is observed and any stress leakage noted.

During the voiding phase, the detrusor pressure and the flow rate are recorded synchronously on the left side of the radiographic image of the contrast-filled bladder and urethra; this synchronous combination of the voiding cystourethrogram and the pressure-flow measurements is often important to the analysis of the bladder/sphincter disturbances.[8,9] When micturition is well established, the stop test is used to assess voluntary efficiency of the urethral and the bladder-neck sphincter mechanisms; and the coincident isometric detrusor contraction pressure rise is noted (Fig. 13–5). Voiding is then restarted, and any vesicoureteral reflux or residual urine is noted.

A few (usually female) patients are unable to void with an audience in the screening room. In such cases, the medical staff leaves after the patient has been assured that, even if she is unable to void, useful information can be gained from the attempts. In particular, the competence of the bladder neck and the extent of vesicourethral descent during abdominal straining are noted. In fact most patients are able to void if treated sympathetically and left in privacy under covert observation. They are asked to call out when micturition is established so that the video system can be switched on. Patients still unable to void are seated on a flow-rate commode in the privacy of an adjacent closet, still connected to the pressure transducers, so that a simple pressure-flow record of the voiding is obtained without video. This is also used to check the finding of residual urine during a screened void.

To minimize the risk of infection, patients are encouraged to increase their fluid intake for a few hours after the examination. Those with a documented infection are given antibiotics.

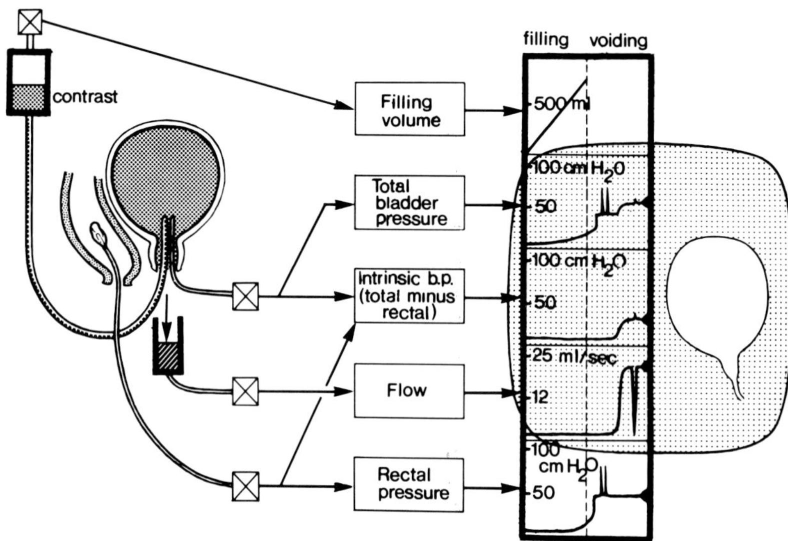

Fig. 13–5. Diagram of the video-pressure-flow study.

All results are tabulated on the reverse side of the history sheet, and a summary report is made. The results and the videotape recordings are discussed at joint weekly urodynamics meetings attended by the whole urologic firm. We have done more than 14,000 of these examinations at Middlesex Hospital during the past 15 years, and the annual number is increasing as their importance is appreciated. For many of these patients, adequate information could have been obtained by the separate performance of the pressure-flow and video studies, both of which should be regarded as essential. Once the system is set up in a referral unit, there is a considerable saving in everyone's time in performing them synchronously, quite apart from the superior diagnostic value and the avoidance of a second catheterization. For a few patients, synchronous studies are essential for the preoperative and postoperative evaluation of some of the complex sphincter reconstructions that the tests have enabled us to develop.[8]

The synchronous video pressure-flow study is an outpatient investigation; it requires no preparation unless an initial IVUD is required to verify the need for detailed urodynamic examination of a patient referred without an appropriate preliminary evaluation. For a few complex problems, and for the accurate evaluation of some functional disorders in children, it is necessary to hospitalize the patient and insert suprapubic filling and pressure catheters to enable truly representative pressure-flow studies to be obtained by repetition without urethral manipulation.

THE USES AND LIMITATIONS OF SOME SPECIAL URODYNAMIC TESTS

Urethral Pressure Profile Studies

Simple perfusion urethral profilometry records the resting closing pressure of the urethra during the filling and the storage phases; in general, its clinical value is limited. The information can be augmented by synchronous intravesical pressure records, by cough-strain pressure records, and by multichannel membrane and microtransducor step-pressure records.[6] The tests have proved particularly disappointing in the selection of female patients for incontinence operations, because continence depends on the relation between the bladder and the urethra, and there is considerable overlap in the range of closing pressures of water-tight and incompetent urethras. Sophisticated profile studies are useful for urophysiologic investigation and research, but accurate clinical interpretation requires an unusual degree of urodynamic expertise and experience.

A particular shortcoming of urethral pressure-profile studies is that bladder-neck function and dysfunction are poorly distinguished. It cannot be assumed that the initial rise in the profile record is located in the true bladder-neck mechanism—this may be incompetent. Furthermore, if the bladder neck is occlusive, it is difficult or impossible to determine from a simple profile record whether it is competent, incompetent, or dyssynergically obstructive. Thus, even an augmented cough-strain profile provides only a fraction of the information that is routinely available from the simple video voiding cystourethrogram (VCUG) available to every urologist.

Electromyography and the Sphincter Mechanism

Although a synchronous electromyographic record of the activity of the perianal and pelvic-floor musculature may be valuable in the functional evaluation of the sphincter mechanism of patients with overt neuropathy, it is important to recognize the record's shortcomings when it is used as a convenient office substitute for the radiographic evaluation of sphincter behavior in patients without obvious neuropathy. For clinical purposes, behavior of the urethral sphincter complex is better evaluated by urography or pressure-profile studies.

The widely held concept of a "urogenital diaphragm" is entirely erroneous; in both male and female, the striated muscle elements of the "external sphincter" that can control the urine passively are located entirely within the wall of the urethra itself. In the male, the only significant paraurethral musculature lies behind the urethra; in the female, there is no significant musculature in the pelvic floor anterior to the vagina within several centimeters of the adult urethra.[1,10,11] Thus, accurate recording of electroactivity of the striated muscle of the urethra requires that the intraurethral or needle electrodes be positioned in relation to the anterior wall of the sphincteric portion of the urethra where there is no significant periurethral musculature.

Electromyographic activity of the pelvic-floor musculature normally ceases during a volitional detrusor contraction unless a synchronous contraction is necessary to prevent the escape of feces or flatus. Under the strange circumstances of urodynamic evaluation, however, it is not unusual for a patient to develop an involuntary contraction of the sphincter mechanisms that prevent volitional voiding. When patients fail to void standing in front of a video screen during voiding cystourethrography, it is generally regarded as a "normal" reaction; however, when similar voiding difficulties occur during electromyographic and pressure studies, synchronous activity is sometimes misinterpreted as detrusor-sphincter dyssynergia.

The appearance of synchronous detrusor and pelvic-floor muscle contractions during the filling phase of a cystometrogram is also sometimes misinterpreted as detrusor–sphincter dyssynergia when it is in reality an entirely normal and appropriate synergic leak-preventing sphincter response to an involuntary unstable contraction if the patient is simply trying to "hold on" to avoid leaking.

Although some degree of dyssynergic bladder-neck dysfunction is a common cause of outlet obstruction in the male, true obstruction of the detrusor by striated urethral sphincter activity is rare in adult men and women in the absence of neuropathy. Thus, in the *absence of neuropathy* and in the *absence of a urodynamically proven bladder outflow obstruction*, the finding of synchronous detrusor–pelvic floor electromyographic activity is rarely of clinical significance in adults. Clinically oriented urodynamic units with facilities for video studies of sphincter behavior rarely use electromyography for the routine evaluation of outpatients unless the findings suggest an underlying neuropathy.

CONCLUSIONS

In our opinion, facilities for the basic urodynamic investigations discussed in this chapter—especially recording uroflowmetry and audiovideo cystourethrography—should be available to every practicing urologist and used routinely in appropriate cases. Subtracted filling-flow pressure studies require a four-channel instrument, special training, and continuing experience to produce clinically useful measurements; whether urologists elect to install facilities for this in their offices will depend on their particular interests and the availability of a local referral center. Air cystometry is not advised, because it is useful only for monitoring the filling phase of the voiding cycle, whereas voiding pressure-flow studies are often critical to the management of inefficient voiding. Sophisticated facilities for synchronous video pressure-flow studies are invaluable for the evaluation of patients who have been shown, by simple urodynamic studies, to have complex problems. Such facilities should be available in referral units specializing in the surgical reconstruction and restoration of the function of the urinary tract.

REFERENCES

1. Turner-Warwick, R., and Whiteside, C.G. (eds.): Symposium on clinical urodynamics. Urol. Clin. North Am., *6*(1):13, 1979.
2. Turner-Warwick, R., et al.: A urodynamic review of clinical problems associated with bladder-neck dysfunction and its treatment by endoscopic incision—trans-trigonal posterior prostatectomy. Br. J. Urol., *45*:44, 1973.
3. Turner-Warwick, R., et al.: A urodynamic view of prostatic obstruction and the results of prostatectomy. Br. J. Urol., *45*:631, 1973.
4. Smith, J.: The measurement and significance of urinary flow. Br. J. Urol., *30*:701, 1966.
5. Arnold, E.P.: Bladder outlet obstruction in the male: a urological analysis of detrusor response. Ph.D. Thesis, London University, 1980.
6. Abrams, P., et al.: Clinical urodynamics. Urol. Clin. North Am., *6*:71, 103, 1979.
7. Turner-Warwick, R., et al.: The intravenous urodynamogram. Br. J. Urol., *51*:15, 1979.
8. Turner-Warwick, R., and Whiteside, C.G.: *In* Scientific Foundation of Urology, 2nd Ed. Edited by G.P. Chisholm and D. Innes Williams. London, Heineman, 1982, p. 442.
9. Bates, C.P., Whiteside, C.G., and Turner-Warwick, R.: Synchronous cine pressure-flow cystourethrography. Br. J. Urol., *42*:714, 1970.
10. Chilton, C.P., and Turner-Warwick, R.: The relationship of the distal sphincter mechanism to the pelvic floor musculature. Br. J. Urol. (in press).
11. Turner-Warwick, R.: The relationship of prostatic enlargement to the distal sphincter mechanism and the bladder neck mechanism: dyssynergic bladder neck obstruction. *In* Benign Prostatic Hypertrophy. Edited by F. Hinman and G. Chisholm. Berlin, Springer-Verlag, 1983.

Section IV

Endoscopy

14

Diagnostic and Therapeutic Applications of Outpatient Cystourethroscopy

RALPH V. CLAYMAN, M.D.

The introduction of long-acting local anesthetics, safer but still potent parenteral analgesics, and recent advances in instrumentation have permitted the transfer of many formerly hospital-based urologic procedures to the ambulatory surgical unit. Today diagnostic cystourethroscopy and many transurethral therapeutic procedures such as relief of urethral strictures and bladder-neck contractures, resection of bladder papillomas, and destruction of bladder diverticula and stones can all be performed without hospitalization.

CYSTOSCOPY

For many years cystourethroscopy has been performed as an outpatient procedure in women and older men but as an inpatient procedure under general anesthesia in younger males. General anesthesia also has been customary for retrograde ureterography.[1] We have found, however, that both procedures can be performed safely and to the patient's satisfaction on an outpatient basis.

Anesthesia and Sedation

For shorter endoscopic procedures we instill 10 ml of 2% lidocaine hydrochloride (Anestacon) jelly into the patient's urethra for 10 to 15 minutes. In men, the pendulous urethra is closed with a Cunningham clamp so the jelly will be retained. For most women and older men, this provides enough anesthesia for comfortable endoscopy. For longer procedures, such as retrograde ureterography, we lengthen the duration of urethral anesthesia by substituting bupivacaine (Marcaine) jelly, which we prepare by mixing 10 ml of 0.5 per cent bupivacaine plus epinephrine with an equal amount of sterile surgical lubricant (Lubafax or K–Y Jelly) in a catheter-tipped syringe. The pharmacology of this long-acting local anesthetic is reviewed in Chapter 8.

In the anxious patient the intravenous injection of 2.5 mg of diazepam (Valium) and 2 mg of butorphanol tartrate (Stadol) produces excellent relaxation and acceptance of the procedure. (Butorphanol tartrate is an analgesic of the narcotic agonist–antagonist class, and respiratory depression may be a prominent side effect, with 2 mg of butorphanol being equivalent in this respect to 10 mg of morphine sulfate; naloxone hydrochloride [Narcan], 0.01 mg per kilogram of body weight, is a specific antidote.) Although the action of butorphanol may last as long as 3 hours after intravenous injection, we have given additional doses of both butorphanol and diazepam as often as every 5 minutes to maintain the patient in a resting, yet arousable condition. When these drugs are used, electrocardiographic monitoring and regular blood pressure measurements are necessary. When diazepam is used, medications and equipment for cardiovascular resuscitation should be readily available. Patients given these two drugs should not leave the ambulatory surgery unit alone.

Instruments

For rigid cystoscopy under local anesthesia, we prefer to use the 17F panendoscope. This smaller cystoscope can also be used for retrograde ureterograms; however, it is then necessary to backload the ureteral catheter if an 8F Foley cone is used.

Recently we have begun using the 16F flexible fiberoptic 33-cm nephroscope (Olympus; ACMI) for cystoscopy. With this instrument, one can view the entire bladder and bladder neck, because the tip can be deflected through a 250° arc (see Chapter 17). The patient is placed in a supine, rather than the dorsolithotomy position, and local urethral anesthesia without intravenous medications is used, because passage of the flexible instrument causes no more discomfort than the insertion of a urethral catheter. An assistant may help by holding the patient's penis erect during the initial passage. Among the 44 patients who have undergone both flexible and rigid cystoscopies at our hospitals, the findings have been similar in 38; but in five patients, the flexible nephroscope revealed features not appreciated with the rigid instrument. (In one case, the converse occurred.) In other words, the flexible nephroscope enables the urologist to perform rapid, comfortable, thorough cystoscopy without the need for general anesthesia, intravenous medications, or stirrups.

TREATMENT OF VESICAL PAPILLOMAS

Many therapeutic endoscopic procedures can be performed on an outpatient basis using the aforementioned combination of local bupivacaine and intravenous butorphanol and diazepam, and this includes removal of small bladder tumors and performance of bladder biopsies.

The patient is instructed to come to the clinic with a companion, who is given an instruction sheet when the patient is discharged that explains what has been done, what problems might arise, and who should be contacted should there be difficulties. If we anticipate any fulguration or cutting within the bladder, we instill a total of 100 ml of 0.25% bupivacaine jelly into the urethra and bladder to provide local anesthesia for the vesical transitional epithelium. After the jelly has remained in the bladder for 15 minutes, the patient is given intravenous diazepam and butorphanol, and the procedure is started. The bladder is inspected, usually with a 21F panendoscope, and any suspicious areas are biopsied with 7F flexible cold cup biopsy forceps (Storz). If a small (< 1 cm in diameter) papillary tumor is seen, its surface is removed with the forceps until the base is revealed. A grounding plate is then placed under the patient's buttocks, and a 9F Bugbee electrode (Greenwald) is passed through the panendoscope and used to fulgurate both the base of the tumor and a 0.5- to 1.0-cm area around the base.

During the procedure urine flow is stimulated by intravenous infusion of 5% dextrose in water at a rate of 200 ml per hour. At the end of the procedure, the patient receives either 4 to 6 g of mannitol or 10 mg of furosemide (Lasix) intravenously to induce further diuresis and thus help prevent the formation of blood clots in the bladder. In healthy patients we prefer to use mannitol, because it causes a longer-lasting diuresis.

After the procedure a Foley catheter is not inserted if the vesical effluent is clear. The patient is kept in the clinic until he voids, and if the urine is also clear, the patient is allowed to go home with the companion and instructed to drink two quarts of fluid during the next 6 hours. If there is significant hematuria at the end of the procedure, however, a Foley catheter is inserted and, if necessary, the patient is admitted to the hospital.

This approach to bladder papillomas and biopsies has been used extensively and successfully by Klein and Whitmore, who describe a series of 36 patients, completed in September 1981, with an average saving per patient of more than 1,400 dollars.[2]

TREATMENT OF URETHRAL, AND VESICAL NECK STRICTURES

The development of the direct-vision cold knife urethrotome (20F from Storz; 22F from ACMI) was a major advance in the treatment of urethral strictures and bladder-neck contractures (Fig. 14–1). For our male patients we use bupivacaine urethral anesthesia supplemented with intravenous diazepam and butorphanol for this procedure. The urine should be sterile beforehand, and an antibiotic, usually a cephalosporin, is given intramuscularly just before the procedure starts. During the procedure and for 2 hours thereafter, the patient is given 200 ml per hour of 5% dextrose in water. Mannitol or furosemide is given at the end of the procedure as described earlier.

Under direct vision the urethral stricture is cut with the cold knife at the 12-o'clock position, the incision being carried 1 cm proximal and 1 cm distal to the area of the stricture. The depth of the incision should be sufficient to divide the scar tissue completely (Fig. 14–2). If the stricture is dense or recurrent, a 40 mg/ml solution of triamcinolone acetonide (Kenalog) is injected with a flexible cystoscopic needle (ACMI; Fig. 14–3) along either edge of the incision to decrease the subsequent scarring. A 20F or 22F catheter is inserted into the bladder, and the patient remains in the recovery room for 2 to 4 hours. A bulky dressing is then placed along the catheter where it exits from the urethral meatus. If the patient's condition is stable and hematuria minimal, he may go home with the companion, to return in two days for removal of the catheter. An oral antibiotic such as a cephalosporin, nitrofurantoin, or trimethoprim/sulfa is continued for six days.

The success rate for resolving urethral strictures of ≤ 2 cm with the direct-vision urethrotome is greater than 90%. Cohen and others have reported the same rates of success using the instrument with local urethral anesthesia as with general or spinal anesthesia.[3] In addition, strictures that are originally refractory can be subjected to a second procedure, with a similar high success rate. Triamcinolone injections during the second session help convert first-time procedural failures into eventual successes.[4,5]

The technique for internal urethrotomy can also be applied to bladder-neck contractures. After local anesthesia has been obtained with bupivacaine jelly, panendoscopy is performed. The bladder neck is infiltrated with 5 ml of 0.25% bupivacaine with epinephrine at the 5- and 7-o'clock positions using the flexible cystoscopic needle. The bladder neck is then incised with the cold knife of the direct-vision urethrotome or the electrosurgical knife at the 5- and 7-o'clock positions, with each incision beginning just distal to the ureteral orifice and continuing through the contracture 1 cm into the prostatic urethra (Fig. 14–4). The incision should be deep enough to reveal the

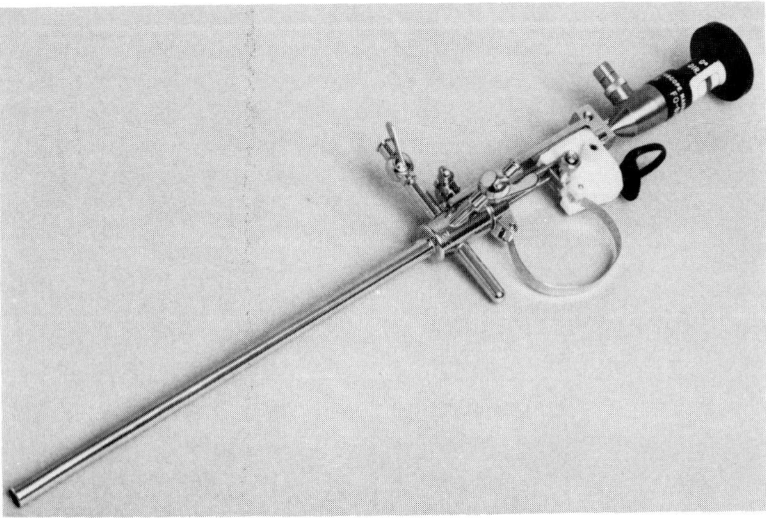

Fig. 14–1. The 22F direct-vision cold knife urethrotome (ACMI).

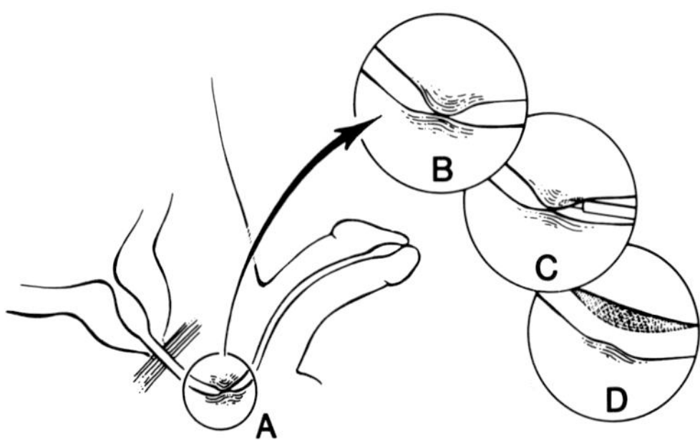

Fig. 14–2. Steps in the incision of a urethral stricture. The incision should extend through all the scar tissue and continue 1 cm proximal and distal to the site.

perivesical fat. Either edge of the incision may then be injected with triamcinolone in order to reduce scarring. Steroid injections also improve the success rate in treating recurrent bladder-neck contracture.[6,7] The diuresis, dressing, postoperative care, and antibiotic usage are as previously described.

TREATMENT OF VESICAL CALCULI

Classically, the removal of bladder calculi has required a general or spinal anesthetic because the instruments were large and the procedure often lengthy. Complete evacuation of the stone and its fragments was not guaranteed, and bleeding and bladder damage were not infrequent. All of this has changed with the advent of electrohydraulic and ultrasonic lithotriptors, which enable the surgeon to destroy and remove bladder stones on an outpatient basis.[8,9]

The electrohydraulic lithotriptor was first described in 1950 by Yutkin and first applied to bladder stones by Goldberg in 1959.[10,11] In one series of 304 patients, the success rate exceeded 90%, with an average procedure time of 21 minutes (range 3 to 60 minutes).[12] To date, we have used this instrument to remove 13 bladder stones.

The machine we have had the most experience with is the SD-1, 120 volt, 60 hertz lithotriptor (Monighan Medical Corporation, Plattsburg, NY), which consists of a generator cabinet, a power cord, an extender cable, a foot pedal, and a 5F or 9F flexible probe (see Chapter 17). The 9F probe is most effective for use in the bladder and can be passed through a 24F cystoscope. The irrigation solution should be $\frac{1}{6}$ to $\frac{1}{7}$ normal saline (Fig. 14–5), because in normal saline or Ringer's lactate the energy from the probe

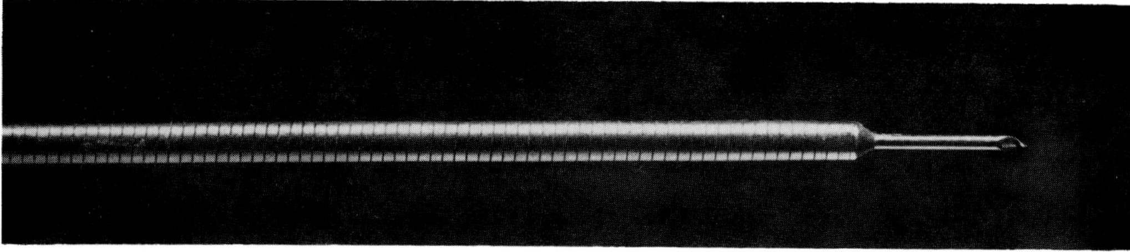

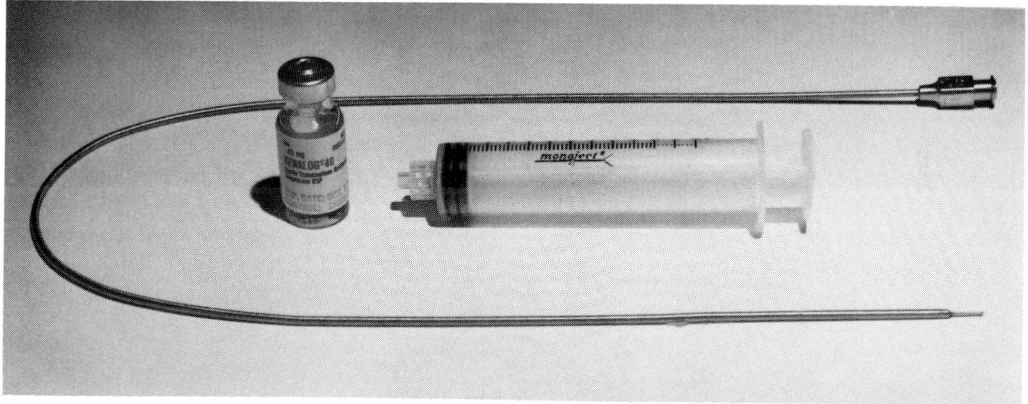

Fig. 14–3. Cystoscopic needle and steroid used to reduce scarring. *(A)* Needle tip on hollow, flexible wire shaft. *(B)* Demonstration of the flexibility of the assembly. A total of 3 to 5 ml of the steroid solution is appropriate for urethral and bladder-neck strictures.

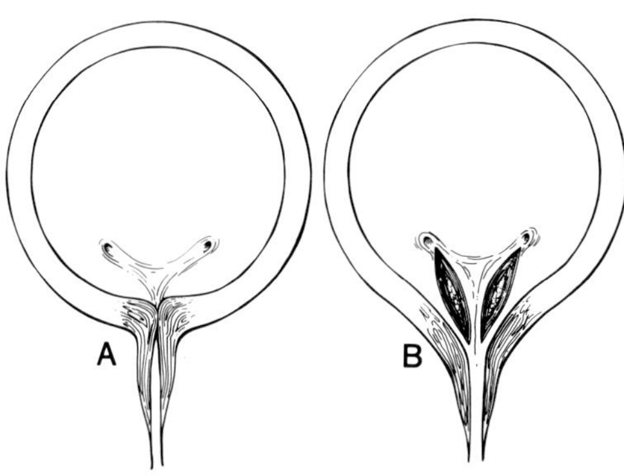

Fig. 14–4. *(A)* Management of bladder-neck contracture. *(B)* The incision begins immediately distal to the ureteral orifice and ends 1 cm into the prostatic urethra. Note that incisions are deep enough to reveal the perivesical fat at the bladder neck.

discharge is scattered and is thus less effective. The patient is not electrically grounded.

The lithotriptor probe is passed through the panendoscope and placed on, or approximately 1 mm from the surface of the most irregular portion of the stone, and at least 5 mm away from the cystoscope lens (Fig. 14–6). The number of discharges per second can be from 50 to 100, and the voltage can be from 90 to 120. We commonly use 50 discharges per second at 100 volts. When the surgeon depresses the foot pedal, there is a small blue flash at the tip of the probe, and the patient may feel a popping, tingling, or mildly uncomfortable sensation. If the stone is not cracked apart, the probe should be discharged again in the same spot. Once the stone has been broken, the jagged surface of the fragments provides an excellent target for further discharges. Fragments are broken into pro-

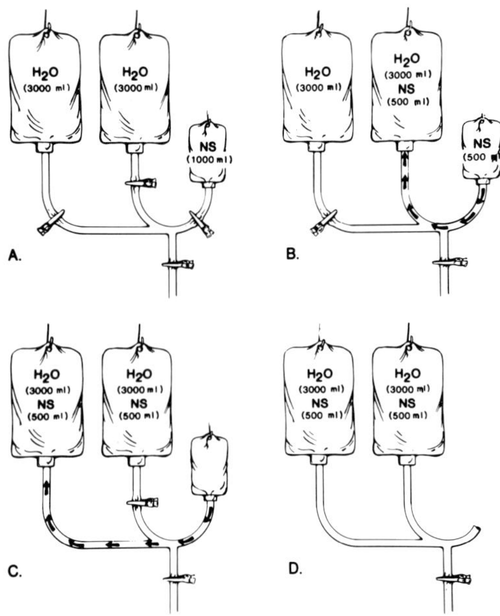

Fig. 14–5. Production of 7 liters of 1/7 normal saline. 500 ml of normal saline (NS) is delivered into each of two 3-liter bags of sterile water, and the contents are mixed.

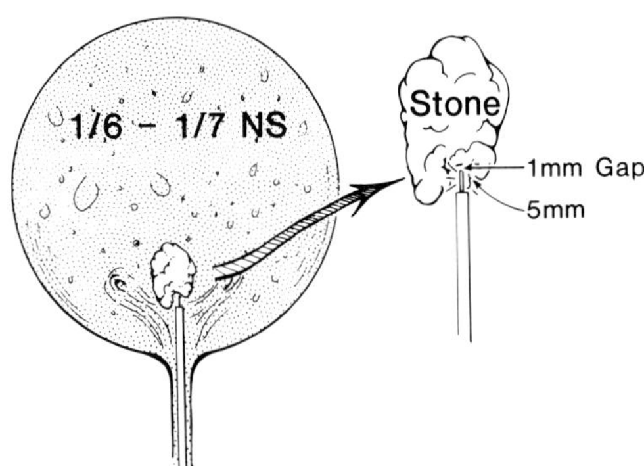

Fig. 14–6. Proper positioning of the electrohydraulic lithotriptor probe. The most irregular area on the stone should be the target, as this maximizes the effectiveness of the force.

gressively smaller pieces until they can be flushed out of the bladder or grasped with alligator forceps and pulled through the cystoscope sheath. Struvite and calcium carbonate stones break up easily, whereas calcium oxalate stones require more effort. Uric acid stones may be refractory to lithotripsy, although we have been successful even with these.

The probe of the electrohydraulic lithotriptor has a life span of 15 to 50 seconds, depending on the strength and duration of the discharges. Therefore, the tip should be checked after each discharge for any wear in the outer insulation, which will make the discharge come from the side of the probe, thereby reducing its effectiveness. For most bladder lithotripsy procedures, two or three probes will be needed.

At the conclusion of the procedure, the bladder mucosa appears undisturbed, and there is usually no need for a Foley catheter. Again, these patients are given oral antibiotics to take for five to seven days.

Other authors have destroyed vesical calculi with the ultrasonic lithotriptor,* albeit usually with the patient under general anesthesia.[13] The machine consists of the ultrasound probe, a sheath, an obturator and suction pump, and the ultrasound generator (see Chapter 17). It is a rigid instrument, and the 12F probe fits through a 24F or 26F sheath. The probe must be in contact with the stone. With a foot pedal, ultrasound waves are directed through the probe and stone, and the stone begins to disintegrate. Both the cystoscope and the probe are connected to wall suction, which evacuates many of the small particles. Because the ultrasonic lithotriptor is not as powerful as the electrohydraulic one, it may take considerably longer to destroy larger, harder bladder stones with ultrasound. The ultrasonic lithotriptor is gentle, however, causing the patient little discomfort. Usually, a Foley catheter is unnecessary after the procedure.

*Karl Storz, 10111 W. Jefferson Blvd., Culver City, CA 90230; R. Wolff, 7046 Lyndon Ave., Rosemont, IL 60018

TREATMENT OF VESICAL DIVERTICULA

Recently, the use of the ambulatory surgery unit has been extended to transurethral resection of the prostate (see Chapter 15) and to the treatment of vesical diverticula.

The idea of treating diverticula transurethrally is not new. In the 1940s, Flocks routinely established transurethral drainage of bladder diverticula by incising their necks, a technique recently revived by Vitale and Woodside.[14] Although this procedure ensures that the diverticular sacs will drain, it does not eliminate them.

In 1977, Orandi described a method for fulgurating the mucosa of vesical diverticula transurethrally.[15] With this method, he was able to reduce the inside of the sacs by 90 to 100% in seven patients and to decrease it by 70% in an eighth patient. Long-term (3 to 49 months') followup of 19 patients showed obliteration of the diverticulum in ten, a significant decrease in size in eight, and no effect in only one.[16] There have been no adverse effects, either immediate or delayed.

Since 1980, we have been combining the techniques of Flocks and Orandi by incising the mouth of the diverticulum and fulgurating the mucosa of the sac (transurethral incision and fulguration of diverticula; TUIFD).[17] To date, we have treated 16 patients who had diverticula 2 to 14 cm in diameter, and in all 16 patients the diverticulum was reduced by 75% or more, with further shrinkage noted on followup radiographs. Our followup experience at 3 to 24 months has been similar to Orandi's, with no enlargement of diverticular remnants and no recurrences. In most patients incision of the bladder neck or transurethral resection of the prostate was performed at the same time without difficulty.

Some of these procedures are carried out with the patient under general anesthesia, but in other patients we have used a 20-minute application of 100 ml of 0.25% bupivacaine jelly to the urethra and bladder and supplemented this with intravenous butorphanol and diazepam. The patient then receives an intramuscular injection of an antibiotic, usually a cephalosporin.

For transurethral management of diverticula, a yellow-roller electrode (ACMI) is used with a 24F continuous-flow resectoscope. This system is helpful because it keeps the same amount of fluid in the bladder at all times, and thus the diverticular wall does not move away from the surgeon. The inside of the diverticulum is first inspected for papillomatous lesions. If the diverticulum will not admit the resectoscope, the roller electrode is connected to the cutting current, and the mouth of the diverticulum is incised at the point farthest from the ureteral orifice. When the resectoscope has been introduced into the diverticulum, fulguration is begun at the apex using the coagulating current set at half power, and the electrode is moved back in an ever-widening spiral (Fig. 14–7*A*). The current should be administered in short bursts in order to preclude damage to extravesical structures and to minimize obturator-nerve spasm. When touched with the roller electrode, the mucosal lining will whiten and shrivel.

After the size of the diverticulum has been reduced as much as possible with this method, a transurethral resection of the prostate or incision of the bladder neck may be performed. The mouth of the diverticulum is then incised in all four quadrants with the roller electrode and cutting current (Fig. 14–7*B*). This divides the muscle fibers that surround and constrict the mouth. If the ureteral orifice is close to the diverticulum, however, that quadrant should not be incised. The most proximal portion of the diverticular mucosa can then be fulgurated (Fig. 14–7*C*).

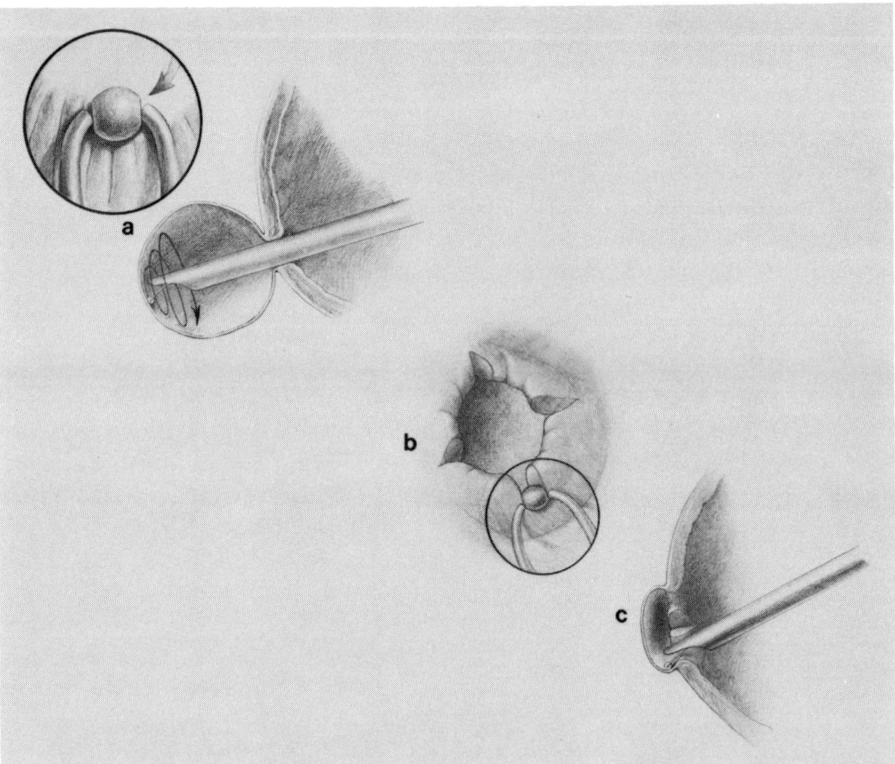

Fig. 14–7. Transurethral incision and fulguration of diverticula. *(A)* The roller electrode is used with coagulating current to fulgurate the diverticular mucosa, which whitens as current is applied. *(B)* The electrode is used with cutting current to incise the diverticular mouth in all four quadrants. *(C)* The proximal portion of the diverticular mucosa can now be fulgurated with the coagulating current. (From Clayman, R.V., et al.: Urology, *23*:573, 1984.)

At the end of the procedure, a three-way Foley Alcock catheter is inserted and connected to low-flow irrigation. In order to avoid undue pressure on the obliterated diverticulum, the bag of irrigating fluid must be no higher than 20 cm above the bedside. Before the patient is discharged, a voiding cystourethrogram is obtained. A small diverticular remnant should not cause concern, as it has been our experience that such remnants shrink during the ensuing two to three months.

We compared our results with this transurethral approach with our recent experiences with open diverticulectomy. With the former, the blood loss has been slight, in contrast to the 400-ml average blood loss associated with the latter technique. Likewise, the operating time for the transurethral procedure is less—1.25 hours on the average, or approximately half the time required for the open technique. There have been no deaths and no complications with the transurethral procedure.[17] We leave the Foley Alcock catheter in place at discharge and ask the patient to return to the clinic in two days for catheter removal. The patient is given an oral antibiotic and an antispasmodic such as belladonna and opium suppositories or hyoscyamine sulfate tablets.

CONCLUSIONS

The urologist can perform many endoscopic procedures in an ambulatory surgery unit without using general anesthesia and without the need for hospitalization. Diagnostic procedures such as cystoscopy and retrograde ureterography can be accomplished easily, as can therapeutic procedures such as bladder biopsy, resection of bladder papillomas, cystolithotripsy, incision of urethral and bladder-neck strictures, and destruction of bladder diverticula. By assimilating these skills into his practice, the urologist can continue to serve the best interests of his patients, both physically and financially.

REFERENCES

1. Hirschhorn, R.C.: Principles of cystoscopy. *In* Handbook of Practical Urology. Edited by R.C. Hirschhorn. Philadelphia, Lea & Febiger, 1965.
2. Klein, F.A., and Whitmore, W.F., Jr.: Bladder papilloma: therapeutic and cost effect of outpatient department management. Urology, *18*:247, 1981.
3. Cohen, E.L.: Urethrotomy and local anesthesia are preferred therapy for strictures. Urol. Times, *10*:9, April 1982.
4. Sacknoff, E.J., and Kerr, W.S., Jr.: Direct vision cold knife urethrotomy. J. Urol., *123*:492, 1980.
5. Noe, H.N.: Endoscopic management of urethral strictures in children. J. Urol., *125*:712, 1981.
6. Malek, R.S., and Greene, L.F.: Corticosteroid therapy of post-operative contractures of the vesical neck. J. Urol., *110*:297, 1973.
7. Farah, R.N., DiLoreto, R.R., and Cerny, J.C.: Transurethral resection combined with steroid injection in treatment of recurrent vesical neck contractures. Urology, *13*:395, 1979.
8. Angeloff, A.: Hydroelectrolithotripsy. J. Urol., *108*:867, 1972.
9. Marberger, M.: Ultrasonic destruction of bladder stones. *In* Ultrasound in Urology. Edited by M. Resnick. Baltimore, Williams & Wilkins, 1979.
10. Comisarow, R.H., and Barkin, M.: Electrohydraulic cystolithopaxy. Can. J. Surg., *22*:525, 1979.
11. Goldberg, V.C.: On the history of the electrohydraulic lithotripsy. Urol. Nefrol. (Moscow), *50*:90, 1974.
12. Bulow, H., and Frohmuller, H.G.W.: Electrohydraulic lithotripsy with aspiration of fragments under vision: 304 consecutive cases. J. Urol., *126*:454, 1981.
13. Terhorst, B., et al.: Die Zerstörung von Harnsteinen durch Ultraschall: Ultraschall Lithotripsie von Blasensteinen. Urol. Int., *27*:458, 1972.
14. Vitale, P.J., and Woodside, J.R.: Management of bladder diverticula by transurethral resection: reevaluation of an old technique. J. Urol., *122*:744, 1979.
15. Orandi, A.: Transurethral fulguration of bladder diverticulum: new procedure. Urology, *10*:30, 1977.
16. Orandi, A.: TUFD effective in followup series. Urol. Times, *7*:12, 1979.
17. Clayman, R.V., et al.: Transurethral treatment of bladder diverticula: safe, cost-effective and therapeutic. Urology, *23*:573, 1984.

15

Outpatient Transurethral Resection of the Prostate

JOSE AMADO PEREZ, M.D., F.A.C.S.

Outpatient transurethral resection of the prostate and of obstructive lesions of the bladder neck can be performed in a secure and effective manner if certain guidelines are followed. First, the obstructive lesion to be treated must be small, so that the area of potential bleeding will not be extensive and so that a short operating time can be expected. Second, hemostasis must be meticulous, so that postoperative catheter drainage may be dispensed with. And third, special measures must be applied upon the patient's discharge from the unit. If these rules are observed, the practicing urologist will be rewarded with a more satisfied patient and a substantial monetary saving.

BACKGROUND AND DEVELOPMENT

Transurethral surgery has been performed on an ambulatory basis since 1912, when the "punch" operation was introduced by Young.[1] Although only a few small pieces of tissue were removed by that procedure, it was still a bold one, because electrocautery was not available. Since then, prostatic surgery has been undergoing gradual modifications to improve hemostasis, avoid infection, make the patient more comfortable, and reduce the hospital stay. Thus, transvesical prostatectomy was perfected with primary closure of the bladder[2] and further modified with emphasis on early removal of the catheter.[3] Transcapsular prostatectomy using a no-catheter technique with[4] and without[5] hypotensive anesthesia produced many successes. Transurethral resection of the prostate is now being performed using the cold punch[6] or the electrosurgical resectoscope[7] without catheter drainage[8] and with good results. The degree of success of any of these procedures is determined by the proper selection of patients and the physician's decision about whether a drainage catheter should be used.

In 1972, Mitchell wrote, "If the true bloodless resection could be achieved without any drop in blood pressure, there would be no contraindication to transurethral resection as an outpatient procedure even in the most decrepit patient."[9] This has now come to pass for selected patients, providing the amount of obstructive tissue to be resected is taken into consideration.

SELECTION OF PATIENTS

In our series the patients who underwent outpatient transurethral resection ranged from 46 to 78 years of age. More important than chronologic age, however, are such factors as the physical, mental, and psychologic condition of the patients.

Indications

Transurethral surgery is appropriate for correction of many obstructive conditions at the bladder outlet, including small (25 to 30 g) fibrous or glandular adenomas, solitary median lobes, median bars, and fibrotic bladder-neck contractures. It also may be useful for managing residual adenomas, apical remnants or tissue tags, and small obstructive carcinomas. In any case, the resection should be confined to prostatic urethras no longer than 2.5 to 3.5 cm, and the expected tissue yield should not exceed 10 to 15 g. The patient's renal function should be normal.

Contraindications

When the prostatic urethra is longer than 3.5 cm, transuretheral prostatic surgery should be performed in the hospital, because the amount of tissue that will be resected will create a large surface of potential bleeding points. Extensive obstructive carcinomatous tissue and obstructive sphincters of neurogenic bladders should also be managed in the hospital.

Medical contraindications to outpatient transuretheral resection include chronic obstructive pulmonary disease, hypertension, cardiovascular disease, blood dyscrasias, diabetes mellitus, or other systemic diseases.

PREOPERATIVE EVALUATION

Clinical and Laboratory Studies

A thorough history (including personal and family data) and physical examination may alert the physician to a systemic disease that would contraindicate outpatient surgery. Particular attention should be given to the genitourinary system. The rectal examination frequently helps define the size of the prostate gland.

Urinalysis, including microscopic examination of the urinary sediment, is essential during the first and subsequent office visits. If the sediment contains bacteria, a quantitative urine culture with sensitivity studies should be done.

Radiologic Studies

An infusion-drip intravenous urogram with nephrotomograms, oblique views, and upright and postvoiding bladder films are usually needed. If the patient is cooperative and can void when instructed, a voiding cystourethrogram may be helpful. I do not believe that most patients should be catheterized to determine the volume of residual urine. Urethrograms may be indicated when an associated urethral lesion is suspected. The examining physician should review all films personally before any further evaluation is undertaken.

Endoscopy

Preliminary cystourethroscopic examinations are not recommended for patients in whom the rectal examination and the intravenous urogram show grade 2 or greater prostatic enlargement. In these cases, endoscopy should be the first step of the surgical procedure. If the clinical and radiologic evaluation suggests bladder-neck obstruction or less than grade 2 prostatic enlargement, a cystourethroscopic examination can be done in the office.

A 17F sheath with a forward oblique 30° telescope is passed under direct vision for evaluation of the entire urethra. The length of the prostatic portion should be measured and the type and degree of obstruction determined. The bladder neck and cavity should be thoroughly inspected with the bladder only partially distended to improve vision. The examiner can kneel with the examining table raised; simultaneous suprapubic compression facilitates observation. If performed gently, these maneuvers should not cause the patient undue discomfort. By simply changing to the lateral 70° telescope, a more complete examination of the bladder can then be made. The initial findings can be verified using a 19F sheath to examine the prostatic urethra when it is more distended.

The final step in the endoscopic examination is a gentle rectourethral palpation with the cystourethroscope in the prostatic urethra. The anal sphincter should be dilated slowly. The amount of tissue between the palpating finger and the instrument can then be estimated. Delicate, gradual movements will result in a brief, almost pain-free examination.

If a soft stricture of the urethra is encountered during the endoscopic examination, the procedure can continue if the lesion can be dilated to 20F, whereas if a hard stricture is present, the examination should stop. A retrograde urethrogram will show the length of the stricture and the prostatic urethra, thereby indicating whether the case is suitable for a combined visual urethrotomy and transurethral resection on an outpatient basis.

Preparation of the Patient

The possible complications and sequelae of the procedure should be explained, including postoperative bleeding, retrograde ejaculation, stricture formation, regrowth of prostatic tissue, and scar formation at the bladder neck. It must be made clear to the patient that in some cases hospitalization will become necessary.

Patients usually are not shaved unless an additional procedure requiring it is planned.

THE OUTPATIENT SURGICAL FACILITY

A conventional operating table with adjustable leg stirrups provides satisfactory positioning of the patient with sufficient padding for the legs. The patient's buttocks should be at the end of the table with the thighs flexed 45° from the horizontal. Resected tissue will not be lost, because with the continuous-flow resectoscope, the bladder is emptied at the end of the operation.

The solid-state 400B Bovie electrosurgical unit is used, with the usual settings being 2 for the cutting current, 6 for the power, and 6 or 7 for the coagulating current.

For the past eight years, I have used the continuous irrigation and suction Iglesias resectoscope for all in-hospital and outpatient transurethral surgery. There is no question that it decreases the operating time significantly, which is particularly advantageous in the outpatient setting. For most resections, a 25F sheath, with the forward oblique 30° telescope, the inner metal tube, and the working element fitted with a 24F yellow cutting loop, is adequate. The universal cold-light fountain (Storz) provides excellent vision. The straight-ahead 0° and retrospective 120° telescopes are helpful at the end of the resection, as will be explained later in this chapter.

Four 3-liter bags of 1.5% glycine irrigating solution with Y connectors provide a constant source of fluid. The primary bottleneck should be adjusted as necessary to keep it 60 to 70 cm above the patient's bladder. The outflow stopcock is connected to a wall suction outlet on a 10 to 25 mm Hg vacuum. After distention of the bladder to approximately 200 ml, the inflow–outflow balance may be disturbed, and the operator will need to correct it. When the bladder wall moves gradually toward the operator, or if there are prostatic chips in the field, distention can be increased by raising the irrigating bag or decreasing the vacuum suction. When the bladder and prostatic urethra become overdistended, the opposite maneuvers can be used to obtain optimal distention of the field.

Because of the imbalance inherent in the present method of continous-flow resection, I have been involved since 1976 in the development of an instrument that will keep the inflow and outflow of irrigating fluid in constant balance, maintain bladder distention, and monitor the intravesicoprostatic pressure and keep it below 15 mm Hg (Fig. 15–1).[10,11] The machine has two smooth peristaltic motorized pumps and can measure the pressure in the prostatic urethra and the amount of urine and blood in the outflow fluid. Originally, the instrument was controlled by printed circuit boards, but the most recent model has a microprocessor (Fig. 15–2*A*). As the new prototypes became available, I used them in both the hospital and the outpatient setting. The inflow–outflow fluid rate can now be regulated with a foot pedal within a range of 200 to 1,000 ml per minute. Bladder distention also can be regulated with a foot pedal that controls both peristaltic pumps. If the surgeon wishes to change the flow rate or the amount of bladder distention, the microprocessor's program memory will change and update the new values accordingly. The front panel of the instrument constantly displays the fluid inflow–outflow rate, the amount of bladder distention in milliliters, the intravesicoprostatic pressure in millimeters of mercury, and the blood-loss contaminant factor (Fig. 15–2*B*). The instrument can also be used with a conventional resectoscope. The inflow pump will deliver the desired amount of irrigant fluid at any set flow rate and stop automatically. After the bladder is emptied, a foot pedal restarts the filling; overdistention of the bladder is thereby avoided.

SURGICAL TECHNIQUE

Anesthesia

We use thiopental for induction, with halothane, nitrous oxide, and oxygen for

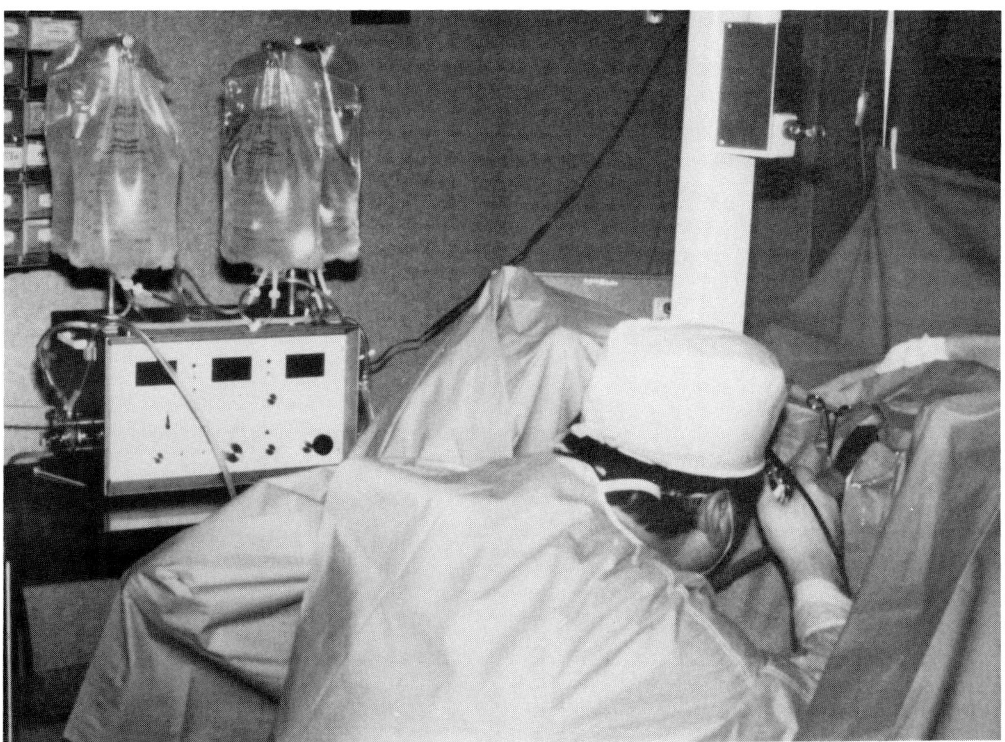

Fig. 15–1. Transurethral resection controller used during a procedure to provide inflow–outflow balance of irrigating fluid and to control and monitor bladder distention and vesicoprostatic pressure.

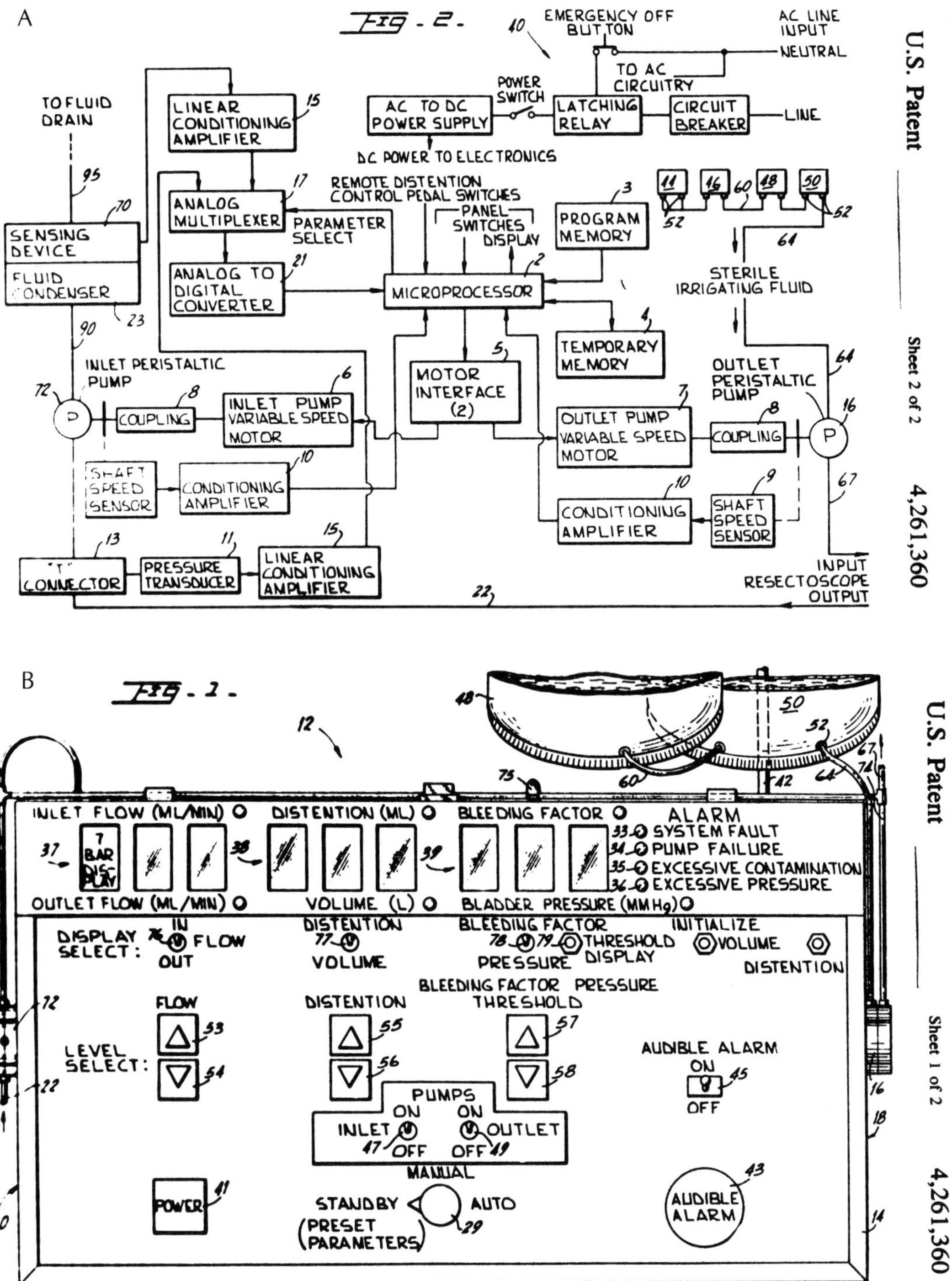

Fig. 15–2. Transurethral pressure controller. *(A)* Schematic block diagram. *(B)* Front view of the control panel.

inhalation anesthesia without an endotracheal tube. Other surgeons have used local anesthesia for selected patients undergoing transurethral prostatic resection.[12,13] For example, in 38 patients, Becher and Peress administered preoperative hydroxyzine (50 mg) and meperidine (pethidine; 25 to 50 mg) intramuscularly. In the operating room, 1 mg of butorphanol and 5 to 10 mg of diazepam were given intravenously. The authors then injected no more than 15 ml of 0.25% lidocaine transperineally through a 20-gauge spinal needle into both lobes of the prostate and its capsule, using an index finger in the patient's rectum as a guide. The urethra was then anesthetized with lidocaine jelly.[13] None of the patients reported discomfort or required general anesthesia. Obviously, the ability to obtain satisfactory anesthesia and analgesia with local agents and intravenous narcotics and sedatives rather than general anesthesia would increase the appeal of outpatient prostatic resection.

Introduction of the Resectoscope

Calibration and dilatation of the urethra to 26F or 28F facilitates passage of the resectoscope sheath. The urethra should not be considered a channel with a caliber, but rather a distensible conduit and should be treated gently.

To ensure that the procedure is accomplished correctly, the resectoscope should be passed under direct vision. It may be necessary to pull up the penis to straighten the urethra, and in this way one prevents damage to the prostatic urethra and bladder neck.

Technique of Resection

Irrigating-Fluid Flow Rate and Pressure. With the outlet of the bag of irrigating fluid 60 cm above the patient's bladder, a constant inflow and outflow of approximately 400 to 650 ml per minute is created, depending on the initial degree of bladder distention and the bladder-wall thickness. This provides adequate vision during the resection. The bladder should be distended initially until its posterior wall and dome are well out of the operating field; in most cases, 200 ml of irrigating fluid is sufficient. With this initial pressure and the continuous flow, the intravesicoprostatic pressure will be below 30 mm Hg.[14]

Sequence of Resection. Whatever the lesion being treated, the actual resection time should not exceed 20 to 30 minutes. Bladder-neck contractures, congenital or postoperative, should be resected around the circumference. Median bars, no matter how high, can be resected from a 7 to 5 o'clock position or a 4 to 8 o'clock position, depending on their lateral extent. Middle-lobe hyperplasia, subcervical or posterior commissural, is amenable to outpatient resection only if it is solitary; if it is associated with lateral-lobe hyperplasia, it will usually yield more than 20 g of tissue and the prostatic urethra may well be longer than 3.5 cm, making it unsuitable for outpatient surgery.

The hyperplastic tissue should be resected to the capsule, avoiding deep cuts in the area of the bladder neck proper in order to save as much as possible of the internal sphincter and prevent undermining of the trigone. All cuts should be made slowly and purposefully with the entire loop, and bleeding vessels should be electrocoagulated as they are encountered, particularly in the 3 to 5 o'clock and 7 to 9 o'clock regions. The resection should be carried distally to the level of the verumontanum. When the floor of the prostatic urethra is well excavated, it is helpful to electrocoagulate any important bleeding vessels and then change to the 0° telescope to determine whether any lateral or anterior tissue has fallen into the prostatic urethra to cause obstruction. The inspection with the 0° lens should be done with the beak of the resectoscope at the mid and distal prostatic urethra.

Small masses of obstructive, recurrent carcinomatous tissue, recurrent or residual small adenomas, apical tissue, and remnants can all be treated. An index finger in the patient's rectum is helpful in controlling the depth of the cuts. Fibrous obstruction with prostatic calculi also can be handled if the stones are not large or numerous. False passages in the prostatic urethra can be corrected if they are not associated with large residual adenomas.

Hemostasis. This task should be performed meticulously. The patient's blood pressure should be stable during the final electrocoagulation. The inflow stopcock is turned off intermittently to facilitate observation for any remaining small bleeders during a slow and thorough inspection of the prostatic urethra. This review should start at the 12 o'clock position on the roof of the prostatic urethra even if this area has not been resected, because the resectoscope may have torn the mucosa, and should continue from the vesicoprostatic border to the verumontanum. In the same manner, it should continue laterally to the 9 o'clock position on the right and the 3 o'clock position on the left. The floor of the prostatic urethra and the apical region around the verumontanum should be inspected also.

Final Inspection of the Operative Field. After all resected tissue has been removed, the operative field should be reviewed, identifying both ureteral orifices. The vesical outlet, the length of the prostatic urethra, the verumontanum, and the apical tissues should be studied for irregularities or bleeding. For reassurance, a final inspection may be made with the 0° and retrospective lenses. Approximately 100 ml of irrigating fluid is left in the bladder when the resectoscope is removed.

Concomitant Surgical Procedures

Bilateral Segmental Vasectomy. Ordinarily, I do not perform this procedure unless the patient has a history of epididymitis.

External Urethral Meatotomy and Meatoplasty. Stenosis and fibrosis of the external urethral meatus are treated by placing two reference anchoring sutures on each side of the stenotic meatus. Ample ventral meatotomy is then performed, and the resection is carried out as usual. After the resectoscope has been removed, the anchored urethral mucosa is approximated to the edges of the glans penis with 4–0 plain or chromic catgut on an atraumatic needle.

Visual Internal Urethrotomy. Short strictures of the urethra may be treated before prostatic resection using a Sachse optical urethrotome. Hard, long, or multiple strictures are best treated in the hospital, with the procedure followed by a short period of small-caliber catheter drainage.

POSTOPERATIVE MANAGEMENT

Recovery Room

Patients should be monitored and given intravenous fluids until they are completely alert and responsive. If the patient feels the urge to urinate, he should be encouraged to do so into a urinal placed between his legs. Alternatively, he can be helped to stand on a high stool by the bed to void into a urinal. After an hour or two, the intravenous fluids can be discontinued and the patient moved to the holding area.

Holding Area

Patients usually stay in this area for 2 more hours. During this period the time and amount of each voiding should be charted and the color of the urine noted. Most patients void with little discomfort, and no medication is needed. After three or four voidings, the urine should be clear and no more than moderately pinkish.

Instructions at Discharge and Followup Care

Any history of urinary-tract infections, as well as inflammatory changes in the bladder or prostatic urethra, or small pockets of purulent material opened intraoperatively, are all indications for antimicrobial drugs.

As after any transurethral prostatic surgery, the patient should remain at home for two to three weeks. He should not drive, and he should have an adequate diet and fluid intake. He should keep a daily record of the time, amount, and color of each voiding, and any alterations should be reported to the physician immediately. In addition, during the first week a daily report should be made to the physician by telephone; thereafter, the progress report can be made less often. Regular bowel movements are facilitated if the patient eats 6 to 8 spoonfuls of whole-wheat bran (available at health-food stores) daily mixed with yogurt or other semisolid food; this should ensure soft stools and defecation without effort. Alcohol, spiced foods, overeating, and sexual intercourse should be foregone until recovery is complete.

At the first postoperative visit to the physician, the patient should bring his voiding records for review. Further measures are based on the results of urinalysis, including a microscopic examination of the urine sediment.

Surgeon's Records

The operative report from an ambulatory surgical unit should be more specific about the indications for the operation than is necessary for a hospital record, since it will be the only available documentation. A brief description should be given of the symptoms, their duration, the significant physical findings (particularly from the rectal examination), the pertinent laboratory results, and the radiologic findings. The physician should also record what the patient was told about his condition, the treatment options, and the need for hospitalization should complications arise.

Scheduling

Because of the length of the procedure and postoperative period and the need to obtain adequate turnover of patients in the recovery room, I no longer schedule more than one outpatient operation per day. It is usually my first scheduled appointment.

RESULTS AND COMPLICATIONS

Transurethral prostatic surgery on an outpatient basis has been accepted enthusiastically by patients. The outpatient environment, which permits more personal attention in pleasant, relaxed surroundings, and the prospect of recovery at home are beneficial to both the patient and his family, and both are delighted with the monetary savings.

Complications have been few. One patient was catheterized to assure him that there was no undue bleeding or urinary retention. He voided spontaneously 90 minutes later. In another case, in which a 26-g prostatic adenoma had been resected, the patient required hospitalization because of blood-clot retention. He was discharged after two days of catheter drainage with continuous irrigation to remove clots; he was then voiding normally.

COST REDUCTION

Particularly in those cases in which the patient has no health insurance, the monetary savings of outpatient transurethral surgery are impressive. More than 25% is saved in operating- and recovery-room charges alone, and added savings accrue because the patient does not require hospitalization and its associated costs.

THE FUTURE

Although my outpatient procedures account for less than 5% of the prostatic resections I perform in a year, that figure could reasonably rise to 10% as more patients with bladder-outlet obstruction become aware of, and accept, outpatient surgery. I believe that urologic residents should be encouraged to assist in performing urologic surgery in ambulatory units. That way, the residents will become familiar not only with the operative techniques but also with the many advantages of outpatient procedures to both patient and physician.

Free-standing, independent ambulatory surgical centers can serve the community in a competent and well-organized manner to the great satisfaction of physicians and patients. As these centers become more numerous, patient-care costs will be reduced significantly. The challenge to hospitals, then, is to create financially independent ambulatory surgical units of their own that can compete with free-standing facilities. With time, this will greatly help to control health-care costs.

REFERENCES

1. Young, H.H.: A new procedure (punch operation) for small prostatic bars and contracture of the prostatic orifice. Am. Med. Assoc. Trans. Sect. Genito-Urin. Surg., 1912, p. 302.
2. Harris, S.H.: Suprapubic prostatectomy with closure. Aust. NZ J. Surg., *4*:226, 1934.
3. Hryntschak, T.: Suprapubic transvesical prostatectomy with primary closure of the bladder. J. Int. Coll. Surg., *15*:366, 1951.
4. Debenham, L.S., and Ward, A.E.: Retropubic prostatectomy using a no-catheter technique. Br. J. Urol., *32*:178, 1960.
5. Macalister, C.L.O.: Retropubic prostatectomy without catheter drainage. J. Urol., *92*:517, 1964.
6. Glaser, S.: Prostatectomy and hypotensive anesthesia: results of no-catheter technique. Proc. Roy. Soc. Med., *57*:1186, 1964.
7. Spooner, J.S.: Report presented to the Northeastern Section, American Urological Association, Canada, 1963.
8. Cass, A.S.: Transurethral prostatic resection without catheter drainage. J. Urol., *101*:750, 1969.
9. Mitchell, J.P.: The Principles of Transurethral Resection and Hemostasis. Baltimore, Williams & Wilkins, 1972.
10. Perez, J.A.: Transurethral resection controller. Presented at the Societe Internationale d'Urologie, 18th Congress, Paris, June 1979.
11. Perez, J.A.: Endoscopic surgical controller: present and future. Presented at the International Society of Urologic Endoscopy, 2nd Congress, Bristol, England, September 1981.
12. Moffat, N.A.: Transurethral prostatic resections under local anesthesia. J. Urol., *119*:141, 1977.
13. Becher, R.A., and Peress, S.A.: Personal communication, 1982.
14. Madsen, P.O., and Naber, K.G.: The importance of the pressure in the prostatic fossa and absorption of irrigating fluid during transurethral resection of the prostate. J. Urol., *109*:446, 1973.

Section V

Endourology

16

Percutaneous Nephrostomy and Insertion of Nephrostomy Tubes and Ureteral Stents

ARTHUR D. SMITH, M.D.

Percutaneous nephrostomy was introduced in 1955 as a means of draining an obstructed kidney,[1] but languished for several years because it was too difficult to perform with the radiographic techniques available. The introduction of fluoroscopy and ultrasonography proved to be the salvation of percutaneous nephrostomy, which began to be used extensively in patients too sick to tolerate anything else. As urologists and interventional radiologists discovered that a percutaneous nephrostomy tract is as useful as the urethra for getting inside the urinary tract to perform various maneuvers, percutaneous nephrostomy became a standard urologic technique. Now it is even being done on fetuses.[2]

This chapter describes the performance of a percutaneous nephrostomy and the insertion of various drainage tubes and stents, all of which can be done as outpatient procedures. I emphasize the use of fluoroscopy as the imaging mode because I have had the most experience with it, and it is essential for most manipulative procedures apart from the actual percutaneous nephrostomy. However, other practitioners prefer to use ultrasonography[3–6] or computed tomography[7] for the percutaneous nephrostomy.

INDICATIONS AND CONTRAINDICATIONS

Percutaneous nephrostomy is indicated to relieve obstruction, to provide access to renal and ureteral calculi, and to study the anatomy and function of the upper tract. In the hands of an experienced operator, a solitary kidney is not a contraindication. It has often been said that infection and bleeding disorders are contraindications, but as Stables has pointed out, in such patients the choice is often between attempting percutaneous nephrostomy and doing nothing at all.[8] Obviously, these patients are not candidates for an outpatient procedure.

There is one contraindication to percutaneous nephrostomy that few would question: widespread carcinoma with ureteral obstruction in a patient to whom no further chemotherapy can be offered (reviewed by Ortlip and Fraley[9]). Again, these patients are unlikely to present to an ambulatory surgical unit.

PREPROCEDURE PREPARATION

A urine culture should be performed so that an appropriate antibiotic can be started before the procedure. If this has not been done, or if no infection is found, a broad-spectrum antibiotic is administered for a few days starting when the patient is admitted.

Approximately an hour before the procedure, the patient is given an injection of a narcotic analgesic such as a combination of fentanyl plus droperidol (Innovar). During the procedure sedation and analgesia can be maintained with intravenous diazepam (Valium), meperidine (Demerol), and pethidine.

The skin around the nephrostomy site is prepared as it would be for a surgical incision, and the subcutaneous tissues are anesthetized with lidocaine (Xylocaine) or bupivacaine (Marcaine).

POSITIONING THE PATIENT

One of the most difficult skills a physician must acquire to take advantage of the percutaneous approach to the kidney is the ability to visualize the collecting system in three dimensions on the basis of the intravenous urogram (IVU). It helps to remember that, except for the uppermost and lowermost calyces, the calyces usually form two distinct rows, being directed anteriorly and posteriorly (Fig. 16–1). Those in the anterior half of the kidney point forward; however, with the rotation of the kidney by the psoas muscle, these calyces are seen from the side and look like stalked cups on the IVU. Those in the posterior half face a line slightly posterior to the lateral convex renal border and again, because of the rotation of the kidney, point almost directly backward and appear on the IVU as round concentrations of contrast medium.[10] Usually, it is the lowermost of these backward-facing calyces that one wishes to puncture for a percutaneous nephrostomy, because this approach brings the needle through the parenchyma in or near the avascular zone called Brödel's line of incision. The patient, therefore, is placed prone on the table, and the side to be punctured is raised approximately 30°. This causes the posterior row of calyces to point almost directly upward, making them easy targets (Fig. 16–2).

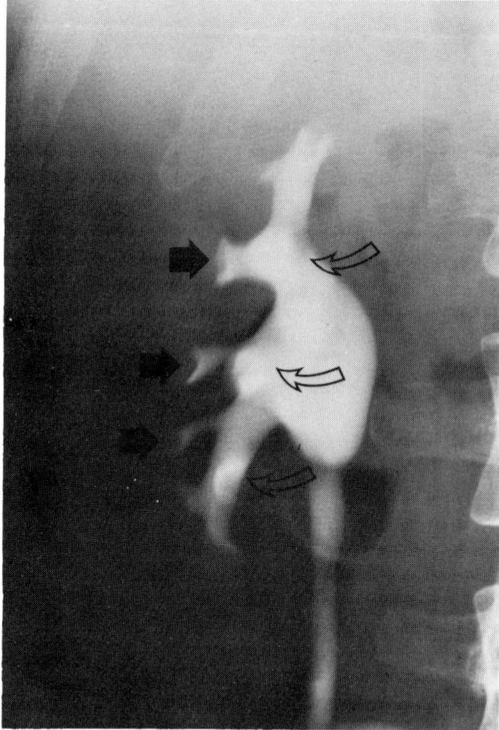

Fig. 16–1. Orientation of the calyces on an IVU. Anterior calyces *(closed arrows)* look like stalked cups, whereas posterior calyces *(open arrows)* look like round concentrations of contrast medium. (Courtesy of Dr. Keith W. Kaye.)

PERCUTANEOUS NEPHROSTOMY

Opacification of the Collecting System for Fluoroscopy or CT

If the collecting system can be sufficiently opacified by the IVU to create an adequate fluoroscopic target, the physician and patient are both fortunate. An obstructed kidney, however, can seldom be opacified in this way, which explains one of the appeals of ultrasound for guiding percutaneous nephrostomy. It is pos-

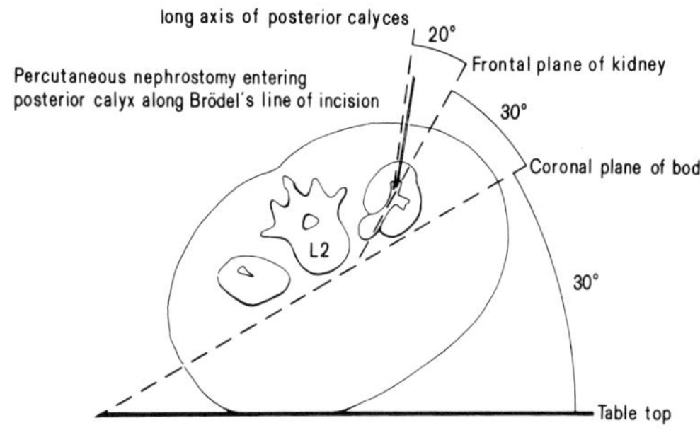

Fig. 16–2. Position of the patient and site of needle entry for percutaneous nephrostomy. (From Kaye, K.W.: J. Urol., *130*:647, 1983.)

sible to insert the trocar needle blindly but better to make what Stables calls a "localization" puncture, at a site slightly away from that chosen for the nephrostomy, through which contrast medium is instilled.

A 22-gauge needle, either a spinal needle or the more flexible Chiba needle, is used. Except in obese adults, for whom a 15-cm needle may be needed, a 10-cm needle is usually appropriate. The patient should be told to breathe quietly and to suspend breathing during passages of the needle.

The needle is inserted vertically through the anesthetized skin to a depth of 8–10 cm lateral to the tips of the transverse vertebral processes in the interspace between the first and second lumbar vertebrae. Return of urine proves that the collecting system has been entered, although it may be necessary to aspirate with tubing and a syringe to get a return through the small needle. If the needle does not enter the collecting system, it is withdrawn and reinserted. Multiple passes cause little trauma.

After the collecting system has been entered, the needle stylet is removed; and an anesthetic extension tube and syringe are attached to the needle hub. Urine is aspirated for culture and replaced with diluted (approximately 17%) contrast medium. The exact percentage is not critical; rather, the intent is to make the renal pelvis sufficiently opaque for the procedure without obscuring the view of the guide wires and instruments. The needle should be left in place until the procedure is complete to make it easy to instill more contrast medium and to prevent leakage of contrast medium. Such leakage causes no harm and soon ceases spontaneously; the extravasation can, however, obscure one's view of the collecting system.

Definitive Puncture under Fluoroscopic Control

We use a posterolateral transparenchymal approach to the collecting system in most cases, because it creates a longer intrarenal course for the guide wires and tubes, thus helping to hold them in place. It also creates an angle with the upper ureter that facilitates manipulation and allows patients to lie on their backs comfortably afterward. Of course, the exact position for the definitive puncture must be chosen with a view to the manipulations one intends to perform through the nephrostomy tract. If one intends to establish U-loop (circle-tube) drainage, a lower calyx should be selected. Also, the skin site must be below the twelfth rib, because transthoracic passage of the needle may cause pneumothorax. In addition, if the tract passes through the diaphragm, this causes marked discomfort when the patient breathes. Finally, the path between the skin site and the calyx should be vertical (it may be necessary to reposition the patient) and should pass medial and cephalad, especially if manipulations in the ureter are planned. The position of the calyx can be indicated by placing the tips of a hemostat on the patient's skin so that they are superimposed on that calyx on the fluoroscope screen.

The skin around the entry site is anesthetized with 1% lidocaine, and a ¼-inch (5-mm) incision is made with a scalpel. Local anesthetic is then infiltrated into the subcutaneous tissues down to the kidney. After it has taken effect, an 18-gauge needle is directed into the collecting system through the chosen calyx under fluoroscopic observation. The needle trocar is withdrawn, and a guide wire is directed through the cannula into the kidney and proximal ureter. The cannula is removed, and 5F, 6F, and 7F dilators are passed in turn over the guide wire to enlarge the tract and permit insertion of the drainage tube. It is imperative that the guide wire be kept taut during these manipulations; otherwise, it and the dilator may slip outside the kidney. Such loss of a percutaneous nephrostomy tract is one of the most vexing complications of this procedure.

Percutaneous Puncture under Ultrasonic Control[3–6,8]

Ultrasound can be used in several ways for percutaneous nephrostomy. However, proper positioning of the drainage catheter requires fluoroscopy.[8]

First, ultrasound may be used to measure the depth of the collecting system from the skin when the patient is lying in the position to be used during the puncture. This is particularly helpful for the novice and for the experienced operator contemplating a difficult puncture. A portable real-time or A-mode machine is the most useful and can be brought into the fluoroscopy suite. The actual depth of the kidney will, however, prove to be approximately 2 cm greater than that determined by ultrasound, in part because the kidney is displaced during puncture by the trocar needle.

Second, some operators prefer to do the localization puncture under ultrasonic rather than fluoroscopic guidance. This is especially desirable in patients with poor renal function whose kidneys are not opacified by intravenous contrast medium. Stables finds it particularly valuable in severely azotemic patients, especially those with diabetes, because such persons are particularly susceptible to kidney damage from contrast medium.[8] The puncture site is chosen after inspection of the image of the collecting system and marked on the skin with indelible ink. The depth of the collecting system and angulation of the path are borne in mind while the 22-gauge needle is being inserted. Alternatively, the needle can be passed through a gas-sterilized aspiration-biopsy transducer under A-mode or, less desirably, B-mode guidance.

Third, the definitive puncture can be performed under ultrasonic guidance if the operator has experience with that modality. Usually, it is not difficult to introduce a percutaneous nephrostomy needle under ultrasonic control. The problem that usually follows is that one often wants to do some additional procedure requiring fluoroscopic control, and unless both facilities are present in the same room, it is advisable to do the whole procedure under fluoroscopic control. Some operators can, however, introduce catheters down the ureter under ultrasonic guidance, but this is the exception rather than the rule.

Percutaneous Puncture under Computed Tomography

Although this is possible, there is little to recommend it unless some other step is planned that requires computed tomography. It does not obviate fluoroscopy.

Intubation of the Tract

Unless one intends to proceed immediately with some endourologic procedure such as stent insertion or nephrostolithotomy, the newly created percutaneous tract is dilated and intubated. Commercial kits for percutaneous nephrostomy contain 5F, 6F, and 7F dilators, which are passed in turn over the guide wire. After dilatation of the nephrostomy tract to 7F, a 7F pigtail catheter can be inserted into the renal pelvis.

For several procedures, however, we prefer to dilate the nephrostomy tract further.

DILATATION OF THE NEPHROSTOMY TRACT

Most of the endourologic procedures described here and elsewhere in this book, including the placement of tubes for long-term drainage, require a tract much larger than 7F. Fluoroscopic control of dilatation is almost always desirable, and if the tract is less than a week old, it is imperative.

The dilatation of the tract, if performed slowly, can be done as an outpatient procedure. If the tract is being markedly dilated, however, as from 12F to 34F in one session, then it is advisable for the patient to be admitted. The procedure can certainly be done under local anesthesia.

A guide wire is first inserted through the nephrostomy tube well into the ureter. If it does not pass spontaneously through the ureteropelvic junction, an angled-tipped polyethylene catheter may be passed over it and directed toward the ureteropelvic junction. The guide wire is then advanced forward gently in probing fashion until it passes into the ureter. Again, the guide wire must be kept taut.

Several dilator sets are available commercially, and others are easily created. The Cook system consists of several interlocking dilators, Vance has a system of followers that will dilate a nephrostomy tract to 36F, as well as a system of dilators to 18F, which are included in the Stamey Malecot nephrostomy kit, and Storz and Wolfe have telescoping metal dilators.[11] Mazzeo et al. have used a series of modified Foley catheters,[12] and Clayman et al. have used Olbert transluminal angioplasty balloon catheters for single-step dilatation.[13] The single-step methods carry less risk of guide wire displacement, but otherwise the most important factor in selecting a method is one's experience.

NEPHROSTOMY DRAINAGE

Drainage via a nephrostomy tract can conveniently be thought of in two ways: as a short-term expedient, for which simple drainage tubes are satisfactory, and as a long-term means of management, for which a U-loop (circle-tube) system is preferable.

Indwelling Nephrostomy Catheters

Several of these catheters are available commercially in kits that contain the necessary equipment and instructions for insertion. These instructions should always be followed, as commercial designs are modified frequently, necessitating changes in technique. Most of these catheters have retention balloons that require frequent monitoring if they are not to compress the renal parenchyma and interfere with drainage. The familiar Foley catheter may also be used, although it is advisable to cut off the tip beyond the balloon to avoid damage to the renal pelvis.

Argyle Ingram Trocar Catheters

This polyvinyl chloride catheter comes in 12F and 16F sizes. It has two lumens, one for drainage and the other for irrigations. There is an end hole and three elliptical side holes large enough to resist obstruction by pus and small calculi. Because of the softness of polyvinyl chloride, the Argyle catheter sometimes resists simple insertion over a guide wire, especially in a fresh nephrostomy tract. It may be stiffened by immersion in sterile ice for several minutes or loaded on a 60-cm translumbar aortography arch needle* for passage over a guide wire.[14] No more than 2–3 ml of fluid should be injected into the retention balloon. In obese patients, the wide disc that is used to anchor this catheter to the skin must be removed so that the catheter will be

*Cook, Inc., 925 Curry Pike, Bloomington, IN 47402

long enough. This should be done by incising the disc with a scalpel, as sliding the disc off may damage the balloon.[14]

Stamey Malecot Nephrostomy Catheter

This system is an adaptation of the well-known Stamey Malecot system for suprapubic cystostomy (see Chapter 24).[15] The original trocar has a cutting edge to puncture the bladder wall; in the system for nephrostomy, this edge has been removed to prevent damage to the renal pelvis (Fig. 16–3A). Also, the shaft of the trocar introducer is a spring that is rigid enough to straighten the wings of the catheter tip but flexible enough to follow the guide wire (Fig. 16–3*B*).[16] After the catheter is in place, the introducer is unlocked and withdrawn, allowing the Malecot wings to re-form. This system is available from Cook Urological.*

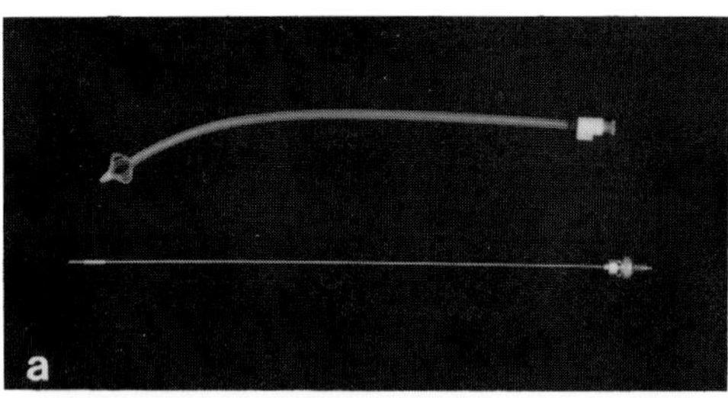

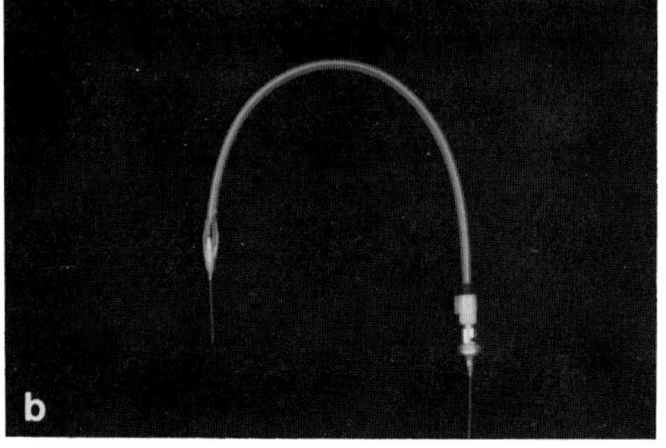

Fig. 16–3. The Stamey Malecot nephrostomy catheter. *(A)* Catheter with wings extended with trocar introducer. *(B)* Catheter with wings closed mounted on flexible trocar.

Whichever catheter is used, it should be fixed to the skin with synthetic suture material or, better, sutured to a plastic retention disc, which is then fastened to the skin. Alternatively, adhesive discs and tape can be used.[17] Fixation is needed even for catheters with a retaining balloon and is critical in a fresh nephrostomy tract.

U-Loop Nephrostomy

The great advantage of the U-loop drainage system is that it is virtually impossible to dislodge accidentally; this makes it particularly desirable for patients who are to be discharged home. The method described here presumes that the patient has one mature nephrostomy tract.[18]

A second nephrostomy site is selected far enough from the first one so that a tube passing between the two will describe a gentle curve through the renal pelvis. A nephrostogram is performed, and a second percutaneous puncture is created as described using the fluoroscopic technique (Fig. 16–4A). A guide wire is passed through the needle. The tube in the original nephrostomy tract is removed, and the tract is dilated to 12F if it is not already this large. The guide wire is then retrieved from the renal pelvis by inserting a Dormia stone basket through the original nephrostomy tract and manipulating it under fluoroscopic observation until it has entrapped the guide wire. After the guide wire has been withdrawn through the original nephrostomy tract, a 7F polyethylene angiogram catheter is passed over the wire until it emerges from the new nephrostomy tract (Fig. 16–4*B*).

The next step is dilatation of the two tracts so that they will admit the large U

---

*Cook, Urological, 1100 West Morgan Street, Spencer, IN 47460

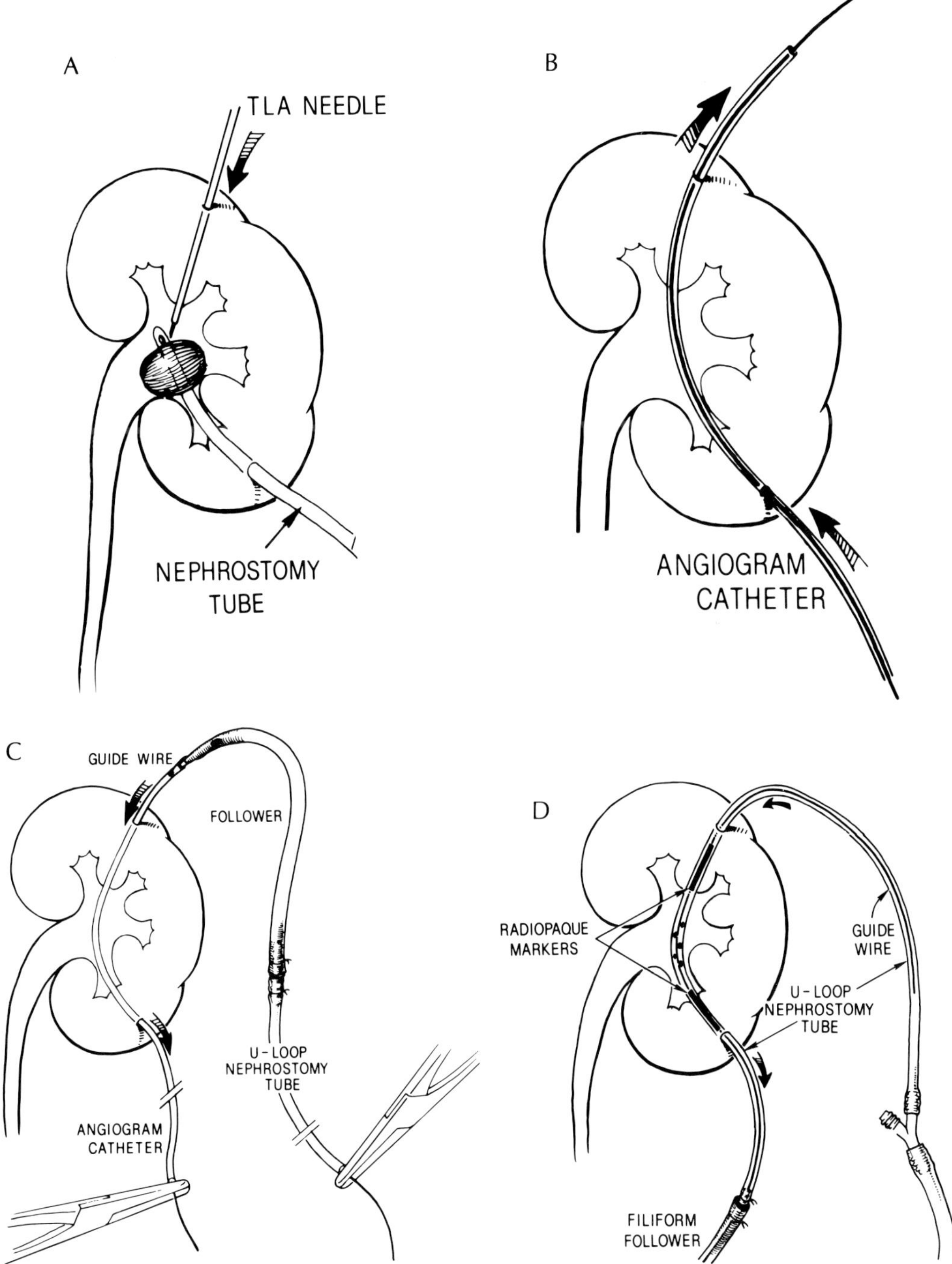

Fig. 16–4. Technique for establishing U-loop nephrostomy drainage. *(A)* Creation of a second nephrostomy puncture; drainage tube is still in place in the first nephrostomy tract. *(B)* Angiogram catheter passed over the guide wire between the two tracts. *(C)* Dilatation of tract with filiform followers; note that guide wire is wrapped around the connection with the angiogram catheter. Hemostats on guide wire help prevent the assembly from separating. *(D)* Positioning of the drainage holes in the renal pelvis.

tube. A side hole is made in the upper end of the angiogram catheter, and the guide wire is passed through it. A series of filiform followers is now attached by inserting the follower tip into the catheter, passing the guide wire around the connection, and inserting the wire through the follower via the side hole (Fig. 16–4*C*). This wrapping of the wire is critical, because if the side holes of the catheter and followers are aligned and the wire passes directly between them, it may cause severe lacerations if the connection buckles during later manipulation. We usually begin with a 10F follower and dilate both tracts to 20F.

When the final follower has been attached, its distal end is cut off, and the U-loop tube is attached with the connectors provided with the kit. The connection is protected from separation by clamping a hemostat on the guide wire at the end of the tube (Fig. 16–4*C*). The U-loop tube is pulled into place with the drainage holes in the renal pelvis. The radiopaque markers on either side of the holes facilitate proper positioning under fluoroscopic observation (Fig. 16–4*D*). The follower is disconnected, the guide wire is removed, and the two ends of the U-loop tube are joined to the Y connector, which is connected to the drainage tube and bag.

When it becomes necessary to change a U-loop tube, the new tube is attached to the old one and pulled into position.

COMPLICATIONS

Stables recently reviewed 1,207 percutaneous nephrostomies, most of them performed in patients with cancer, and found that there had been significant, but usually not life-threatening, complications in 48 cases (4%). Bleeding, especially into the retroperitoneum where it may be undetected for several hours, is the most serious complication; and in two patients, it was fatal. Two other reports of fatal hemorrhage after percutaneous nephrostomy have been published since Stables' article appeared; all four patients had some coagulopathy and thus would not have been candidates for outpatient nephrostomies.

There has been a recent spate of reports of delayed bleeding after percutaneous nephrostomies as the result of formation and rupture of renal pseudoaneurysms or arteriovenous fistulas.[18–21] In many of these cases, it is clear that the nephrostomy tube was removed before the tract had matured. Once a nephrostomy tract has been established, it should not be extubated, except to change tubes, for at least six days. The patient must be instructed to report any hematuria or bleeding from the nephrostomy site to the physician immediately. Most of the other complications of percutaneous nephrostomy, such as infection, urine leakage, and pneumothorax, are the result of improper techniques.

URETERAL STENTS

Traditionally, ureteral stents have been inserted intraoperatively to protect a repair. Now, however, they are far more likely to be inserted transcystoscopically or endourologically; that is, with the aid of a percutaneous nephrostomy tract. This can be done on an outpatient basis unless the patient requires hospitalization for some other reason.

Types

Gibbons Stents.[22] This is the original indwelling ureteral stent (Fig. 16–5). It is made of silicone rubber tubing and designed to resist radial compression. It has tooth-like protrusions to prevent it from migrating in the ureter and has a distal collar with a tail to facilitate its removal. The proximal end has drainage holes, and its protrusions and the collar and tail are radiopaque. The principal advantages of this stent are its larger internal diameters, the small amount of potentially irritating foreign body it leaves in the blad-

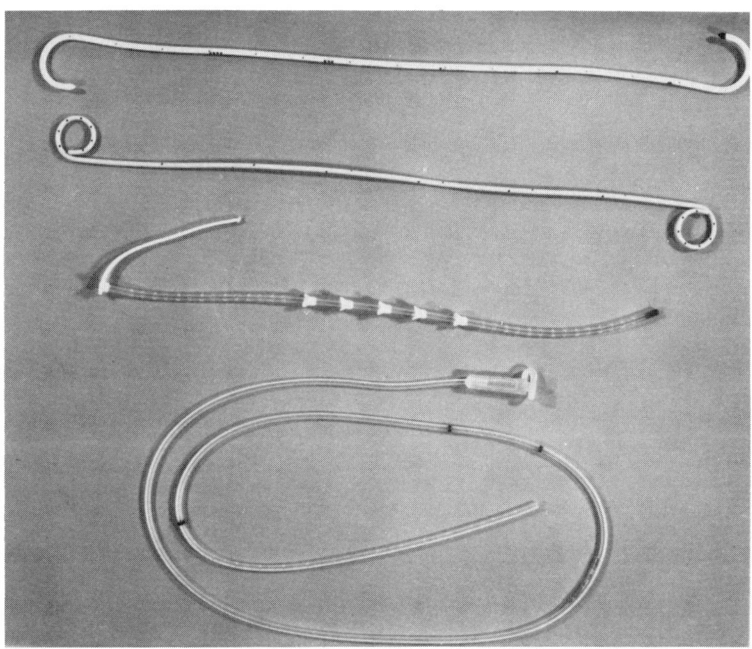

Fig. 16–5. Popular ureteral stents. From top to bottom: Double-J (Finney), Double-Pigtail, Gibbons; and Universal (Smith).

der, and the fact that one need not measure the ureteral length as precisely as is necessary with stents that have retention devices such as pigtails in the renal pelvis. The Gibbons stent is most effective in patients with obstructions in the lower ureter, below the protrusions, but also may be useful in patients in whom the double-J or double-pigtail stents cause irritative bladder symptoms. It is not as effective when the obstruction is physiologic (e.g., hydronephrosis of pregnancy) and, because of the protrusions, probably should not be used if there is a ureteral fistula. Gibbons stents are usually inserted transcystoscopically but can also be inserted endourologically, as will be described.

Double-J (Finney) Stents.[23] The Finney stent has a J or shepherd's crook at either end, which is both its greatest advantage and its greatest disadvantage. The advantage of the design is that, because there are retention devices in both the renal pelvis and the bladder, the stent seldom migrates. The disadvantages are that one must measure the length of the ureter exactly and that, in some patients, the distal J irritates the bladder. The stent is made of radiopaque silicone elastomer in diameters of 6F, 7F, and 8.5F and in four lengths from 16 to 30 cm and has drainage holes throughout most of its length. A guide strip, marked in centimeters, is imprinted at the proximal end in such a manner as to be visible through the cystoscope, which is the easiest way to insert this stent (Fig. 16–5). Less readily, it can be inserted endourologically.

Double-Pigtail Stents.[24] These stents are made of radiopaque polyethylene and are prevented from migrating by a large open coil at either end (the "pigtail"). They have side holes (Fig. 16–5) and are manufactured with diameters to 5F to 8F and lengths of 8 to 30 cm. The double-pigtail stent has the fastest flow rate of the available stents, which may prolong its useful life.[24] It can be inserted transcystoscopically or by percutaneous antegrade methods, and the designers recommend that equipment for endourologic insertion be available even when endoscopic insertion is planned in case the latter fails.

Universal (Smith) Stents.[25]* This silicone rubber stent is highly cost effective, because it comes in only one size that is cut to fit the patient, thus reducing inventory. It is an 8F tube, 80 cm long, with a proximal 3.5-cm zone of side holes, marked on both sides with radiopaque material (to make it easier to position in the renal pelvis) and distal drainage holes (Fig. 16–5). The proximal end has a Luer-Lok connector that can be used to attach an irrigation apparatus. The stent is inserted by endourologic techniques with the proximal end protruding from the percutaneous nephrostomy. The end can be clamped or not, depending on whether one wants nephrostomy drainage. The universal stent has been particularly useful in outpatients who do not have ready access to a hospital, because if the intraureteral portion becomes occluded, the stent can be unclamped at the nephrostomy site to provide drainage until the patient visits the physician.

*Cook Urological, 1100 West Morgan Street, Spencer, IN 47460

Techniques for Insertion of Ureteral Stents

Endoscopic Methods. With the exception of the Smith stent, all of these ureteral stents were designed to be inserted transcystoscopically and, therefore, are sold in kits that include the necessary dilators, guide wires, etc. Both the stents and the insertion equipment are evolving, so the manufacturer's instructions should always be consulted before a kit is used.

The protrusions of the Gibbons stent can interfere with insertion, so the ureter must be dilated until a catheter the size of the stent will pass. The stent should be the largest that will pass the obstruction and must be long enough to extend at least 3 cm proximal to the obstruction.[22] A helpful booklet, *An Illustrated Technical Manual for Insertion of Gibbons Ureteral Stents*, is available from the manufacturer.*

The greatest difficulty in the placement of the double-J stent is usually in selecting the proper length. (In measuring the length of the ureter on a radiograph, one must include an allowance for the magnification effect of approximately 10%). The distal tip of the stent is cut off with scissors so that the stylet wire can be inserted, and the stent is passed up the ureter via the cystoscope with the help of a push catheter. It is easier to do this if the inside and outside of the stent are lubricated with sterile mineral oil. The stent is held in place with the push catheter while the stylet wire is removed. The J's then form automatically.

Precise measurement of ureteral length is as necessary for the double-pigtail stent as it is for the double-J stent. It is helpful to dilate the narrowed area before passing the stent, and it is essential that the guide wire be passed well beyond the lesion into the renal pelvis to prevent ureteral perforation.

Endourologic Methods. These techniques take advantage of a percutaneous nephrostomy performed through a posterolateral approach into a lower or middle calyx and can be classified as either retrograde, in which the stent is pulled up through the urethra and bladder, or antegrade, in which the stent is pulled or pushed down the ureter through the nephrostomy tract. The former approach is necessary for the Gibbons and Finney stents, the latter for the Smith stent. Endourologic methods often succeed where

*Cook Urological, 1100 West Morgan Street, Spencer, IN 47460

cystoscopic methods have failed, because it is usually easier to bypass a ureteral obstruction from above than from below.

For the retrograde method of inserting Gibbons stents, an angiographic guide wire is passed down the ureter into the bladder. We prefer the 210-cm, 0.035-inch TSFB wire,* which is flexible and straight-tipped. Rarely is an obstruction so severe as to prevent guide wire passage, although it may be necessary to instill contrast medium and examine the area fluoroscopically. After the guide wire has entered the bladder, a 7F or 8F polyethylene angiographic catheter is passed over the guide wire into the bladder. The guide wire should always precede the catheter, which should never be used alone as a probe.[26]

The guide wire and angiographic catheter are retrieved from the bladder transcystoscopically with Bumpus, biopsy, or alligator forceps. The end of the catheter is cut off, a hole is punched in the new end, and the guide wire is routed out through it. The end of a 10F filiform follower is screwed into the lumen of the catheter so that the hole on the follower is on the side opposite the one in the catheter, and the guide wire is passed through the hole. The guide wire is passed through a Gibbons stent cut to the proper length and then through the distal half of a whistle-tipped ureteral catheter, and hemostats are clamped on the wire at both ends to keep the parts of the apparatus in apposition (Fig. 16–6). Traction on the apparatus at the nephrostomy site now pulls the Gibbons stent up into the ureter. The operator should confirm cystoscopically that the distal collar is flush against the vesicoureteral junction. The proximal hemostat is removed, allowing the angiographic catheter and filiform follower to be pulled off the guide wire.

*Cook, Inc., 925 Curry Pike, Bloomington, IN 47402

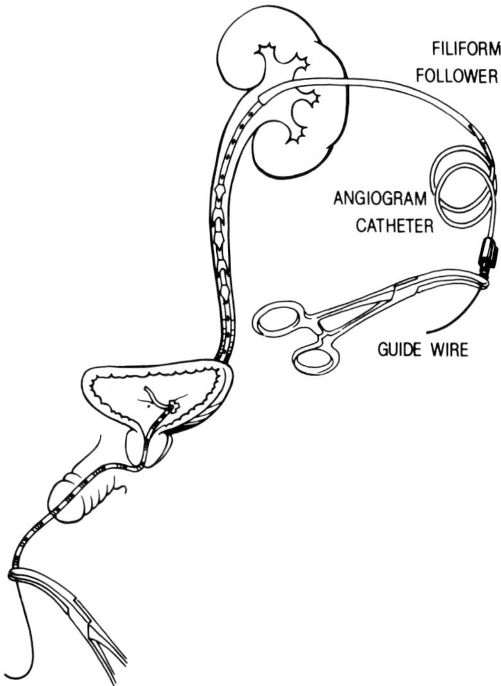

Fig. 16–6. Endourologic insertion of a Gibbons stent. The stent has been pulled up into the ureter; note hemostats keeping assembly from separating.

The unused proximal half of the whistle-tipped catheter can now be passed over the guide wire as a temporary nephrostomy tube if one desires. The guide wire is then withdrawn through the cystoscope while the stent is stabilized by pressing the distal portion of the whistle-tipped catheter against its flange. A cystogram is performed to ensure that free reflux is occurring.

Antegrade endourology techniques are used for the double-pigtail and Smith stents. The former is sufficiently stiff that it can be pushed down the ureter over a guide wire (Fig. 16–7).

The Smith stent is softer and thus its insertion is more complex. A guide wire and angiographic catheter are passed down the ureter and retrieved as in the retrograde method. The length of the ureter is measured on a nephrostogram (with allowance for the magnification ef-

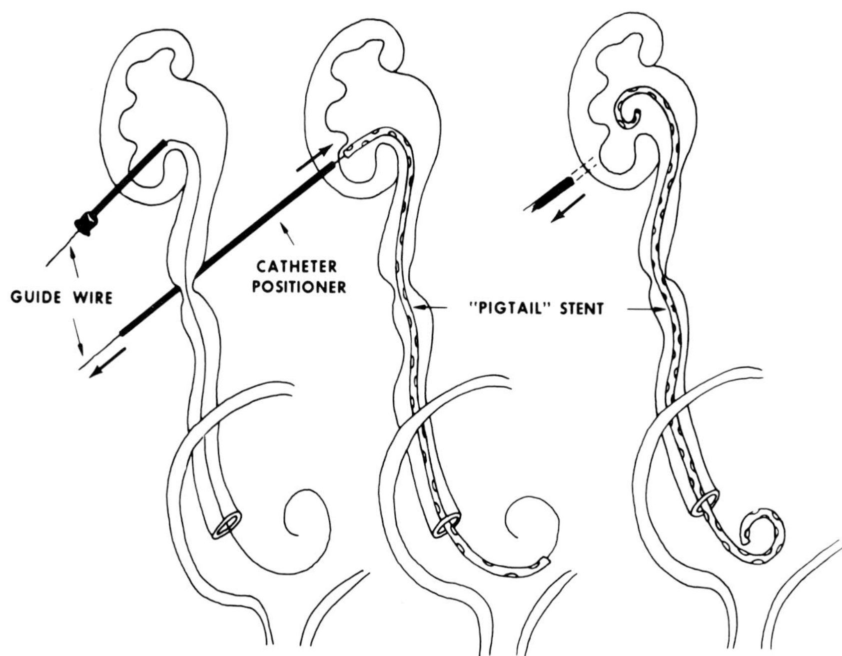

Fig. 16–7. Antegrade insertion of the double-pigtail stent. (From Mardis, H.K., et al.: Urol. Clin. North Am., 9:95, 1982.)

fect), and the portion of the stent beyond the renal pelvic drainage holes is cut to this length plus 2 cm. The stent is passed over the guide wire and coated with a water-soluble lubricant. Hemostats clamped on the guide wire at both ends of this apparatus hold it together and permit the Smith stent to be pulled down into the ureter until the tip emerges from the urethral meatus (Fig. 16–8). The hemostats are unclamped, and the guide wire is pulled out, releasing the angiographic catheter. The tip of the stent is pulled back into the bladder, where its position is checked cystoscopically. The proper positioning of the drainage holes in the renal pelvis is confirmed fluoroscopically. If nephrostomy drainage is not desired, the proximal end of the stent is clamped, sutured to the skin, and buried in a small Betadine ointment dressing.

I recently devised a method for the antegrade noncystoscopic insertion of the universal stent,[27] which lends itself more

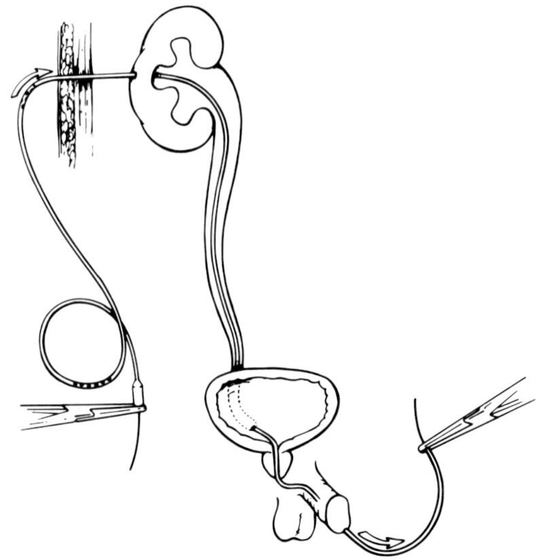

Fig. 16–8. Insertion of the Smith universal stent. Hemostats prevent separation of catheter and stent during passage down the ureter.

readily to the outpatient setting. After the nephrostomy tract has been dilated to 8F and a guide wire has been advanced into the bladder, an 8F vessel dilator is passed over the guide wire into the upper ureter. A Lunderquist guide wire is then introduced through the dilator and passed into the bladder. This steel wire does not have an outer spiral layer, and thus the silicone rubber stent is less likely to bind to it than to a standard guide wire. A 12F coaxial dilator is advanced over the 8F dilator to stretch the nephrostomy tract and ureteropelvic junction, and the dilators are withdrawn. A universal stent, cut to the proper length and lubricated with sterile mineral oil, is then passed over the Lunderquist guide wire until the radiopaque markers are in the upper ureter. The guide wire is then removed while the stent is held in position. Contrast medium is instilled through the stent to assist in the accurate positioning of the drainage holes within the renal pelvis. The stent is then fixed to the skin. When hematuria has stopped, the proximal end of the stent is flushed with 20 ml of sterile water or saline and plugged. (The stent must not be plugged when the end is full of urine, as this predisposes the stent to occlusion). The excess stent is curled on the skin and covered with a Betadine dressing that is changed twice a week.

CONCLUSIONS

In most cases, percutaneous nephrostomy and insertion of drainage tubes or stents can be done as an outpatient procedure. In other instances, one may wish to do the percutaneous nephrostomy on an outpatient basis and then admit the patient to the hospital after the tract has matured for the endourologic procedures, thus shortening the hospital stay and reducing the cost. Some of the useful things that can be done via a percutaneous nephrostomy tract are described by Doctor Clayman in Chapter 17.

REFERENCES

1. Goodwin, W.E., Casey, W.C., and Woolf, W.: Percutaneous trocar (needle) nephrostomy in hydronephrosis. J. Am. Med. Assoc., *157*:891, 1955.
2. Vallancian, G., et al.: Percutaneous nephrostomy in utero. Urology, *20*:647, 1982.
3. Pedersen, J.F., et al.: Ultrasonically guided percutaneous nephrostomy. Radiology, *119*:429, 1976.
4. Sadlowski, R.W., et al.: New techniques for percutaneous nephrostomy under ultrasound guidance. J. Urol., *121*:559, 1979.
5. Baron, R.L., et al.: Percutaneous nephrostomy using real-time sonographic guidance. AJR, *136*:1018, 1981.
6. Stables, D.P., and Johnson, M.L.: Percutaneous nephrostomy: the role of ultrasound. Clin. Diagn. Ultrasound, *2*:73, 1979.
7. Haaga, J.R., et al.: CT-guided antegrade pyelography and percutaneous nephrostomy. Am. J. Roentgenol., *128*:621, 1977.
8. Stables, D.P.: Percutaneous nephrostomy: techniques, indications, and results. Urol. Clin. North Am., 9:15, 1982.
9. Ortlip, S.A., and Fraley, E.E.: Indications for palliative diversion in patients with cancer. Urol. Clin. North Am., 9:79, 1982.
10. Kaye, K.W., and Goldberg, M.E.: Applied anatomy of the kidney and ureter. Urol. Clin. North Am., 9:3, 1982.
11. Rusnak, B., Castanada-Zuniga, W.R., and Smith, A.D.: An improved dilator system for percutaneous nephrostomy. Radiology, *144*:74, 1982.
12. Mazzeo, V.P., Jr., Pollack, H.M., and Banner, M.P.: A technique for percutaneous dilatation of nephrostomy tracts. Radiology, *144*:175, 1982.
13. Clayman, R.V., et al.: Rapid balloon dilatation of the nephrostomy tract for nephrostolithotomy. Radiology, *147*:884, 1983.
14. Gerber, W.L.: Use of the Argyle catheter for nephrostomy drainage. Urol. Clin. North Am., 9:61, 1982.
15. Smith, A.D., et al.: A modified Stamey catheter kit for long-term percutaneous nephrostomy drainage. Radiology, *139*:230, 1981.
16. Castaneda-Zuniga, W.R., et al.: A flexible trocar for percutaneous nephrostomy. AJR, *136*:434, 1981.
17. Shoenfeld, R.B., et al.: Stabilization of percutaneous catheters. AJR, *138*:972, 1982.
18. Smith, A.D., et al.: Percutaneous U-loop nephrostomy. J. Urol., *121*:355, 1979.
19. Gavant, M.L., Gold, R.E., and Church, J.C.: Delayed rupture of renal pseudoaneurysm: complication of percutaneous nephrostomy. AJR, *138*:948, 1982.
20. Cope, C., and Zeit, R.M.: Pseudoaneurysms after nephrostomy. AJR, *139*:255, 1982.
21. Clayman, R.V., et al.: Vascular complications of percutaneous nephrostomy. J. Urol., *132*:228, 1984.
22. Gibbons, R.P.: Gibbons ureteral stents. Urol. Clin. North Am., 9:85, 1982.

23. Finney, R.P.: Double-J and diversion stents Urol. Clin. North Am., 9:85, 1982.
24. Mardis, H.K., et al.: Polyethylene double-pigtail ureteral stents. Urol. Clin. North Am., 9:95, 1982.
25. Smith, A.D.: The universal ureteral stent. Urol. Clin. North Am., 9:103, 1982.
26. Miller, R.P., et al.: Percutaneous approach to the ureter. Urol. Clin. North Am., 9:31, 1982.
27. Smith, A.D., and Lee, W.: Characteristics and uses of the universal (Smith) ureteric stent. Brit. J. Urol., Supplement 79, 1983.

17

Nephroscopy and Nephrostolithotomy

RALPH V. CLAYMAN, M.D.

The development of percutaneous nephrostomy has provided the urologist with a conduit for the examination, diagnosis, and treatment of renal disorders, much as the urethra provides access to the bladder.[1] In this chapter, I describe our methods for examining the renal pelvis through a percutaneous nephrostomy tract (nephroscopy), along with our techniques for using the tract to extract renal and ureteral stones (nephrostolithotomy).

At present, percutaneous nephroscopy is usually performed in the hospital, and to date we have performed nephrostolithotomy only on inpatients. Both of these techniques are new, however, and we expect that certain aspects may soon be performed in the ambulatory care center. In a patient with a previously established nephrostomy tract, we have performed nephroscopy with a flexible instrument and removed small stone remnants during outpatient clinic visits. In addition, in some highly motivated patients, percutaneous nephrostomy, tract dilation, and stone removal have been completed on the first hospital day in a single session in the angiography suite using only local anesthesia, the patients being discharged the following morning.

Within the next year, we believe that some patients will undergo nephrostolithotomy without hospitalization.* In these first cases, the patient will probably have a percutaneous nephrostomy tract created and dilated with tube insertion during the first visit to the ambulatory care center (see Chapter 16). Three to five days later, he would return to the unit for stone removal through the now-mature tract, after which he will be observed for several hours and then sent home. Two to ten days after stone removal, the nephrostomy tube will be removed during an office visit. In our judgment, this day is close at hand.

*We now know of five patients who have had their renal calculi removed on an outpatient basis.

NEPHROSCOPY

Preoperative Preparation

The patient's urine should be sterile. In all cases, antibiotic coverage is used: intravenous ampicillin and an aminoglycoside (usually gentamycin) if the nephrostomy tract is fresh, and oral nitrofurantoin or trimethoprim–sulfa if the tract is more than four days old. Before the patient is sent to the radiology suite, a Foley catheter is inserted.

Provided that the patient's cardiac and renal function is adequate, we recommend inducing diuresis with 4–6 g of mannitol intravenously and an infusion of 200–300 ml of Ringer's lactate per hour. This makes it easier to see the infundibula and calyces and helps keep the field free of debris. In addition, the diuresis may protect the kidney by helping to prevent pyelotubular backflow.

Position of the Nephrostomy Tract

Successful nephrostolithotomy requires proper placement of the nephrostomy tract. For stones in the middle and lower-pole calyces, we usually place the nephrostomy through the infundibulum of the stone-containing calyx, thereby trapping the stone. Stones in upper-pole calyces are approached through the lowermost calyx, so that there is a straight or gently curved path from the tract across the pelvis to the stone. We rarely place the nephrostomy tract in an upper-pole calyx, because in our experience placement of the tract between the eleventh and twelfth ribs causes the patients much discomfort.

Calculi in the renal pelvis can be approached either through the middle or lower portion of the kidney. The advantage of the lower-pole approach is that it provides a longer nephrostomy tract through which to work, thereby decreasing the chance of losing the passage, whereas the advantage of the mid-kidney approach is that it provides a more direct route to the stone and access to the upper ureter. Thus, for stones at the ureteropelvic junction or in the upper ureter, the path is usually through a middle calyx. If one attempts to approach a ureteral or ureteropelvic stone through the lower pole, the acute angulation necessary to gain access to the stone is usually such as to prevent stone extraction.

Radiologic Control of the Procedure

Nephroscopy is best performed in the radiology suite with a fluoroscopy unit, preferably one with a C arm. The endoscopist can see only the area near the instrument lens, and fluoroscopy helps orient him to the rest of the renal field. Fluoroscopy can also help in guiding the nephroscope to a desired location, such as to a stone trapped in an upper-pole calyx. As the endoscopist's experience increases, the need for fluoroscopy decreases; and we sometimes perform nephroscopy without fluoroscopic control in a well-established nephrostomy tract.

If a nephrostolithotomy is planned, anteroposterior and oblique nephrostograms must be examined beforehand to determine the relation of the several calyces to the renal pelvis and to pinpoint the location of the stone. A thorough understanding of the three-dimensional renal anatomy is essential[2] (see Chapter 16).

Anesthesia and Analgesia

Before the patient is sent to the radiology suite, he or she is given 50–100 mg of meperidine (pethidine; Demerol) and 25–50 mg of hydroxyzine pamoate (Vistaril) intramuscularly. Further relaxation and analgesia can be obtained with 2.5 mg of intravenous diazepam (Valium) and 2 mg of butorphanol tartrate (Stadol). This may be repeated until the patient is relaxed but still arousable (see Chapter 8). All procedures are performed under the designation: "anesthesia standby."

If the nephrostomy tract is well established, it does not need to be anesthetized. If the tract is fresh, however, or if considerable intrarenal manipulation is expected, the tract should be infiltrated with 30–50 ml of 0.25% bupivacaine without epinephrine. This takes effect within 5 minutes and lasts from 40 to 630 minutes.[3,4]

Topical anesthesia may be obtained inside the renal pelvis and collecting system by instilling 30 ml or more of 0.25% bupivacaine slowly by gravity flow and clamping the nephrostomy tube for 5 to 10 minutes. As much as 90 ml of bupivacaine has been used without difficulty.

Monitoring

All patients are connected to a cardiac monitor during nephroscopy and nephrostolithotomy, and their pulse and blood pressure are checked regularly. Sudden dilatation of the renal pelvis sometimes causes a vasovagal response.

The resulting bradycardia can be controlled with intravenous atropine sulfate, 0.3 mg, and *immediate* drainage of the renal pelvis.

Preparation and Draping of the Patient

The patient is placed prone on the fluoroscopy table. Because the irrigating solution creates an electrical hazard on a fluoroscopy table, special precautions are needed to evacuate the solution efficiently. This can be accomplished by placing an angiogram drape over the patient with the precut hole positioned over the nephrostomy site. The skin around the tract is then prepared with a benzoin solution to make the drape more adherent, and a 3M aperture drape or Steri-drape with a hole cut in it is placed over the nephrostomy tube and secured to the benzoin-coated skin. The apron of the plastic drape is then led onto the outer portion of the angiogram drape, and the latter is formed into a trough (Fig. 17–1). At the bottom of the trough, a pool suction apparatus or a Jackson–Pratt drain is placed and attached to wall suction. Alternatively, a cranial incise drape* may be used; it comes with its own reservoir for fluid collection. A urethral catheter is placed.

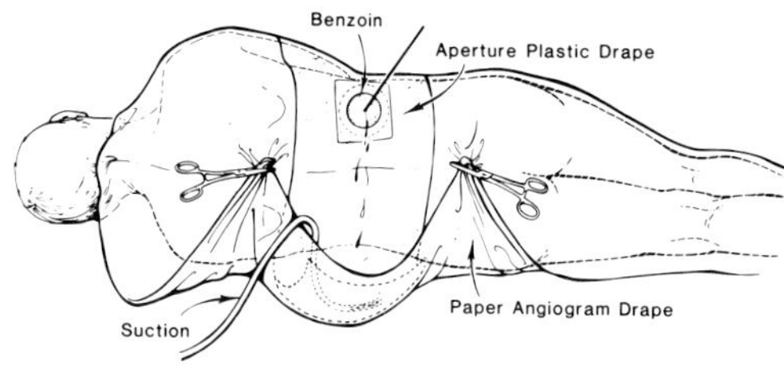

Fig. 17–1. Drape arrangement to avert leakage of irrigant. (From Clayman, R.V., et al.: J. Urol., *31*:864, 1984.)

*Surgikos, Arlington, TX 76010.

Irrigation

A regular 3-liter bag of normal saline is used as the irrigant during nephroscopy. We often attach a 30-ml syringe to one side of the rigid panendoscope so that a forceful blast of fluid can be introduced when desired to help identify intrarenal structures or a clot-laden stone or to dislodge clots.

Rigid Instruments for Nephroscopy

With a rigid nephroscope, the smaller the diameter of the instrument, the greater its mobility within the collecting system. Examination is usually limited to the renal pelvis and ureteropelvic junction; but with a 20F instrument, one can sometimes enter an upper- or lower-pole infundibulum or even the proximal portion of the ureter. Inspection with the 70° lens increases the area of the collecting system that can be examined.[5,6]

A 20F McCarthy panendoscope is sufficient for viewing and grasping small stones. It has a straight beak that protrudes 1 to 2 cm beyond the microlens, a feature that must be remembered to avoid perforating the renal pelvis. The Woppler system is less desirable, because its curved beak can abrade the friable tissue lining the nephrostomy tract and thus cause bleeding. An excellent alternative to the McCarthy instrument is the 20F or 22F direct-vision urethrotome, which has a smooth end without a beak. The 24F Wolf and 26F Storz nephroscopes also work well, although their size constrains their movement within the kidney (Fig. 17–2).

As a rule, the nephrostomy tract should be 4F (1.3 mm) larger than the rigid instrument selected to afford maximum comfort for the patient and easy outflow of the irrigating solution. When a long procedure is planned, we place a 24F to 30F Amplatz Teflon sheath* (Fig. 17–3)

*Cook Urological, 1100 West Morgan St., Spencer, IN 47460.

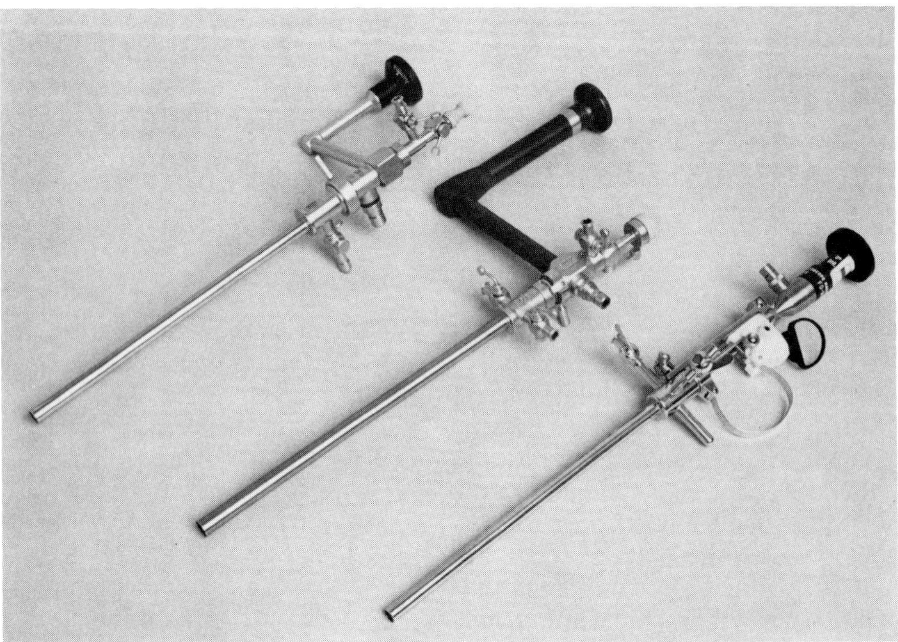

Fig. 17–2. Rigid nephroscopes. *From left to right:* 24F Wolf nephroscope, 26F Storz nephroscope, and 22F ACMI direct-vision urethrotome. (From Clayman, R.V.: Br. J. Urol. (Suppl.),11, 1983.)

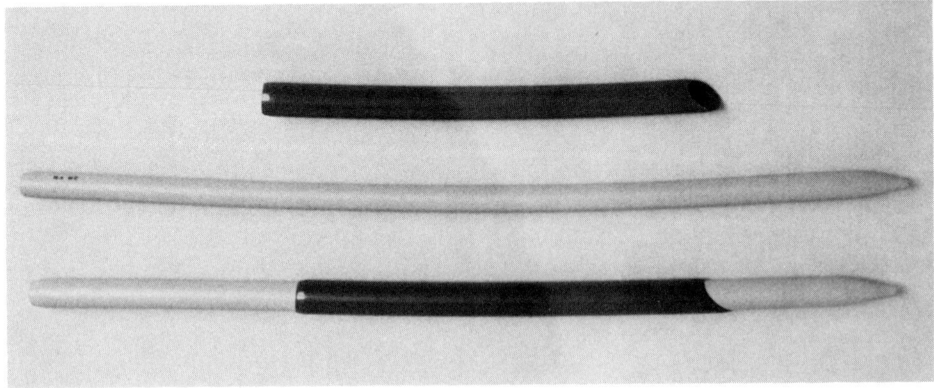

Fig. 17–3. Amplatz sheath system. The 32F radiopaque sheath at top fits snugly over the 28F fascial dilator in center; the assembly is then passed into the renal pelvis over a guide wire, and the dilator is withdrawn.

in the tract to keep it open and to protect it from abrasions and trauma during instrument passage. Force must never be used to pass an instrument, as it will inevitably lead to a false passage or to perforation of the renal pelvis.

Flexible Instruments for Nephroscopy

The flexible nephroscopes (Olympus, ACMI, Pentax) are ideal for nephroscopy and do not require a working sheath (Fig. 17–4). They are 30 to 35 cm long and 15F or 16F in diameter and have a 250° viewing arc and a 6F port for the passage of instruments such as graspers. They are fragile and are best used after the nephrostomy tract has matured, as bleeding from a newly created tract is usually too brisk to permit adequate observation

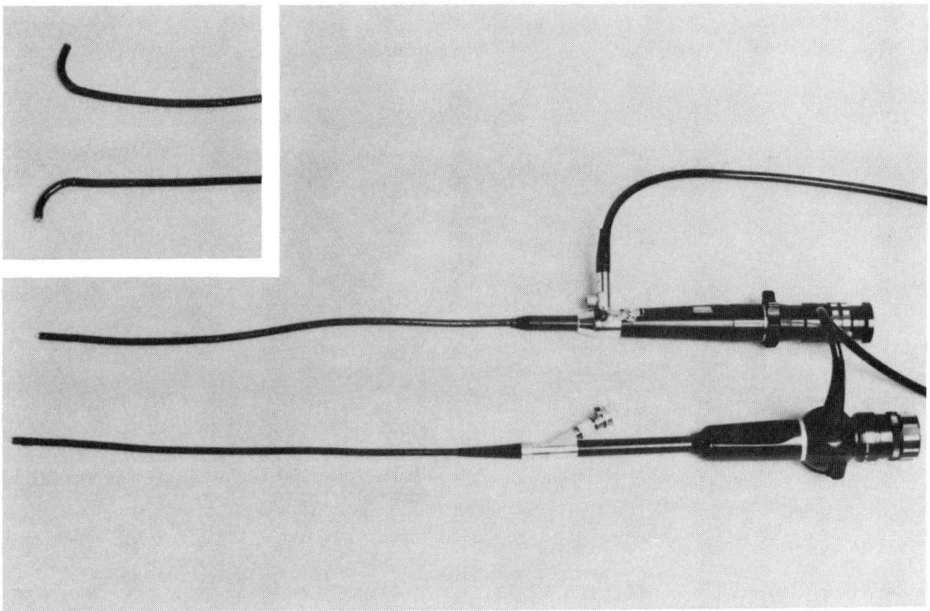

Fig. 17–4. Flexible nephroscopes. *(A)* Tip of instrument being deflected through 250° arc. *(B) Above,* 15F, 35-cm ACMI choledocho/nephroscope. *Below,* 15F, 33-cm Olympus choledocho/nephroscope. (From Clayman, R.V.: Br. J. Urol. (Suppl.)11, 1983.)

with a flexible instrument. There is no need for a local anesthetic, and only rarely will the patient require diazepam.

With flexible nephroscopes, the upper- and lower-pole infundibula and calyces can be entered easily, as can the proximal, and occasionally the middle, portion of the ureter. Examination of the middle calyces can be difficult, but with 160° deflection, even these calyces are accessible. A simple maneuver for obtaining entry into a sharply angled infundibulum is shown in Figure 17–5.

Mastery of the flexible instrument requires some practice. Sheep or pig kidneys from the market are excellent for this purpose after a nephrostomy tract has been punched in them with blunt-tipped forceps. If desired, stones can be inserted via the ureter for subsequent removal. The ureter is then clamped or ligated to keep the system water tight. It is helpful to have another person hold the kidney steady so the examiner can use both hands to guide the nephroscope. During one's first clinical efforts with the instrument, it is helpful if the radiologist passes a yellow, red, or gray 5F angiographic catheter down into the ureter and a different-colored catheter into the infundibulum and calyx of interest. The examiner can then follow the colored catheter to the stone and can also orient himself cephalad and caudad by reference to the catheter in the ureter.

After an instrument has been passed through the working channel of the flexible nephroscope, pressure on the bag of irrigating fluid is usually needed to maintain an adequate flow rate. A 500-ml bag of normal saline can be placed in a blood pump bag and the pressure increased to 150 mm Hg. Alternatively, a blood pressure thigh cuff can be wrapped around a 3-liter bag of irrigating fluid and inflated to 150 mm Hg. As long as there is sufficient space between the nephroscope and the wall of the nephrostomy tract to allow free efflux of the fluid, patients have little discomfort.

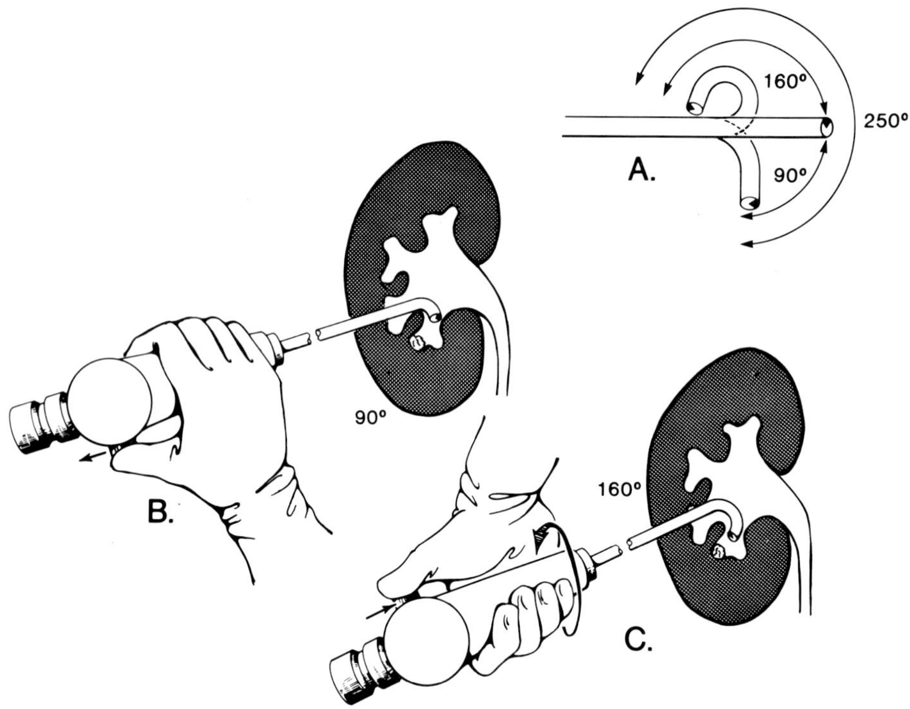

Fig. 17–5. *(A)* Flexible nephroscope tip reveals a black arrowhead that is at 12 o'clock when the instrument is held in the usual manner with hand pronated. This arrowhead indicates the point of maximum flexibility. *(B)* With this maneuver the instrument can be deflected only 90° downward, which is not enough to enter the stone-containing calyx. *(C)* When the wrist and thus the nephroscope is turned 180°, the arrowhead moves to 6 o'clock, and the examiner can move the tip of the instrument 160° downward.

Indigo Carmine

Occasionally, 10 ml of indigo carmine given intravenously will help the examiner by revealing previously unseen calyces. We have seldom needed this technique, however, as use of the C-arm fluoroscopy unit and contrast medium not only outlines all calyces but also enables one to define their anteroposterior relation to the renal pelvis.

Postprocedure Care

After nephroscopy, the Foley catheter is withdrawn and the nephrostomy tube reinserted (Fig. 17–6). Replacement of the tube is essential to tamponade the tract if there is bleeding. If one elects not to replace the tube, the tract will seal within three to four days in most cases. All patients are given an oral antibiotic for 48 hours, and if the tube is not replaced, the drug is continued for four to seven days, after which a urine culture is obtained.

NEPHROSTOLITHOTOMY

Percutaneous nephrostomy has been used most often simply as a method for draining an obstructed kidney, and the application of the technique to therapeutic maneuvers within the urinary tract has been slow in developing. Although the first report of the establishment of a nephrostomy tract percutaneously appeared in 1955,[7] it was not until 1976 that anyone reported removing a renal calculus through a percutaneously placed nephrostomy tract.[8] Since then, there have been additional case reports and series with over 2,000 cases completed.[7–15]

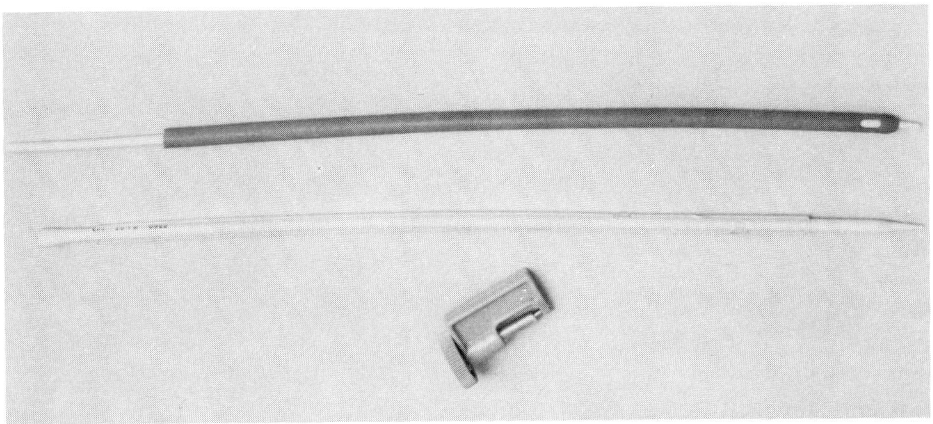

Fig. 17–6. Apparatus for replacing nephrostomy tube. *(Below)* The Cook Urological punch, which creates a smooth beveled opening in the end of any catheter. All nephrostomy tubes must have an end hole to provide easy passage of a guide wire. *(Center)* A 24F chest tube (inner diameter 16F), which can be stiffened by passage of a 16F dilator as shown. The chest tube provides excellent drainage, and it has a radiopaque stripe on its distal tip. *(Top)* 24F Red rubber Robinson catheter, which is softer and lacks radiopaque markings. Its internal diameter is 12F.

At the Veterans Administration Medical Center in Minneapolis, we performed our first nephrostolithotomy in 1977. Since that time, more than 140 stones have been removed in this way from all areas of the kidney and ureter in 122 patients. The calculi ranged in size from 3 mm to 4 to 5 cm, and in six patients, staghorn stones were removed.[16] All but one of our cases were completed with local anesthesia supplemented with intravenous diazepam and butorphanol. The success rates have been 92% for renal stones and 67% with ureteral stones. Stone remnants < 3 mm have been noted in 6% of patients.[17]

Instruments

The instruments selected for percutaneous stone removal are very much dependent on the size of the stone.

Three basic techniques are available: flushing, grasping, and fragmentation. Stones 0.5 cm in diameter or smaller can be either flushed from the renal pelvis or grasped; for the latter, grasping forceps passed through the 16F flexible nephroscope are usually sufficient. Stones between 0.5 and 1.0 cm can be grasped under direct vision with 7F Storz alligator forceps passed through a 20F rigid panendoscope, although occasionally these stones can be flushed from the kidney or basketed. Stones in the 1.0- to 1.5-cm range can be basketed or grasped under direct vision with Bumpus forceps passed through a 24F McCarthy panendoscope or with rigid forceps (e.g., Randall's) under fluoroscopic observation. Stones between 1.5 and 2.0 cm can also be removed with rigid forceps under fluoroscopic control and are usually too large for any of the grasping instruments used under direct vision. Calculi larger than 2.0 cm require destruction with either the electrohydraulic lithotriptor* or the ultrasonic lithotriptor.† The fragments are then removed with any of the aforementioned tools.

Each of these methods will now be described in more detail.

Flushing Techniques

A special set of Teflon irrigating catheters, designed by Amplatz and manu-

---

*A.C.M.I., 300 Stillwater Avenue, Stamford, CT 06902
†Karl Storz, 10111 W. Jefferson Blvd., Culver City, CA 90230; R. Wolf, 7046 Lyndon Ave., Rosemont, IL 60018

factured by Cook, can be used to flush stones from the renal pelvis (see Fig. 17–3).[18] The internal diameter of these sheaths ranges from 0.5 to 1.5 cm. A Grüntzig, or Olbert balloon catheter is usually passed into the ureter either antegrade or retrograde before the procedure to prevent the escape of stones into the ureter.

Irrigation can be direct or indirect. For direct flushing, the sheath is connected to large-bore polyvinyl tubing, which is then attached to a 60-ml plunger syringe. Diluted (16%) contrast medium is instilled into the renal pelvis through the tubing and then sucked forcefully back into the syringe, thereby drawing the stone and any blood clots out of the collecting system. For indirect flushing, a small-bore tube may be placed through the existing nephrostomy tract or a second tract, or a balloon catheter with an irrigating lumen may be passed up the ureter transcystoscopically. Fluid is then instilled into the renal pelvis through this smaller tube in the hope of washing the stone out of the collecting system via the large sheath.

The appealing simplicity of the flushing techniques is offset by their lack of utility for stones > 1 cm in diameter.[19] We rarely use flushing now because of the improvements in our ability to see and remove the stones directly via nephroscopy.

Grasping Techniques

Various instruments are available for grasping stones under fluoroscopic control or direct vision. Stone baskets, as well as Randall's, nasopharyngeal, and Mazzariello–Caprini forceps, may be used under fluoroscopic control,[19,20] whereas alligator and Bumpus forceps and three- or four-pronged graspers are used under direct vision (Fig. 17–7).

When grasping instruments are necessary to remove a stone, we prefer to begin with those that can be used in conjunction with a nephroscope. Removal of a stone under direct vision causes the least renal trauma, whereas manipulation under fluoroscopic control may cause intrarenal bleeding.

The problem of trauma during manipulation under fluoroscopy is least serious with the Mazzariello–Caprini forceps, which can be passed down a 20F tract and opened maximally without significant increase in shaft diameter because of their rotational opening action. We have modified this instrument by cutting a 0.05-inch groove in the grasping end to permit its passage over a guide wire that has been placed in the kidney. This decreases the chance of renal trauma.[20] (A similar groove can be cut in the grasping end of Randall's forceps.) The position of the forceps must be checked in anteroposterior and lateral views both before the jaws are opened and upon engaging the stone.

Fragmentation Techniques

Two instruments have greatly aided the advance of nephrostolithotomy for stones ≥ 2 cm: the electrohydraulic lithotriptor and the ultrasonic lithotriptor.[11,12,21] Both of these instruments can be used through a rigid nephroscope, and the electrohydraulic probe can also be used with a flexible nephroscope.

The electrohydraulic lithotriptor was first described by Yutkin in 1950 and was first used in 1959 to destroy bladder stones.[22,23] Raney and Handler introduced the use of the instrument for renal stones,[24] and we have used it successfully even for branched and staghorn renal calculi.[16] The probe of the instrument creates an electrical discharge, which, in an irrigating fluid, is transformed into an hydraulic shock wave. When this discharge is close to a calculus, the force of the shock is sufficient to fragment a stone.

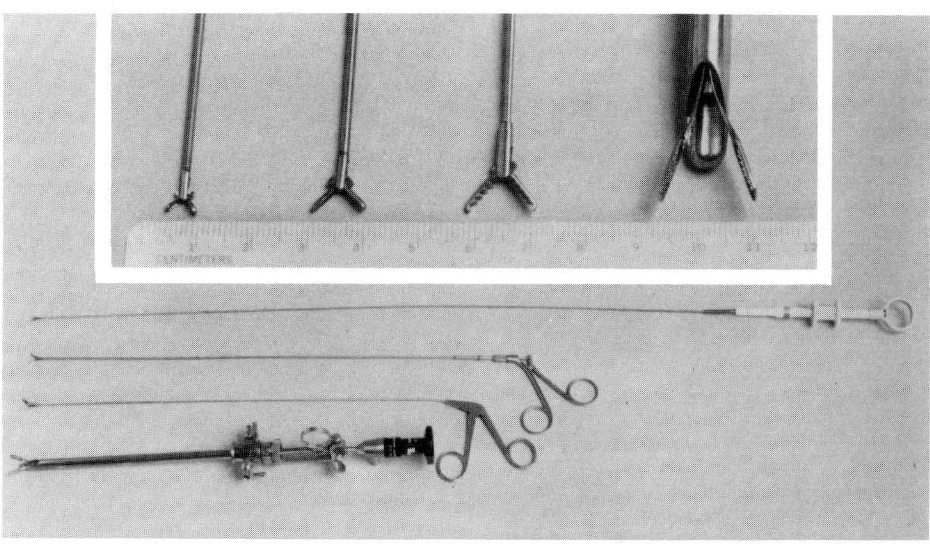

Fig. 17–7. Graspers. *From top to bottom:* 5F biopsy forceps for flexible nephroscope, 7F Storz alligator forceps for a 20F nephroscope, 9F rigid Wolf alligator forceps for a 24F nephroscope, and Bumpus forceps for a 24F McCarthy panendoscope. Inset shows open span of jaws.

The machine we use* consists of the probe, a generator cabinet, a power cord, a foot switch, and an extender cable and permits the strength of the discharge to be varied from 0 to 120 volts and the pulse frequency to be set at either 50 or 100 per second (Fig. 17–8). We usually use 100 volts and 50 discharges per second.

The probes are available in 9F and 5F sizes suitable for passage through a 21F rigid or 16F flexible nephroscope, respectively. The 9F probe has been the most satisfactory because of its greater power. Each probe can be used only once, as it has a life span of 15–50 seconds, depending on the duration and strength of the discharge, and the tip must be examined frequently for wear in the insulation. When the metal beneath the insulation becomes visible, the electrical discharge comes from the side rather than the tip of the probe, and this makes the shock wave less effective. If the operator continues to use the worn probe, the metal tip may separate from the shaft (Fig. 17–9).

Electrohydraulic lithotripsy requires either sterile water or a $\frac{1}{6}$–$\frac{1}{7}$ normal saline solution (see Chapter 14), which should flow rapidly to dissipate the heat generated by the probe. The probe is placed in contact with or approximately 1 mm away from the surface of the most irregular portion of the stone and at least 5 mm from the lens of the panendoscope, and the discharge is created by pressing the foot switch. The probe must never be discharged unless the operator can see its proximity to the stone, as inadvertent discharge near tissue may cause damage or perforation.

When working with hard stones, such as those of calcium oxalate or uric acid, several discharges may be needed before the stone cracks. These discharges must be delivered at the same site for maximum effectiveness.

Once the stone has broken apart, the

*We use the SD–1 120-volt, 60-hertz machine produced by the Monighan Medical Corporation, Plattsburg, New York, and distributed by American Cystoscope Makers, Inc. This machine and its attachments cost $6,000 (1982), and the probes cost $40–80, depending on the size.

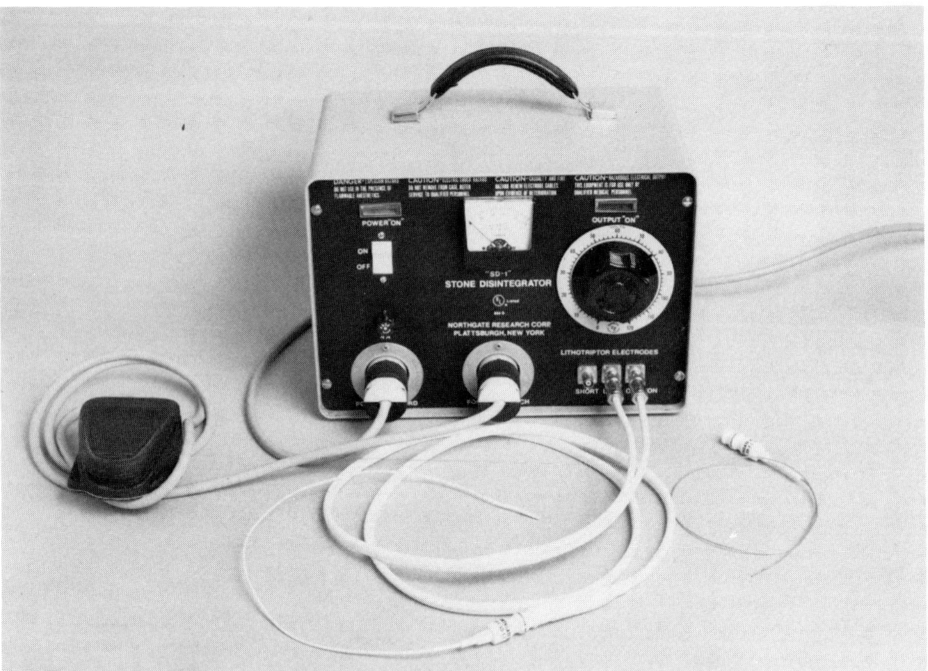

Fig. 17–8. Electrohydraulic lithotriptor. *In foreground from left to right on the machine.* Power cord and foot switch, generator cable attached to a 9F probe, unattached 5F probe.

ragged surfaces of the pieces make an ideal target for further discharges of the probe that reduce the stone to small pieces. This debris can be removed by flushing, with a 7F Storz grasper through a 20F panendoscope, or by a combination of methods.

The ultrasonic lithotriptor is marketed by both the Wolf and the Storz companies and consists of a sheath (24F for Wolff, 26F for Storz), telescope, ultrasound transducer, suction pump, foot switch, and 12F probe (Fig. 17–10). The stone is destroyed by placing the probe in direct contact with the stone and pressing the foot switch; a high-pitched sound is emitted as the stone is ground into small particles. The hollow center channel of the probe, as well as the panendoscope, are connected to suction; and thus the particles of the stone are sucked from the renal pelvis.

Most investigators have used general or epidural anesthesia for ultrasonic lithotripsy, but we have used local anesthesia with intravenous diazepam and butorphanol. There have been no reported long-term complications, and patients tolerate the procedure well.[11,12,15] The drawbacks are that the method is sometimes slower than electrohydraulic lithotripsy; the rigidity of the probe restricts its use to rigid nephroscopes, thus preventing one from destroying stones that are not in the direct path from the nephrostomy tract; and the instrument is two to three times as expensive as the electrohydraulic lithotriptor. One important advantage is the continuous suction evacuation of particles by the ultrasonic instrument.

Aids to Nephrostolithotomy

There are a variety of devices and maneuvers that are valuable aids to the expedient extraction of stones percutaneously. These are: ureteral catheterization, safety guide wires, tract dila-

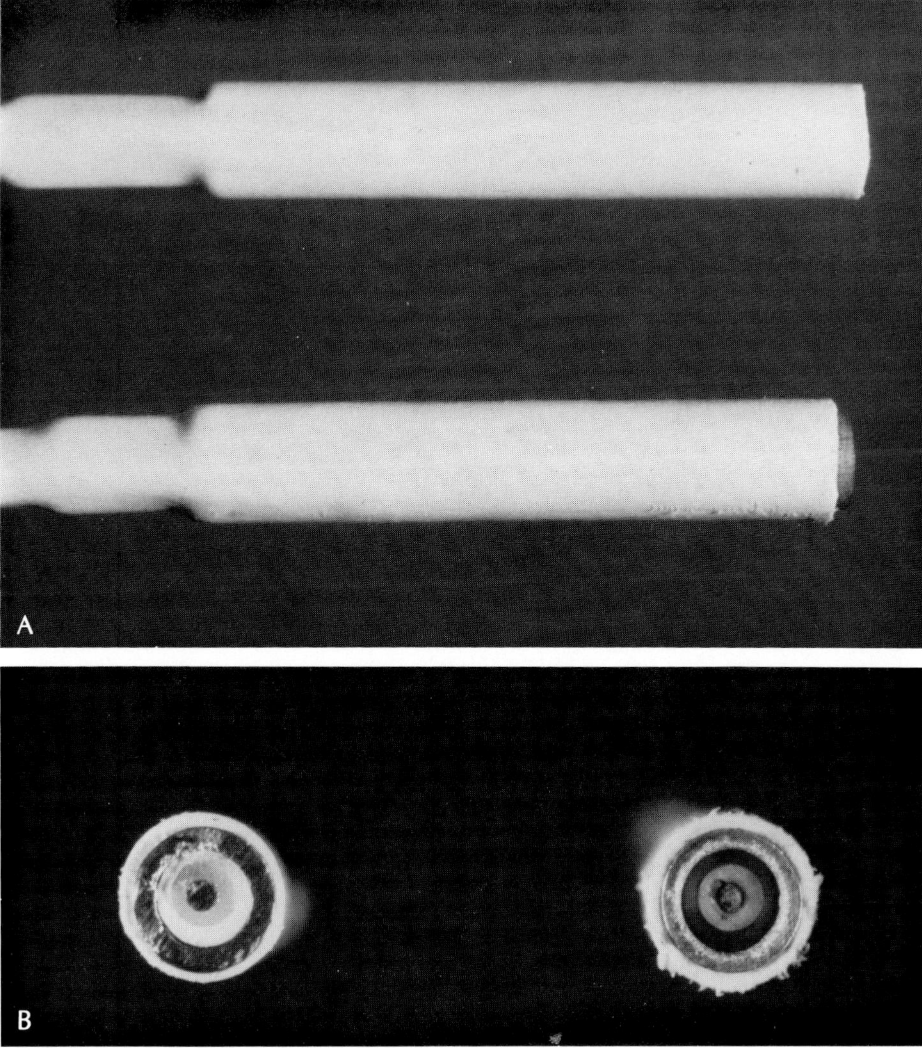

Fig. 17–9. New and worn lithotriptor probes. *(A)* Side view; new *(top)* and worn probe *(bottom)*. *(B)* End view; new *(right)* and worn probe *(left)*.

tation with a balloon catheter, stone dislodgement with a Fogarty balloon catheter, percutaneous renal surgery, and chemolysis of stones or fragments.

Ureteral Catheters. Retrograde transurethral placement of a ureteral catheter immediately before percutaneous nephrostomy is helpful. Through this catheter, contrast medium can be infused to opacify and distend the renal pelvis, thus eliminating the need to opacify the collecting system via a Chiba needle, which sometimes causes extravasation of contrast medium, necessitating postponement of the procedure. Passage of a ureteral catheter may also be helpful in patients with a ureteral calculus, as the catheter may dislodge the stone upward into the renal pelvis, making it easier to remove. Also, in patients undergoing lithotripsy, the catheter can be used both to prevent fragments from entering the ureter and to irrigate fragments backward toward the nephrostomy tract.

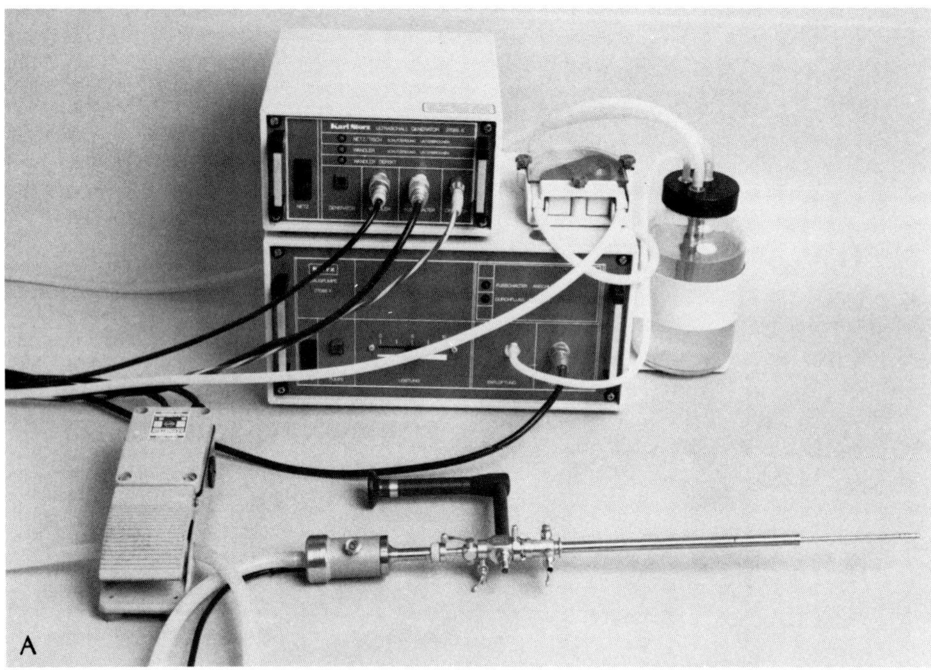

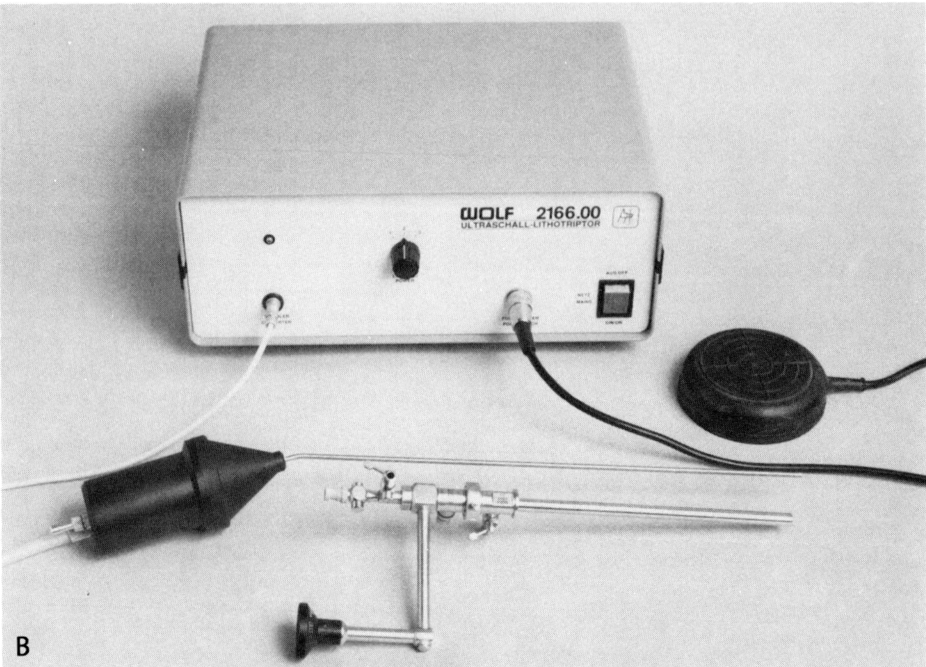

Fig. 17–10. Ultrasonic lithotriptors. *(A)* Storz instrument. *Above*, Generator and suction pump. *Below*, foot switch with 26F nephroscope sheath; ultrasound probe protrudes from the end of the sheath. *(B)* Wolf instrument. *Above*, Generator and foot switch. *Below*, 24F nephroscope. Suction pump not shown.

The choice of a ureteral catheter depends on the size of the stone. For stones ≤ 1.5 cm in the renal pelvis, we use an 8F or 10F flush-ending angiographic catheter, whereas for larger stones, a Grüntzig or Olbert balloon catheter is inserted. With the latter types, the balloon can be inflated to occlude the ureter, and irrigation fluid can be infused through the catheter's central lumen.

Safety Wire. When working through a fresh nephrostomy tract, placement of a safety wire is essential. After the definitive puncture of the renal pelvis, a 0.035-inch floppy-tip guide wire is passed through the translumbar aortogram needle and manipulated until it has been threaded down the ureter. The needle is removed, and the tract is dilated by passing a series of 7F–10F Teflon dilators over the guide wire. After the 10F dilator has been removed, a 10F embolization catheter is passed over the guide wire, and a second 0.035-inch guide wire is passed through its lumen into the renal pelvis. The embolization catheter is removed, and a 5F catheter is passed over the first guide wire down the ureter. The entire catheter–guide wire assembly is then sutured to the skin; this constitutes the safety guide wire. Subsequent dilatation and placement of the working sheath are done over the second, or working, guide wire (Fig. 17–11), with the assurance that if this wire becomes displaced, the operator will not have lost the nephrostomy tract.

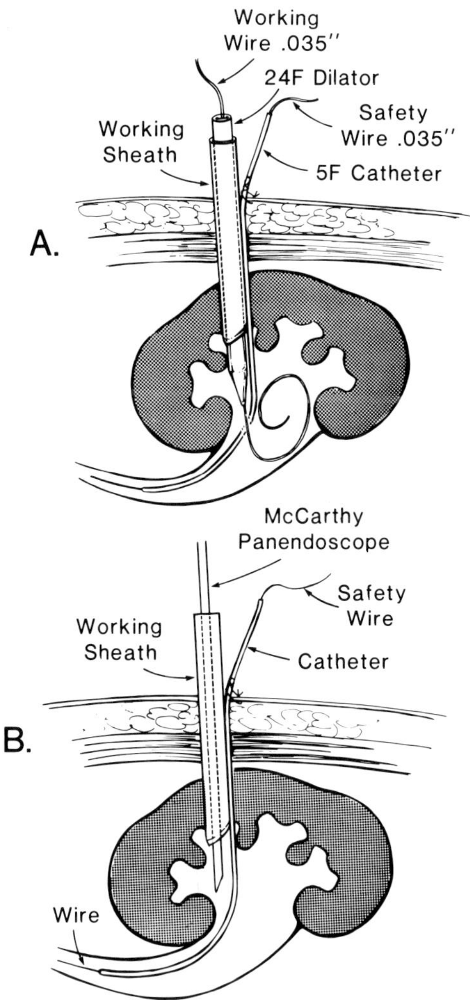

Fig. 17–11. Safety and working guide wires and working sheath. *(A)* Passage of working sheath (see Fig. 17–3). *(B)* Passage of panendoscope.

Balloon Dilatation of Nephrostomy Tract. Dilatation of a nephrostomy tract can be time-consuming and difficult and cause marked bleeding that interferes with nephrostolithotomy. Instead of the conventional dilator systems, we have found it simpler to use a 9F Olbert catheter with a 4-cm long, 10-mm balloon, which is passed over the working guide wire and inflated to dilate the surrounding tissue to 30F (Fig. 17–12).[25] After several minutes, the balloon is deflated, pulled back slightly, and reinflated. This is repeated until the entire tract has been dilated. The 10-mm balloon can withstand pressures as great as 9 atmospheres, whereas the 8-mm balloon can withstand as much as 12 atmospheres. This is usually sufficient to dilate the renal capsule, Gerota's fascia, and the lumbodorsal fascia. Balloon dilatation is rapid, comfortable for the patient, and associated with minimal bleeding.

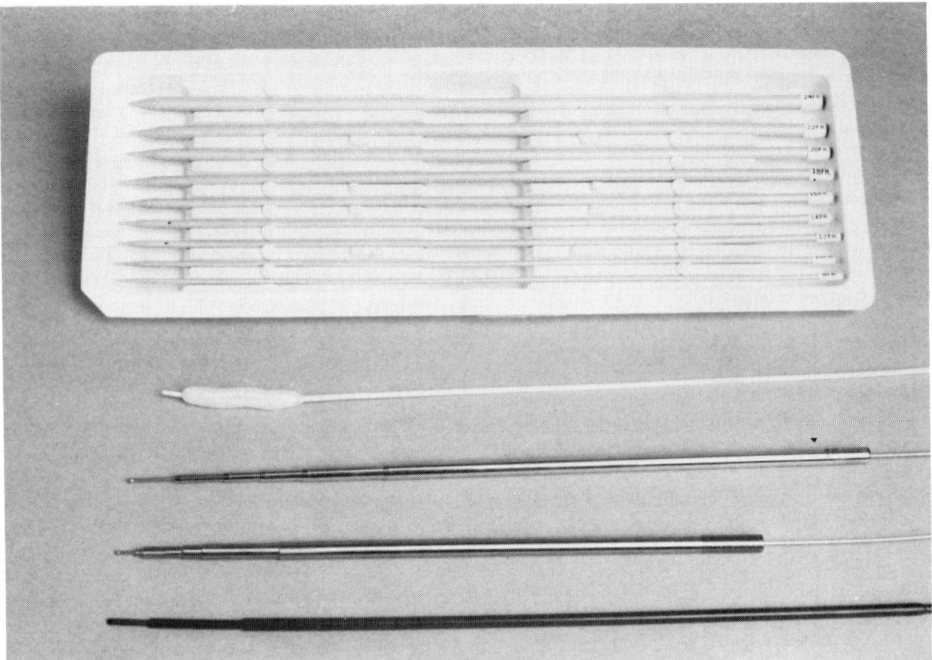

Fig. 17–12. Several ways to dilate a nephrostomy tract. From *top to bottom:* A set of fascial dilators, a 10-mm Olbert balloon catheter, two sets of metal coaxial dilators, and flexible coaxial dilators.

Balloon catheters are also useful for gaining access to some stones. Thus, a Fogarty balloon catheter can be used to dilate a narrowed infundibulum that has trapped a stone in a calyx. The Fogarty catheter also can be used to dislodge a ureteral or calyceal stone. For this maneuver the catheter is passed beyond the stone, and the balloon is inflated, trapping the stone between the balloon and the introducing catheter. Gentle traction often delivers the stone into the renal pelvis, from which it can be removed with the methods described earlier.

Intrarenal Electrosurgery. For the retrieval of other trapped stones, percutaneous renal surgery is helpful. A 4F whistle-tip ureteral catheter is cut off approximately 4 cm from its distal end, and a thin wire is passed through it and connected to a power cord, which in turn is attached to the cautery unit. This assembly is passed into the kidney through a 16F flexible nephroscope (Fig. 17–13). Under direct vision, a narrowed portion of an infundibulum can be incised to a depth of 1–2 mm to allow passage of a calculus into the renal pelvis, or a stone impacted at the ureteropelvic junction can be cut free. The area to be incised should be examined first for arterial pulsations, and any minor bleeding can be controlled with a coagulation current. We have not had any instances of significant bleeding with this method but believe that it could be controlled by inserting a balloon catheter and inflating the balloon to tamponade the area.[26]

Chemolysis. This stone-removal method is used primarily in patients with infection stones that have been largely removed with lithotripsy in combination with various grasping instruments. These methods may leave minute (< 1-mm) fragments that cannot be picked up with instruments, and we have used irrigation with 10% hemiacidrin (Renacidin) to dissolve or flush them out.[27]

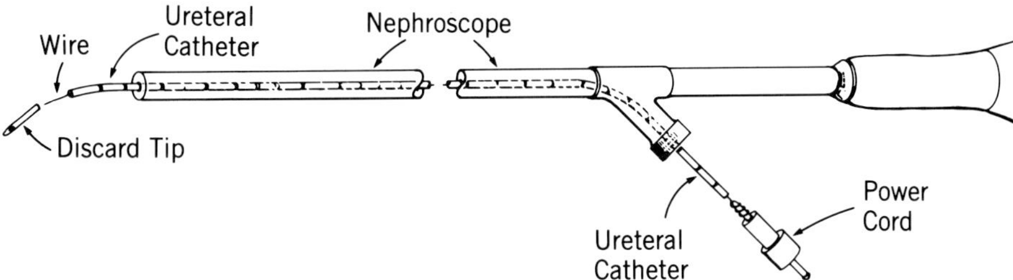

Fig. 17–13. Tip of 4F whistle-tipped catheter has been cut off. Thin wire inserted through catheter is connected to power cord from the electrocautery unit to create instrument for intrarenal electrosurgery. (From Clayman, R.V., et al.: J. Urol., *31*:864, 1984.)

The urine must be sterile. A nephrostogram is performed to ensure that there is no extravasation or pyelovenous or pyelosinus backflow. Irrigation is then started at the rate of 25–50 ml per hour, gradually increasing to 100 ml per hour. Usually, the solution is introduced through a ureteral catheter and drained through a nephrostomy tube, although other arrangements are also satisfactory.[28] The ureteral catheter system does have the advantage, however, of preventing stones from escaping into the ureter and permitting thorough bathing of the renal pelvis. For chemolysis with hemiacidrin, it is important that the solution is directed in by gravity, not by a pump, and that the solution is no more than 20–25 cm above the patient's bed in order to prevent renal backflow and absorption of the solution, which can have serious, even fatal, effects. Electrolytes, especially magnesium, and blood cells should be measured daily, and the urine should be cultured daily. Irrigation must be stopped if the patient has flank pain, fever, bacteriuria, or hypermagnesemia.[28]

After two or three days of irrigation, tomograms of the kidney are obtained without contrast medium. If no stones are seen, nephroscopy is performed with a flexible instrument to search for particles.

RESULTS

The probability of success in nephrostolithotomy is directly dependent on the size and location of the stone. For stones ≤ 1.5 cm located in the renal pelvis or calyces, the success rate in our series is 89%. The average hospital stay has been seven days, but this figure includes our first cases, many of whom were poor operative risks. Some of our recent, healthier patients have been hospitalized for as little as a day and a half. For larger (> 1.5 cm) renal pelvic and calyceal stones, the success rate is even higher: 92%. In this group, however, the hospital stay averages 17 days, because it takes one session to insert the nephrostomy tube, another session to break up the stone, and one or two more sessions to remove all the fragments. At present, the time required to remove these larger stones exceeds that of an open stone operation, and hence the percutaneous approach to staghorn calculi is warranted only when the surgical risk is high. For example, we have used the percutaneous approach in paraplegic and quadraplegic patients, some of whom had urinary infections or long histories of stone disease, sometimes with several previous open operations.[16]

The success rate for ureteral calculi has been less impressive: 67%, with a hospital stay of 6–25 (average 16) days. However, within this group there is considerable variation. If the stone is freely moveable, the chances of extracting it are high. Problems occur when the stone is embedded in the ureteral wall; and therefore in patients who desire a percutaneous approach to their ureteral stone, we first pass a balloon catheter up the ureter. If the stone cannot be moved either by fluid flushed through the catheter or by direct pushing, we recommend ureteroscopy.

COMPLICATIONS

Serious complications of nephrostolithotomy are rare. Early in our series, serious complications, such as hypotension and bleeding from the nephrostomy tract, occurred in 6 of 112 patients. In one case, an emergency nephrectomy was needed to control the bleeding; but the other patients were managed satisfactorily by tamponade and blood transfusion. No patient has had gram-negative septicemia, and there have been no deaths.

Early minor complications occurred in 40% of patients and consisted of blood clots obstructing the renal pelvis, transient fever, small perforations of the renal pelvis, ileus, nephrostomy tube displacement, and flank discomfort lasting longer than 24–36 hours. If the renal pelvis has been perforated during the procedure, we leave a ureteral catheter as well as a nephrostomy tube in place to ensure complete drainage. In our experience, the perforation invariably heals within two to three days, as documented by subsequent nephrostograms.

Delayed complications are unusual and consist of bleeding, persistent nephro-cutaneous fistulae, stricture, sepsis, and residual or recurrent calculi. In one of our patients, there was massive hematuria approximately seven days after removal of the nephrostomy tube that resulted from formation of a pseudoaneurysm.[29] A few similar cases of delayed bleeding have been reported after percutaneous nephrostomy.[30,31] This complication appears to be associated with early removal of the nephrostomy tube, so we now leave the tube in for two weeks, the patient being discharged with the tube clamped and bandaged to the flank. We have had no cases of ureteral stricture; and in two patients, upper ureteral strictures associated with ureteropelvic junction stones resolved after percutaneous dilatation of the area and nephrostolithotomy. We give patients an oral antibiotic, usually nitrofurantoin or trimethoprim–sulfa, to take while the nephrostomy tube is in place and for seven days after its removal. With this regimen, bacteriuria has been found in only 4% of our patients, and there have been no episodes of sepsis or renal abscess formation.

Residual and recurrent calculi are a major concern after nephrostolithotomy. We obtain nephrotomograms without contrast medium before the patient is discharged from the hospital and try to remove any remnants thus discovered with the flexible nephroscope. Our residual stone rate has been 4% and limited to patients whose stones initially were > 1.5 cm. No remnant has been > 4 mm. Recurrent stones have been found in 6% of our patients, but this cannot be taken to be the recurrence rate, as many of our patients have undergone nephrostolithotomy less than one year ago.

FOLLOWUP

A nephrostogram is performed in the outpatient clinic approximately two weeks after the procedure to rule out stricture and obstruction. If contrast medium flows readily into the bladder, the nephrostomy tube is removed. (No anesthetic is necessary.) Drainage from the flank has usually ceased within two days, and we have seen no persisting pyelocutaneous fistulas. Patients are seen three to six months later for an intravenous urogram.

Nephrostolithotomy does not result in significant functional kidney damage. Followup measurements of serum urea nitrogen and creatinine showed either no change or a slight improvement, and renal nuclear scans in 21 of our patients were normal and the site of the nephrostomy could not be seen. In the other patient, the sole abnormality was a small area of poor perfusion in the lower pole where the nephrostomy tract had been.

CONCLUSIONS

The percutaneous approach to the removal of renal calculi is a rapidly advancing technique. Within the past four years, it has become the primary method for removing upper urinary tract calculi at our institution. All the methods described in this chapter can be performed with assisted local anesthesia, and nephroscopy may be performed on an outpatient basis. At present, the safety of nephrostolithotomy has been proved only in the hospital setting. Presumably, the next advance will be the development of methods and expertise that permit its transfer to the ambulatory surgery center.

ACKNOWLEDGMENTS

All of the techniques described in this chapter are the outgrowth of close collaboration between the Departments of Radiology and Urologic Surgery at the University of Minnesota and the Sections of Diagnostic Radiology and Urology at the Minneapolis Veterans Administration Medical Center. Accordingly, I am happy to acknowledge the pioneering contributions and continued support of Doctors Paul H. Lange, Elwin E. Fraley, and Arthur D. Smith* of the urology services and Doctors Wilfrido R. Castaneda–Zuniga, Kurt Amplatz, and Robert P. Miller of the radiology services.

REFERENCES

1. Stables, D.P., Ginsberg, N.J., and Johnson, M.L.: Percutaneous nephrostomy: a series and review of the literature. AJR, *130*:75, 1978.
2. Kaye, K.W., and Goldberg, M.E.: Applied anatomy of the kidney and ureter. Urol. Clin. North Am., 9:3, 1982.
3. Caputo, L.J., Hembree, J.L., III, and Dobbs, B.M.: Two long acting anesthetics: etiodocaine HCl and bupivacaine HCl. J. Podiatr. Assoc., 72:186, 1982.
4. Moore, D.C., et al.: Bupivacaine hydrochloride: a summary of investigational use in 3274 cases. Anesth. Analg., *50*:856, 1971.
5. Clayman, R.V., et al.: Nephroscopy: advances and adjuncts. Urol. Clin. North Am., 9:51, 1982.
6. Gittes, R.F.: Nephroscopy. Urol. Clin. North Am., 6:555, 1979.
7. Goodwin, W.E., Casey, W.C., and Woolf, W.: Percutaneous trocar (needle) nephrostomy in hydronephrosis. J. Am. Med. Assoc., *157*:891, 1955.
8. Fernström, I., and Johansson, B.: Percutaneous pyelolithotomy. Scand. J. Urol. Nephrol., *10*:257, 1976.
9. Rupel, E., and Brown, R.: Nephroscopy with removal of stone following nephrostomy for calculous anuria. J. Urol., *46*:177, 1946.
10. Harris, R.D., McLaughlin, A.P., and Harrell, J.H.: Percutaneous nephroscopy using a fiberoptic bronchoscope for removal of a renal calculus. Urology, 6:367, 1975.
11. Alken, P., et al.: Percutaneous stone manipulation. J. Urol., *125*:463, 1981.
12. Marberger, M., Stackl, W., and Hruby, W.: Percutaneous litholapaxy of renal calculi with ultrasound. Eur. Urol., 8:236, 1982.
13. Wickham, J.E.A., and Kellet, M.J.: Percutaneous nephrolithotomy. Br. Med. J., *283*:1571, 1981.
14. Castaneda–Zuniga, W.R., et al.: Nephrostolithotomy: percutaneous techniques for urinary calculus removal. AJR, *139*:721, 1982.
15. Segura, J.W., et al.: Percutaneous removal of kidney stones. Mayo Clin. Proc., *57*:615, 1982.
16. Clayman, R.V., et al.: Percutaneous lithotomy: an approach to branched and staghorn renal calculi. JAMA, *250*:73, 1983.
17. Clayman, R.V., et al.: Nephrostolithotomy: percutaneous removal of renal and ureteral calculi. Br. J. Urol., (Suppl.):6, 1983.
18. Rusnak, B., et al.: An improved dilator system for percutaneous nephrostomies. Radiology, *144*:174, 1982.
19. Castaneda–Zuniga, W.R., Miller, R.P., and Amplatz, K.: Percutaneous removal of kidney stones. Urol. Clin. North Am., 9:113, 1982.
20. Clayman, R.V., et al.: Percutaneous nephrolithotomy with Mazzariello–Caprini forceps. J. Urol., *129*:1213, 1983.
21. Angeloff, A.: Hydroelectrolithotripsy. J. Urol., *108*:867, 1972.
22. Comisarow, R.H., and Barkin, M.: Electrohydraulic cystolitholapaxy. Can. J. Surg., *22*:525, 1979.
23. Goldberg, V.V.: On the history of electrohydraulic lithotripsy method. Urol. Nefrol. (Mosk.), *50*:90, 1974.
24. Raney, A.M., and Handler, J.: Electrohydraulic nephrolithotripsy. Urology, 6:439, 1975.
25. Clayman, R.V., et al.: Rapid balloon dilatation of nephrostomy track for nephrostolithotomy. Radiology, *147*:884, 1983.

---

*Now Chief, Division of Urology, Long Island Jewish Hospital–Hillside Medical Center, New Hyde Park, New York.

26. Clayman, R.V., et al.: Percutaneous intrarenal electrosurgery. J. Urol. *31*:864, 1984.
27. Blaivas, J.G., Pais, V.M., and Spellman, R.M.: Chemolysis of residual stone fragments after extensive surgery for staghorn calculi. Urology, *6*:680, 1975.
28. Sheldon, C.A., and Smith, A.D.: Chemolysis of calculi. Urol. Clin. North Am., 9:121, 1982.
29. Clayman, R.V., et al.: Vascular complications of percutaneous nephrostomy. J. Urol., *132*:228, 1984.
30. Gavant, M.L., Gold, R.E., and Church, J.C.: Delayed rupture of renal pseudoaneurysm: complication of percutaneous nephrostomy. AJR, *138*:948, 1982.
31. Cope, C., and Zeit, R.M.: Pseudoaneurysms after nephrostomy. AJR, *139*:255, 1982.

Section VI

Radiologic Procedures

18

Spermatic Vein Embolization in the Treatment of Infertility

WILFRIDO R. CASTAÑEDA–ZUÑIGA, M.D., RICARDO GONZALEZ, M.D., and KURT AMPLATZ, M.D.

The relation between male sterility and varicocele was first postulated in 1929 by Macomber and Sanders[1] and later confirmed by the finding of improved semen quality after correction of the abnormality.[2–5] With a physical examination during the Valsalva maneuver, varicocele can be detected in 24 to 39% of infertile men, being three times more common on the left side of the scrotum.[6,7] By using thermography, Chatel et al. found left-sided varicocele in 70% of infertile men.[8] Recently, Dopper ultrasound has proved to be very useful in detecting a large number of varicoceles.[9]

The incidence of subclinical varicocele (asymptomatic reflux into the internal spermatic vein) in patients with primary sterility varies according to the method used in the diagnosis. With the use of thermography or Doppler ultrasound, the detection of subclinical varicocele in infertile men has become common. The role of subclinical varicocele in producing infertility is not clear, but because the size of a clinical varicocele does not correlate with the degree of testicular and epididymal dysfunction,[10] and because testicular temperature can be increased even by small varicoceles it has been suggested that subclinical varicoceles may be a significant cause of infertility.[11] Certainly, spermatic venography reveals varicocele in 76 to 81% of infertile men,[7,8] and thus this diagnostic technique may be indicated in patients with infertility.

Several surgical techniques have been developed for the ligation of the spermatic vein for the treatment of varicocele, all of which have negligible morbidity but usually require general anesthesia and hospitalization. In recent years, techniques for the therapeutic transcatheter obliteration of the spermatic vein have been developed.[12–18] In most cases, transvenous embolization can be performed immediately after venography, providing diagnosis and treatment in a single sitting. This method also avoids one of the shortcomings of the surgical ligation, namely recurrence, which results from failure to ligate all of the communicating venous channels. In contrast, the nonsurgical approach places occluding devices precisely in accordance with the variable anatomy of the spermatic vein. The procedure can be performed on an outpatient basis under local anesthesia provided it is done early in the day to allow 3 to 4 hours of observation of the patient in the radiology department before discharge. The procedure itself takes approximately 2 hours.

INDICATIONS

Therapeutic embolization of the spermatic vein is indicated in patients with clinical or subclinical varicoceles who have been infertile for at least two years and who have oligoasthenospermia and no other apparent cause of infertility. A large number of patients with clinical left-sided varicocele will have right-sided subclinical varicocele detected during spermatic venography;[19] and they are also candidates for embolization.

SELECTION OF PATIENTS

The patient is evaluated initially by the urologist, who obtains a fertility history and performs the physical examination, which should be conducted in a warm room. Both sides of the scrotum are palpated while the patient is upright with and without the Valsalva maneuver and are examined with the Doppler stethoscope. Thermography also may be helpful in detecting subclinical varicocele. At least two, preferably three, semen analyses are performed one month apart, and whatever other blood, urine, and semen studies appear to be indicated are completed (see Chapter 27). If no other cause for the infertility is found, spermatic venography is considered.

The urologist then explains the nature of the spermatic venography and embolization procedure, its possible risks, and the expected results. Patients with obvious varicocele are given the option of embolization or operation and nearly always choose the former, especially as it can be done on an outpatient basis under local anesthesia and does not create a large scar.

TECHNIQUE

A coagulation profile is obtained one or two days before the procedure. On the day the procedure is scheduled, the patient is admitted to the radiology suite early in the morning, so that he may discuss the procedure with the radiologist.

For nonsurgical occlusion of the internal spermatic veins, most investigators use a femoral approach, demonstrating incompetent venous valves angiographically and then occluding the vessels with sclerosing agents,[12–14] coils,[15,16] or balloons.[17,18] We have found, however, that the transjugular approach facilitates the introduction of a catheter deep into the spermatic vein, a necessary maneuver for the correct placement of mechanical obstructing devices. It probably also permits the right spermatic vein to be catheterized more consistently.[15,19]

The right internal jugular vein is punctured 5–6 cm above the right clavicle. To do this, the patient's head is turned 45° to the left, and the carotid artery is palpated. A sheathed needle is introduced just lateral to the artery and directed to a point 4–5 cm lateral to the external clavicular joint, at an angle of 20–30° to the surface of the skin (Fig. 18–1). If venous blood is aspirated, a guide wire is introduced, and a sheath introducer is inserted. Through this sheath, a specially

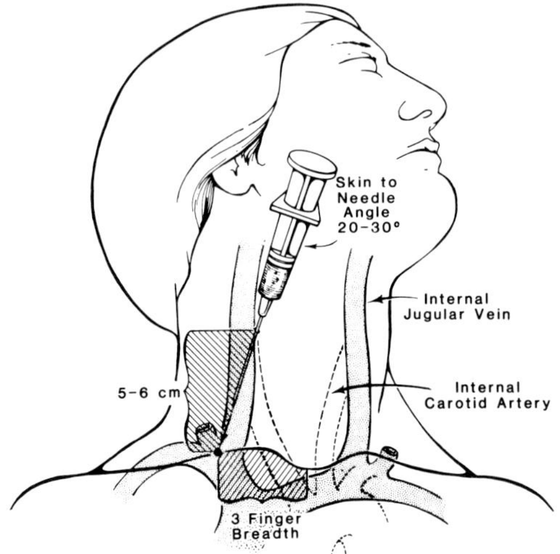

Fig. 18–1. Method of puncture of the right internal jugular vein.

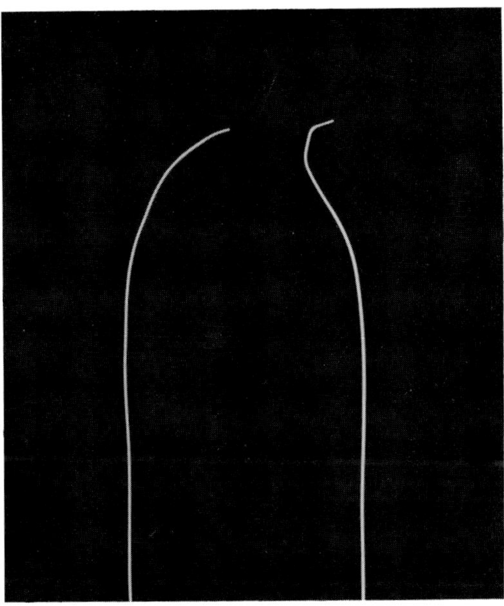

Fig. 18–2. Catheters used in the transjugular approach to the internal spermatic veins. The gently curved one is used on the right side, the other on the left side.

curved 7F catheter (Fig. 18–2) is passed into the inferior vena cava. Under fluoroscopic control, the left renal vein is entered, and the mouth of the left spermatic vein is catheterized. A test injection of 3–5 ml of contrast medium is made and recorded on film to assess the competence of the venous valves.

If they are found to be incompetent, a guide wire is passed into the distal spermatic vein. The catheter is advanced over the wire until it is just above the level of the iliac crest, and a venogram is performed by injecting 20 to 40 ml of contrast medium at the rate of 5 ml per second and obtaining 10 films at the rate of one per second to determine the exact venous anatomy (Fig. 18–3). This is critical, because there may be venous duplications or branches that communicate with the hypogastric or epigastric veins, and if these communication channels are not occluded, the varicocele will not be obliterated.

Occluding Devices

We have used the following occluding devices: compressed Ivalon plugs, modified stainless steel coils with a barb,* coilons, spiders, and spiderlons. In all cases, dislodgment of the occluding device is prevented by the modification of the Gianturco coil or coilon or by using spiders or spiderlons. One device is usually sufficient. In most cases, it is placed at the level of the iliac crest, which is the most common site of bypassing channels. If communicating channels are more proximal, an additional device must be placed as close as possible to the origin of the spermatic vein in the renal vein or inferior vena cava or both channels must be occluded (Fig. 18–4).

Ivalon, a polyvinyl alcohol open-pore sponge, is a good occluding material, because it is nonabsorbable and does not produce a local reaction. It heals firmly in place by fibrocytic invasion. However, the sponge has to be compressed before it is introduced through small catheters. Once in contact with blood, the plug expands to its original size.[20] Ivalon is not available in its compressed form and is difficult to introduce. For this reason, we have developed techniques for embolization with spring coils, which are economical and readily available and can be introduced rapidly.

The size of the coil needed depends on the size of the spermatic vein. In order to prevent migration and embolization of the coil,[21] it is modified by stretching its end. The stretched wire is cut with scissors to form a sharp barb, which engages the venous wall (Fig. 18–5*A*). The modified coil or coilon (coil with compressed Ivalon) is then mounted on a special wire introducer and delivered through the catheter (Fig. 18–5*B*).[22] Usually, two or three coils are placed.

*Gianturco-Wallace-Chuang spring embolus; Cook, Inc., 925 Curry Pike, Bloomington, IN 47402

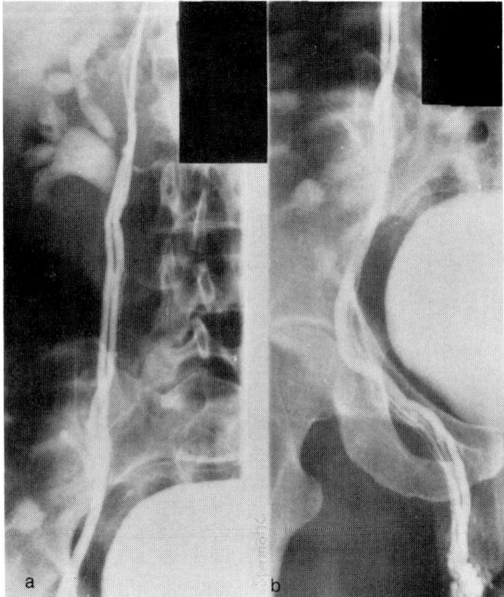
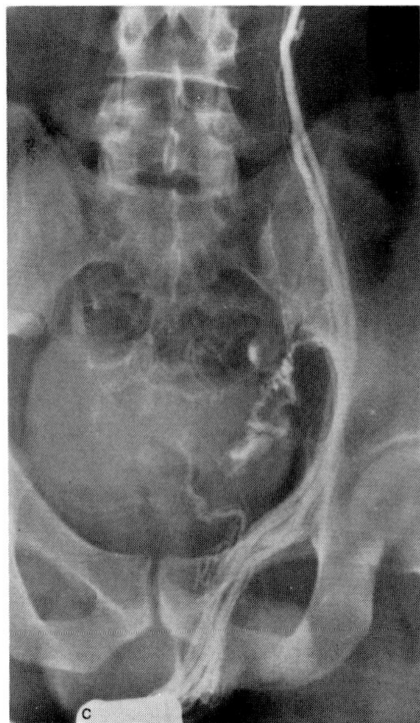

Fig. 18–3. Spermatic venograms revealing unusual anatomic features. *(A)* Paired veins on the right joining close to the junction with the inferior vena cava. *(B)* Incompetent venous valves allow reflux of contrast medium into the scrotum. *(C)* Paired spermatic veins on the left unite at the level of the iliac crest; small communicating channels join the common trunk more proximally, and there are communications with the pelvic, hypogastric, and presacral venous systems.

Another technique for preventing coil migration is the placing of a steel spider (Fig. 18–5*C* and *D*) or spiderlon (spider with compressed Ivalon; Fig. 18–5*E* and *F*).[23,24]

Completion of Procedure

A postembolization angiogram is performed to prove complete obliteration of the left spermatic vein.

The same catheter can sometimes be used to enter the right spermatic vein, but usually a specially shaped catheter is needed (see Fig. 18–2). In 85% of cases, the right spermatic vein enters the vena cava along the right anterolateral wall at the level of L-1 or L-2. In the remainder of cases, it may enter the right renal vein (5 to 10%) or the vena cava at a more inferior location. Rarely, the right spermatic vein joins the vena cava on the left side. Once the catheter engages the mouth of the right spermatic vein, a test injection is made to assess the competence of the venous valves. If the valves are found to be incompetent, the procedure used on the left side is repeated on the right side.

COMPARISON OF METHODS

At present, there is great controversy about which method is best for nonsurgical obliteration of veins, about whether sclerosing agents should be used, as described by Lima and others,[12–14] or whether permanent occluding devices, such as detachable balloons[17,18] or Gianturco coils,[15,16] should be placed. One disadvantage of sclerosing agents is the potential for recanalization of the vein after a period of time, with recurrence of varicocele. Also, if there is venous perforation, the agent may escape into the retroperitoneal space and cause tissue irritation.[13] One of the major drawbacks of this technique is that large communicating channels with the renal vein may be present, in which case thrombosis of

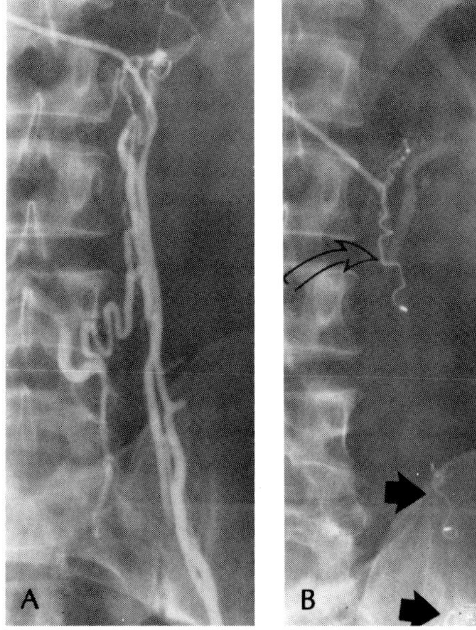

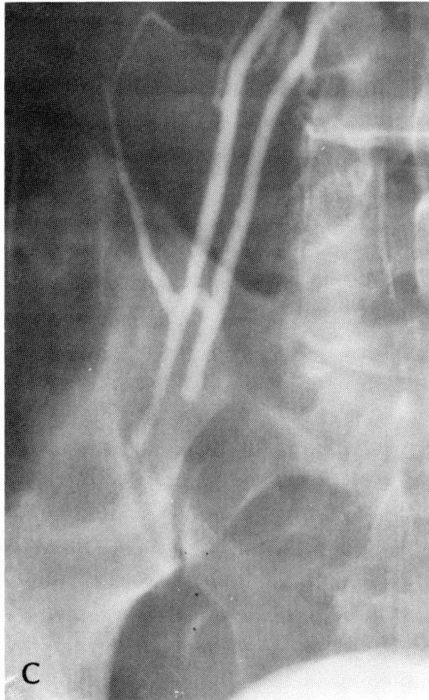

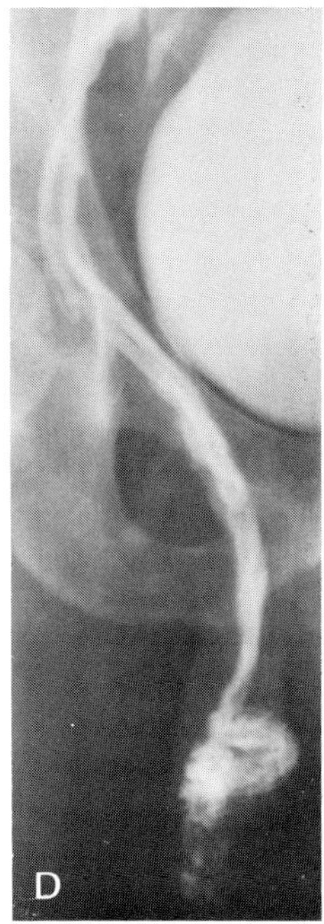

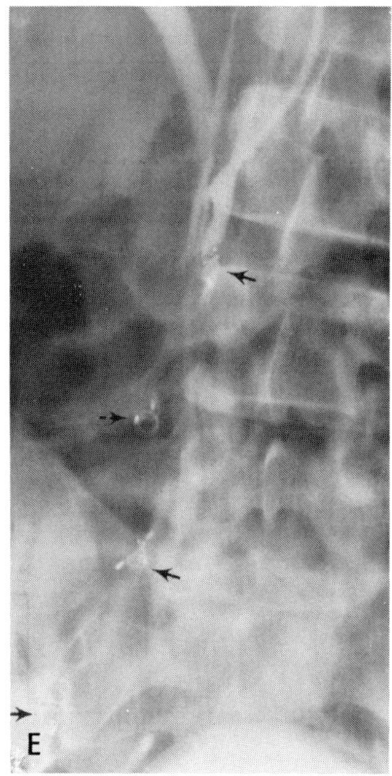

Fig. 18–4. Placement of occluding devices in anatomically unusual veins. *(A)* Venogram shows paired veins joining above the iliac crest, with a communicating channel arising at that level and joining the common trunk near the renal vein. *(B)* Springs have been placed in each of the paired veins *(black arrows)*, and a modified spring has been placed in the most proximal segment to abolish all collaterals *(open arrow)*. *(C)* Paired veins and several interconnecting channels on the right. *(D)* Large venous trunks are opacified together with the enlarged pampiniform plexus. *(E)* Selective obliteration of all channels; two springs have been placed in the medial vein and one in the lateral vein, and one modified spring has been placed in the most proximal common trunk.

the renal vein is a possibility. Therefore, Zeitler prefers not to use such agents in patients with large channels communicating with the renal vein.[26] Admittedly, however, in patients with small incompetent spermatic veins or multiple small veins arising from a common or dual trunk, the injection of sclerosing agents is the simplest procedure. In addition, this procedure is faster than the placement of several spring coils or detachable balloons.

With spring coils, there is more danger of erosion and perforation of the venous wall. However, because this is a low-pressure system, perforation is of no clin-

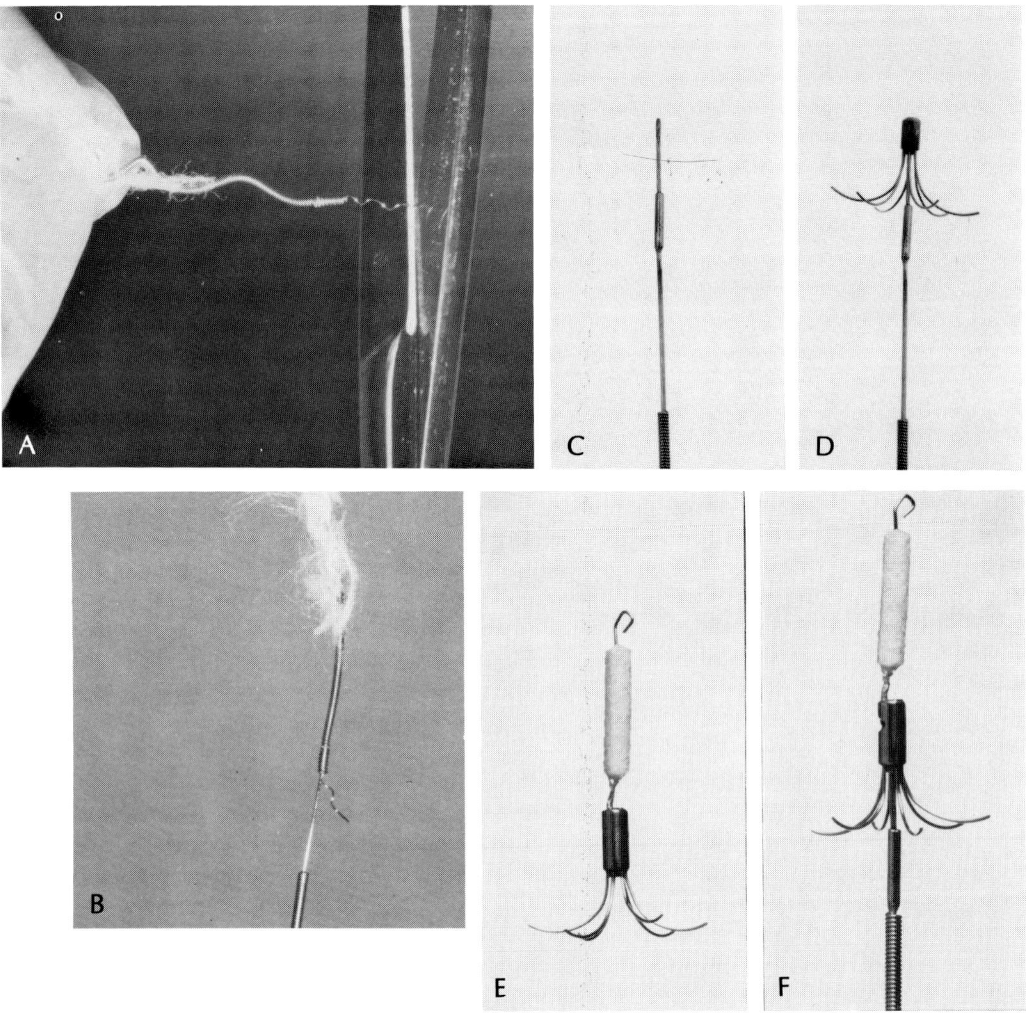

Fig. 18–5. Occluding devices. *(A)* Cutting tip of commercial Gianturco-Wallace-Chuang coil with scissors. *(B)* Modified spring mounted on a coil introducer; note barb created by procedure shown in A. *(C)* Spider introducer. *(D)* Introducer with mounted spider. *(E)* Spiderlon (stainless steel spider with compressed Ivalon). *(F)* Spiderlon mounted on introducer.

ical consequence. In addition, it has been demonstrated in experimental animals that coils heal in place by a firm fibrous reaction, thus preventing erosion and perforation.[25] The principal objection to coils is fear that they will migrate into the renal vein and embolize to the pulmonary artery. However, the simple modification described here apparently prevents such complications.[22] It is likely that the pressure in the spermatic vein rises considerably during straining or coughing. A sharp barb on the coil prevents dislodgment despite such sudden pressure changes, but the smooth inflated balloon may not be as resistant to dislodgment. Furthermore, use of detachable balloons requires extensive previous experience in the laboratory, and balloons are more expensive than coils.

POSTPROCEDURE CARE

Patients are transferred to the recovery area, where their vital signs are monitored every half hour until stable and hourly thereafter. When the signs have been stable for 3 to 4 hours, the puncture site and abdomen are examined. If no problems are detected, the patient is discharged. No medication is needed. Patients are told to report any fever, pain, or testicular swelling.

COMPLICATIONS

To date, more than 100 patients have undergone spermatic venography and embolization in our hospital, with few complications. One patient had avulsion of the spermatic vein as a result of entrapment of the catheter by venous spasm. There were no adverse clinical effects. One patient had a three-day fever of unknown origin that subsided without treatment. Three patients had small asymptomatic hydroceles that resolved spontaneously in a few months. In one of the first patients in the series, a fragment broke off the catheter and lodged in the lung without apparent ill effect. Subsequent modifications in catheter design and the technique have prevented recurrences of this complication.[19] Early in our experience, we admitted patients to the hospital overnight, but since we began performing venography and embolization as an outpatient procedure, no patient has required hospital admission.

FOLLOW-UP AND RESULTS

The patient is seen by the urologist one week after the procedure. The first semen analysis is performed three months later. The effects on the sperm count have been similar to those of successful open varicocelectomy. In patients whose pretreatment sperm counts were $< 4 \times 10^7$ per milliliter, the mean increase in the count was 4×10^7 per milliliter, and the mean increase in the motility index was 32%. In those with pretreatment counts of $1–4 \times 10^7$ per milliliter, the mean increase was 2.6×10^7 per milliliter, with a 16% increase in motility. In those whose initial sperm counts were $> 4 \times 10^7$ per milliliter, the mean increase was 2.72×10^7 per milliliter, with a mean increase in motility of 20%. Only two patients failed to show considerable improvement in sperm count, motility, or both after occlusion.

CONCLUSIONS

Much work remains to be done to clarify the relation between varicocele and subfertility. In the meantime, the technique described here is safe and effective for proving the presence of the condition and for correcting it in most cases, and our early results suggest that transvenous embolization restores fertility in a significant number of patients with clinical or subclinical varicocele.

REFERENCES

1. Macomber, D., and Sanders, M.D.: The spermatozoa count. N. Engl. J. Med., *200*:981, 1929.
2. Charny, W.C.: Effect of varicocele on fertility. Fertil. Steril., *13*:47, 1962.
3. Dubin, L., and Amelar, R.D.: Varicocele size and results of varicocelectomy in selected subfertile men with varicocele. Fertil. Steril., *21*:606, 1970.
4. MacLeod, J.: Seminal cytology in the presence of varicocele. Fertil. Steril. *16*:735, 1965.
5. Tulloch, S.: Considerations of sterility, subfertility in the male. Edinburgh Med. J., *59*:29, 1952.
6. Howards, S.S., Lipschultz, L.I. (eds.): Symposium on male infertility. Urol. Clin. North Am. 5:433, 1978.
7. Narayan, P., Amplatz, K., and Gonzalez, R.: Varicocele and male subfertility. Fertil. Steril., *36*:92, 1981.
8. Chatel, A., et al.: Intérêt de la phlébographie spermatique dans le diagnostic des stérilitiés d'origine circulatoire (varicocèle): comparison avec les données cliniques, thermographiques et anatomiques. Ann. Radiol. (Paris), *21*:565, 1979.
9. Greenberg, S.H., et al.: The use of the Doppler stethoscope in the evaluation of varicoceles. J. Urol., *117*:296, 1977.
10. Coolsaet, B.R.R.A.: The varicocele syndrome: venography determining the optimal level for surgical management. J. Urol., *124*:833, 1980.
11. Zorgniotti, A.W., MacLeod, J.: Studies on temperature, human semen quality and varicocele. Fertil. Steril., *24*:854, 1973.
12. Lima, S.S., Castro, M.D., and Costa, O.F.: A new method for the treatment of varicocele. Andrologia, *10*:103, 1978.
13. Zeitler, E., et al.: Selective sclerotherapy of the internal spermatic vein in patients with varicoceles. Cardiovasc. Intervent. Radiol., *3*:166, 1980.

14. Seyferth, W., Eddehard, J., and Zeitler, E.: Percutaneous sclerotherapy of varicocele. Radiology, *139*:335, 1981.
15. Formanek, A., et al.: Embolization of the spermatic vein for treatment of infertility: a new approach. Radiology, *139*:315, 1981.
16. Gonzalez, R., et al.: Transvenous embolization of internal spermatic veins: nonoperative approach to the treatment of varicocele. Urology, *17*:246, 1981.
17. Riedl, P., Lunglmayr, G., and Stackl, W.: A new method of transfemoral testicular vein obliteration for varicocele using a balloon catheter. Radiology, *139*:325, 1981.
18. White, R., Jr., et al.: Occlusion of varicoceles with detachable balloons. Radiology, *139*:127, 1981.
19. Gonzalez, R., et al.: Transvenous embolization of the internal spermatic veins for the treatment of varicocele scroti. Urol. Clin. North Am., 9:177, 1982.
20. Zollikofer, C., et al.: Therapeutic blockage of arteries using compressed Ivalon. Radiology, *136*:635, 1980.
21. Mazer, M., Baltaxe, H., and Wolf, L.G.: Therapeutic embolization of the renal artery with Gianturco coils: technical pitfalls. Radiology, *138*:37, 1981.
22. Castaneda, W.R., et al.: Single barbed stainless steel coils for venous occlusion: a simple but useful modification. Invest. Radiol., *17*:186, 1982.
23. Castaneda, W.R., et al.: "Spiderlon": new device for fast arterial and venous occlusion. AJR, *136*:627, 1980.
24. Castaneda-Zuniga, W.R., et al.: Experimental venous occlusion with stainless steel spiders. Radiology, *141*:238, 1981.
25. Barth, K.H., et al.: Chronic vascular reactions to steel coil occlusion devices. AJR, *131*:455, 1978.
26. Zeitler, E.: Personal communication, 1982.

19

Renal Cyst Puncture and Needle Aspiration Biopsy

ROBERT P. MILLER, M.D.

Percutaneous aspiration biopsy of cystic and solid lesions of the genitourinary tract can be performed on ambulatory patients with little risk. The necessary equipment is readily available in most clinics.

RENAL CYST PUNCTURE

The introduction of ultrasound has greatly reduced the need for an open operation to determine the nature of a renal mass.[1-3] There are a few cases that require further studies, however, and percutaneous cyst aspiration with fluid analysis is an accurate method for resolving the question of whether a mass is truly a cyst or a tumor.[4,5] For more than 30 years, such punctures have been done as an office procedure.[6]

Indications and Contraindications

Most renal masses detected at intravenous urography can immediately be classified as probably tumorous or probably cystic. For the former, we perform angiography; for the latter, we perform ultrasonography.

The ultrasonic characteristics of a benign renal cyst are enumerated in Table 19–1. If all of these criteria are met by a given lesion, no further studies are necessary, although we usually repeat the scan 6 months to a year later as a precaution. Such an approach will detect virtually all of the rare tumors within a cyst while they are still small and premetastatic.[4] If the ultrasound scan shows a complex or solid lesion, we perform angiography.

TABLE 19–1. Ultrasound Characteristics of a Benign Renal Cyst

Mass in same position as that on intravenous urogram
No internal echos
Sharply defined posterior wall
Zone of increased echogenicity beyond the lesion (through transmission)

Cyst puncture under fluoroscopic control with fluid analysis is indicated if the results of the scan are indeterminant or if clinical findings such as hematuria suggest a tumor. The only contraindications are bleeding diatheses, lack of patient cooperation, and allergy to contrast medium. Because the first two are correctable problems and because the use of contrast medium can be avoided by doing the puncture under ultrasound or computed axial tomography (CT), virtually all patients can be made suitable for cyst puncture. If it is desirable to avoid ionizing radiation (e.g., in pregnant patients), ultrasonic guidance should be used.

Preparation of Patients

The patient is interviewed and the medical history is reviewed. The procedure and its risks are explained to the patient, and oral and written consent are obtained. The laboratory studies must include assessment of clotting factors.

The patient should receive nothing by mouth for 4 to 6 hours before the procedure. Sedation is used only for unusually anxious patients. Local anesthesia is used.

Technique

We prefer to perform this procedure under fluoroscopic guidance, as do some other investigators.[7] Methods for puncture under ultrasonic or CT guidance are also available.[8,9]

The location and diameter of the cyst and its depth below the skin are determined from the available radiographic films or ultrasonic scans. The volume is then estimated according to the formula $V = 4r^3$. When using fluoroscopy, it is invaluable to note the position of the cyst in relation to the parts of the collecting system. With experience, even small lesions can be located accurately (Fig. 19–1).

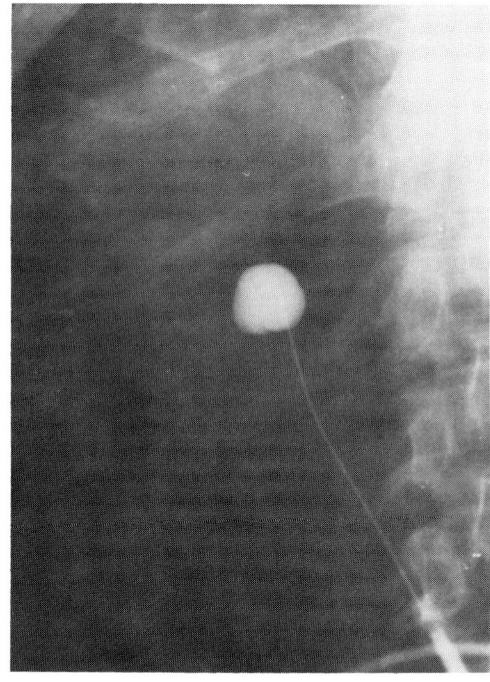

Fig. 19–1. A 10-ml upper-pole cyst being aspirated under fluoroscopic control. Location was determined by intravenous urography and ultrasound.

The patient is placed prone on the fluoroscopy table, and the lumbar vertebrae are counted. This is important, as some patients with six lumbar vertebrae have only 11 ribs, and a puncture immediately below the last rib may then lead to pneumothorax. The kidney and collecting system are then opacified with intravenous contrast medium; and, under fluoroscopic observation, a point caudal to the twelfth rib is marked on the skin. For lesions above the twelfth rib, it will be necessary to angle the biopsy needle cephalad (Fig. 19–2). The chosen area is scrubbed and draped, and the skin and subcutaneous tissues at the point of needle entry are infiltrated with 1% lidocaine (Xylocaine).

A small incision is made in the skin, and the biopsy needle is introduced. We prefer the 15-cm, 22-gauge, thin-walled needle. Under intermittent fluoroscopy (to minimize the radiation exposure of the operator's hands), the needle is advanced. When it is aimed in the proper direction, the patient is asked to suspend breathing while the needle is advanced quickly into the cyst. Movement of the needle with inhalation and exhalation confirms the needle's position in the kidney.

The needle stylet is removed, and a clear extension tube and syringe are attached to the needle. Gentle suction is applied with the syringe; and if fluid appears, the patient is asked to breathe quietly while aspiration continues. If no fluid appears, the needle is drawn back 1 cm

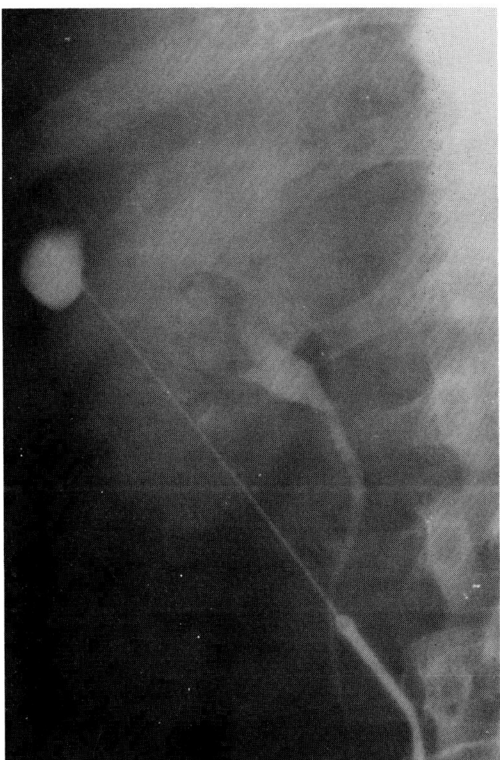

Fig. 19–2. A 12-ml cyst being drained. Note angled course of needle from point below the twelfth rib. Approaching perpendicular to the rib shortens the needle's path to the cyst.

and aspiration is repeated. This step can be repeated as necessary. If no fluid appears on the initial pass, additional passes are made, with the needle directed to a slightly different location on each attempt. Fresh blood is sometimes seen if the wall of the cyst is touched with the needle.

Fluid Analysis

The appropriate studies depend on the appearance of the fluid. If it is crystal clear, cytology study and measurements of lactic dehydrogenase (LDH), protein, and fat are appropriate (Table 19–2). If it is cloudy or purulent, it also should be gram-stained and cultured for both aerobes and anaerobes. If it is turbid or contains necrotic or other solid material,

TABLE 19–2. Normal Limits in Laboratory Analysis of Fluid From Benign Cyst

LDH	136–309 units/litre
Protein	< 3 g/dl
Fat	None
Cytology:	Normal

it is smeared on a glass slide, fixed immediately in 95% ethanol, and stained for cytology study. Large pieces of tissue are placed in saline for preparation of a cell block for histopathologic analysis.

It is imperative that the operator observe the fluid being obtained during the aspiration. In our experience with more than 260 masses, crystal clear fluid always means that the lesion is benign. However, we observed clear fluid during the initial stage of aspiration of a large cystic carcinoma; and only when continued aspiration produced debris-filled fluid from the dependent, tumorous part of the lesion did the diagnosis of malignancy become obvious. Thus, a small volume of fluid from a large mass should not be relied on for diagnosis of benign disease. A small amount of fresh blood followed by continued clear fluid is evidence of a traumatic puncture, not proof of malignancy, especially if the data from the fluid analysis are within normal limits.

Radiographic Confirmation

If the lesion proves benign, water-soluble contrast medium is instilled into the cyst, the volume being the same as the amount of fluid aspirated. A cystogram is obtained to confirm that the lesion corresponds to the mass detected by earlier studies (Fig. 19–3). The film also serves as a useful reference if further studies are needed later. The contents of the cyst are then aspirated completely as a precaution against infection, and the needle is removed.

A chest radiograph is obtained during exhalation if an upper-pole cyst has been

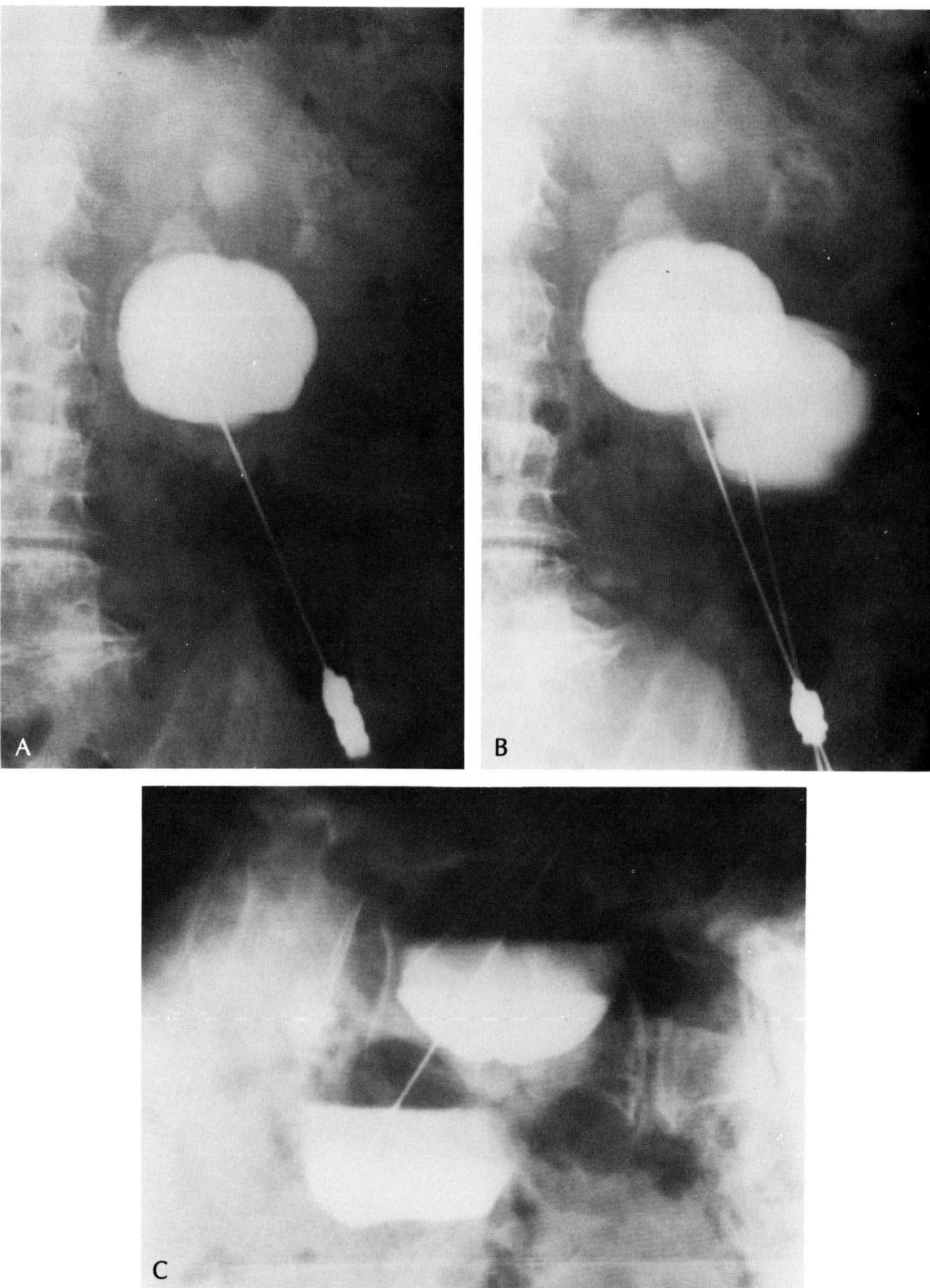

Fig. 19–3. Importance of radiographic confirmation. Ultrasound scan indicated a bilobular cystic mass. *(A)* Initial cystogram. *(B)* A second needle was inserted and a cystogram performed, which corresponded to the ultrasound scan. As a lateral film *(C)* shows, the two cysts do not communicate. Note anterior flattening of one cyst by abdominal contents.

punctured and examined for evidence of pneumothorax.

Use of Sclerosing Agents

We do not use sclerosing agents routinely in asymptomatic cysts, as we share Mindell's opinion[10] that this technique often causes more morbidity than it prevents. If the patient has cyst-related symptoms, we perform the aspiration as described to confirm that the symptoms were caused by the lesion. We repeat the aspiration if the symptoms and cyst recur, and only if symptoms and cyst recur rapidly do we consider obliterating the lesion.

Postprocedure Care

Ambulatory patients remain in the area for 3 hours and are discharged if they are asymptomatic and there is no gross hematuria in a voided urine specimen. They are instructed to return if they have flank pain, fever, chills, or blood in their urine. Patients who have been sedated are released only in the company of a responsible adult.

Complications

The potential complications of percutaneous renal cyst puncture are perirenal hemorrhage, pneumothorax, infection, and seeding of the needle track with tumor cells. In 5,674 cases compiled from 84 institutions, the incidence of serious complications was 1.4%, with no deaths.[11]

Bleeding is more common when the ultrasonic transducer, with its more rigid needle, is used than when the more flexible thin-walled needle is used.[11] Our two instances of hemorrhage occurred in patients in whom cyst puncture was necessary despite the existence of bleeding diatheses.

Pneumothorax occurs only when the puncture is made above the twelfth rib. As noted, even upper-pole cysts can be punctured from below the rib with proper angulation of the needle. In obese patients, it is necessary to start well below the twelfth rib during cephalad angulation because of the longer path the needle must make; and in our series, failure to appreciate the length of the tract led to punctures between the eleventh and twelfth ribs with pneumothorax in three patients. However, none had symptoms or required a chest tube. In Lang's series, pneumothorax most often occurred during ultrasonic guidance, because with this technique the approach to upper-pole lesions is a direct one between the eleventh and twelfth ribs.[11]

Infection is uncommon unless there are lapses in technique. The single instance in our series was, we believe, the result of failure to drain the cyst adequately after cystography.

According to our analysis, the risk of seeding a needle tract with carcinoma cells has been greatly exaggerated. The reported cases generally occurred before the introduction of present ultrasound technology and thus may well have involved lesions that today would not be aspirated because the accuracy of ultrasound in identifying tumors is so high. For example, in our series of 260 renal masses, there were only two instances in which the ultrasound scan was falsely believed to indicate a benign cyst, and in both cases a review of the scans showed errors in interpretation. Second, a recent case of needle-track seeding involved use of an 18-gauge needle,[12] and it is possible that the use of smaller needles will make seeding less likely, although there has been a report of seeding during thin-needle aspiration biopsy of a pancreatic carcinoma.[13] Furthermore, in a series of 150 patients with renal cell carcinoma, there was no difference in the survival rates of the 77 who had undergone needle aspiration and the others who had not.[14] We do not advocate puncture of obviously malignant lesions but believe that the danger of tract seeding during puncture of cystic lesions is minuscule and that the reduction in morbidity and mortality when cyst puncture is used in lieu of more invasive methods more than justifies the approach described in this chapter.

ASPIRATION BIOPSY OF PERIRENAL, PELVIC, AND RETROPERITONEAL MASSES

This technique requires the help of an experienced and enthusiastic cytopathologist to be useful, and we routinely discuss techniques and cases with this person. Several reviews and large series have been reported,[7,9,15,16] including some in which the procedure was done on outpatients.[17,18]

Imaging Techniques

Some practitioners prefer fluoroscopic guidance after lymphography;[7,19] others favor CT.[9,20] Although CT can be useful for locating small, deep-seated lesions, we question its cost-effectiveness in most cases, especially in view of the longer time needed and the fact that fluoroscopy is so much simpler and so effective. Ultrasound is not used routinely because of the difficulty in imaging the needle tip once it is in the mass and because of the interference with the image by bowel gas when an anterior approach is used.

Technique

Informed consent is obtained and the patient is prepared as described earlier in this chapter, observing the same precautions and contraindications. For aspiration of lymph nodes, lymphangiography is performed by the route appropriate to opacify the masses one wishes to examine (Fig. 19–4). Most lesions adjacent to the kidneys and ureters can be located with the aid of the far simpler method of intravenous urography (Fig. 19–5). The patient is placed on the fluoroscopy table supine for aspiration of lower periureteral, retroperitoneal, or pelvic masses and prone for perirenal or upper periureteral masses. The skin at the chosen site is anesthetized, and a 22-gauge 15–20-cm Chiba needle is advanced into the lesion under intermittent fluoroscopic control. The stylet is removed, and an extension tube with a 10-

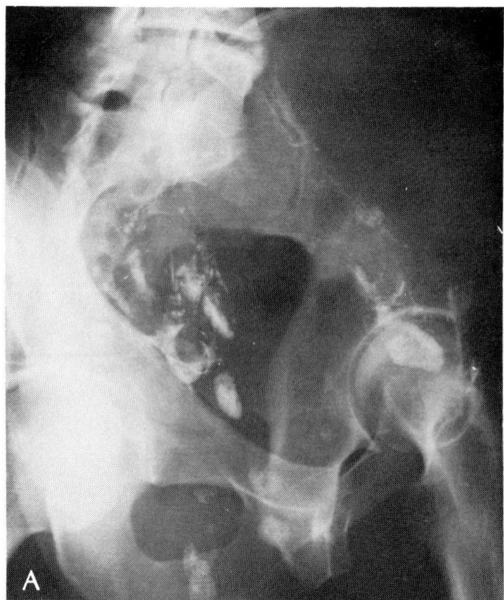

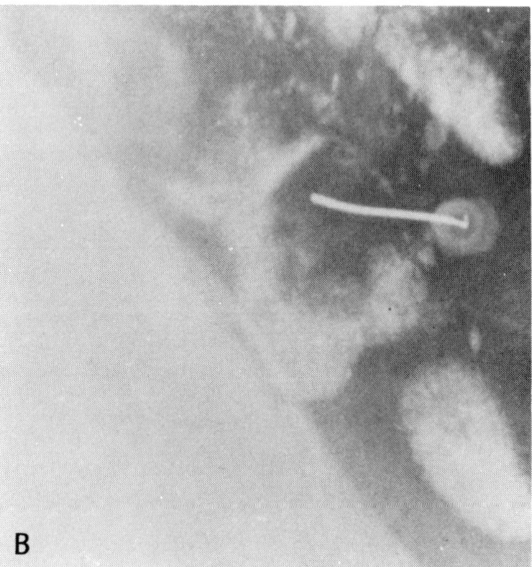

Fig. 19–4. Aspiration with the aid of lymphangiography. *(A)* Oblique view of pelvis; note nodal filling defects. *(B)* With patient in the supine oblique position, the biopsy needle has been directed into an abnormal lymph node.

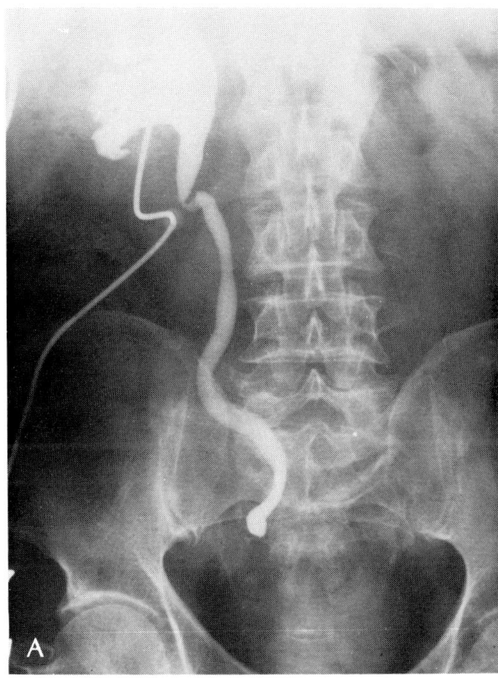

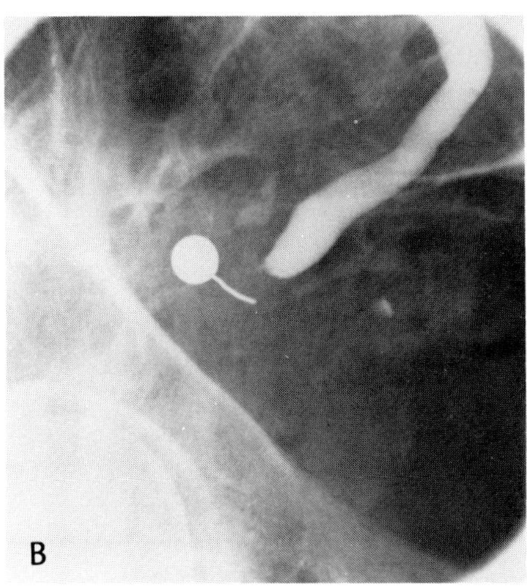

Fig. 19–5. Aspiration with the aid of urography. *(A)* Patient with total ureteral obstruction has undergone percutaneous nephrostomy for decompression; contrast medium has been instilled through the tract. *(B)* Contrast medium in ureter used to guide Chiba needle for aspiration biopsy. Lesion was carcinoma of the prostate.

ml syringe is attached to the needle. Suction is then applied while the needle is moved up and down and rotated in the lesion.

The material obtained is squirted onto a slide, smeared, and fixed in 95% ethanol. If a large amount of tissue is obtained, the contents of the syringe may be placed in saline and centrifuged for preparation of a cell block. The needle is rinsed in saline, with the material being added to the slide or block. Aspiration is then repeated; two to four passes are usually sufficient.

Postoperative Care

This is as described for cyst puncture.

Interpretation of the Results

An unfortunate and unavoidable feature of aspiration biopsy for cancer staging is the fact that, whereas there are virtually no false-positive diagnoses, there are many false-negative ones. Thus, although the physician can rely on the results if the cytopathologist reports that cancer was found, a report that only benign tissue was found does not mean that the patient does not have cancer. The frequency of false-negative staging studies can be reduced by obtaining samples from several lymph nodes. For example, in staging prostatic carcinoma, Correa found a false-negative rate of 17%, which is similar to the 20% false-negative rates found with some staging lymphadenectomy techniques with frozen-section biopsy.[21]

However, in many of the aspiration biopsy procedures performed on an outpatient basis, staging is not being attempted. Rather, the identity of a particular mass, discovered by ultrasound or CT scan, is sought in a patient already known to have cancer; and in these cases, aspiration biopsy is very accurate.

Complications

Bleeding and infection are the principal complications of percutaneous aspiration biopsy. Provided one does not use the technique on a hypervascular mass, the use of a 22-gauge needle rarely causes significant bleeding in a patient with a normal coagulation profile. There have been reports of single cases of needle-tract seeding after 10 needle passes in a pancreatic carcinoma,[22] intra-abdominal hemorrhage,[23] and puncture of an aortic dissection without sequelae.[24] Pneumothorax is an occasional complication of adrenal gland biopsy.[15]

CONCLUSIONS

Outpatient cyst puncture and aspiration biopsy can save many patients the trouble and costs of hospital admission. Even in those cases in which patients must later be admitted for treatment of their disease, the previous outpatient procedure will shorten the stay, with a commensurate lowering of the cost.

REFERENCES

1. Lindblom, K..: Diagnostic kidney puncture in cysts and tumors. Am. J. Radiol. Rad. Ther., *68*:209, 1952.
2. DeWeerd, J.H.: Percutaneous aspiration of selected expanding renal lesions. J. Urol., *87*:303, 1962.
3. Clayman, R.V., Williams, R.D., and Fraley, E.E.: The pursuit of the renal mass. N. Engl. J. Med., *300*:72, 1979.
4. Clayman, R.V., et al.: Renal cyst or renal tumor? Definitive nonoperative evaluation of the renal mass. Am. J. Med., (in press)
5. Pollack, H.M., Banner, M.P., and Arger, P.H.: The accuracy of gray scale renal ultrasonography in differentiating cystic neoplasms from benign cysts. Radiology, *143*:741, 1982.
6. Ainsworth, W.L., and Vest, S.A.: The differential diagnosis between renal tumors and cysts. J. Urol., *66*:710, 1951.
7. Pereiras, R.V., et al.: Fluoroscopically guided thin needle aspiration biopsy of the abdomen and retroperitoneum. Am. J. Roentgenol., *131*:197, 1978.
8. Goldberg, B.B., and Pollack, H.M.: Ultrasonically guided renal cyst aspiration. J. Urol., *109*:5, 1973.
9. Sundaran, M., et al.: Utility of CT-guided abdominal aspiration procedures. AJR, *139*:1111, 1982.
10. Mindell, H.J.: On the use of Pantopaque in renal cysts. Radiology, *119*:747, 1976.
11. Lang, E.K.: Renal cyst puncture and aspiration: a survey of complications. Am. J. Roentgenol., *128*:723, 1977.
12. Gibbons, R.P., Bush, W.H., Jr., and Burnett, L.L.: Needle tract seeding following aspiration of renal cell carcinoma. J. Urol., *118*:865, 1977.
13. Ferrucci, J.T., Jr., et al.: Malignant seeding of the tract after thin-needle aspiration biopsy. Radiology, *130*:345, 1979.
14. von Schreeb, T., et al.: Renal adenocarcinoma: is there a risk of spreading tumor cells in diagnostic puncture? Scand. J. Urol. Nephrol., *1*:270, 1976.
15. Ferrucci, J.T., Jr., et al.: Diagnosis of abdominal malignancy by radiologic fine-needle aspiration biopsy. AJR, *134*:323, 1980.
16. Stabb, E.V., Jaques, P.F., and Partain, C.L.: Percutaneous biopsy in the management of solid intra-abdominal masses of unknown etiology. Radiol. Clin. North Am., *17*:435, 1979.
17. Zornoza, J., et al.: Transperitoneal percutaneous retroperitoneal lymph node aspiration biopsy. Radiology, *122*:111, 1977.
18. Göthlin, J.H., and Macintosh, P.K.: Interventional radiology in the assessment of the retroperitoneal lymph nodes. Radiol. Clin. North Am., *17*:461, 1979.
19. Göthlin, J.H.: Post-lymphographic percutaneous fine needle biopsy of lymph nodes guided by fluoroscopy. Radiology, *120*:205, 1976.
20. Haaga, J.R.: New techniques for CT-guided biopsies. AJR, *133*:633, 1979.
21. Correa, R.J., Jr.: Lymphangiography with fine-needle aspiration biopsy of pelvic and abdominal lymph nodes in cancer staging. Urol. Clin. North Am., 9:153, 1982.
22. Ferrucci, J.T., et al.: Malignant seeding of the tract after thin needle aspiration biopsy. Radiology, *130*:345, 1979.
23. Holm, H.H., et al.: Ultrasonically guided percutaneous puncture. Radiol. Clin. North Am., *13*:493, 1975.
24. Jaques, P.F., et al.: CT-assisted pelvic and abdominal aspiration biopsies in gynecological malignancy. Radiology, *128*:651, 1978.

20

Renal-Artery Angioplasty in the Management of Renovascular Hypertension

WILFRIDO R. CASTAÑEDA-ZUÑIGA, M.D., and
KURT AMPLATZ, M.D.

Renovascular causes are believed to be responsible for 1 to 2% of the cases of hypertension in the United States.[1] Classically, such renovascular hypertension has been treated with surgery, which usually produces good results, but has considerable morbidity and a mortality rate of 3%.[2]

The introduction of the Grüntzig catheter with a nonexpandable balloon made it possible to dilate stenotic renal arteries percutaneously,[3] and the first reports of success in treating atherosclerotic and fibromuscular dysplastic lesions appeared in 1977.[4–6] Since then, numerous reports have shown that transluminal renal-artery angioplasty can be performed with little morbidity, virtually no risk of death, and results comparable to those of open operation. Two- and three-year follow-up data show that the results of angioplasty are superior to those of surgery for dysplastic lesions, being successful in controlling hypertension in 90% of patients.[7,8] The success rate is lower for atherosclerotic lesions, especially when bilateral or ostial lesions, or those without renin lateralization, are dilated.[7–9] Transluminal angioplasty is an excellent alternative to surgery for many of these patients also.

Transluminal angioplasty cannot be performed on an outpatient basis, particularly in a free-standing unit, because some of the rare complications necessitate immediate vascular surgery. Also, if the procedure is successful in relieving the stenotic obstruction, profound hypotension may occur; thus the patient must be monitored closely for the first 6 to 12 hours. However, much of the preprocedural evaluation, such as angiography, does not require hospitalization and can be performed on an outpatient basis. The Northland Vascular Clinic, for example, has done this in more than 800 patients and found it safe and reliable for the evaluation of vascular disease.[10] Katzen, of George Washington University Medical Center, routinely performs digital subtraction angiography, and obtains renal-vein renin levels with the same venous catheter, as a single outpatient screening procedure before doing the transluminal angioplasty.[11] Furthermore, followup angiography may be required to assess continued patency, and this can also be performed on an outpatient basis. Thus, although at present transluminal angioplasty itself is not being performed on outpatients, the preliminary evaluation is being done in this way. Also, transluminal angioplasty is cost effective in comparison with standard surgery because of the short (one- or two-day) hospital stay, the low morbidity and mortality rates, the high success rates, and the fact that it is performed with only local anesthesia. Thus, we have included this chapter in *Outpatient Urologic Surgery*.

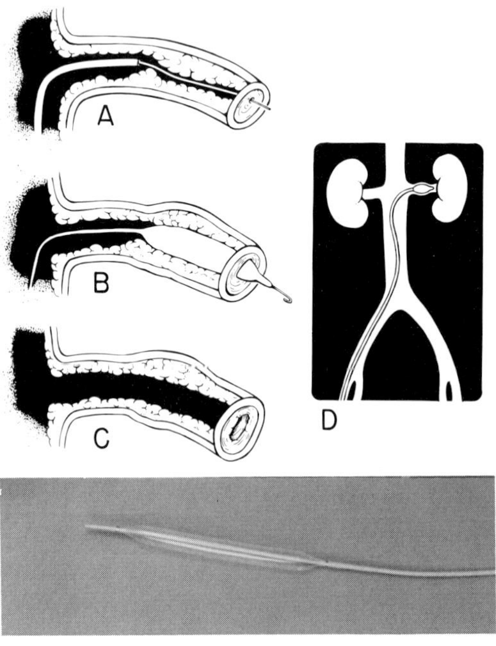

Fig. 20–1. Transfemoral approach with a Grüntzig balloon catheter. *(A)* The guide wire has been passed across the stenosis. *(B)* The balloon has been passed across the area and inflated. *(C)* Increase in lumen size after procedure. *(D)* Overview of the transfemoral approach. *(Inset)* The Grüntzig catheter.

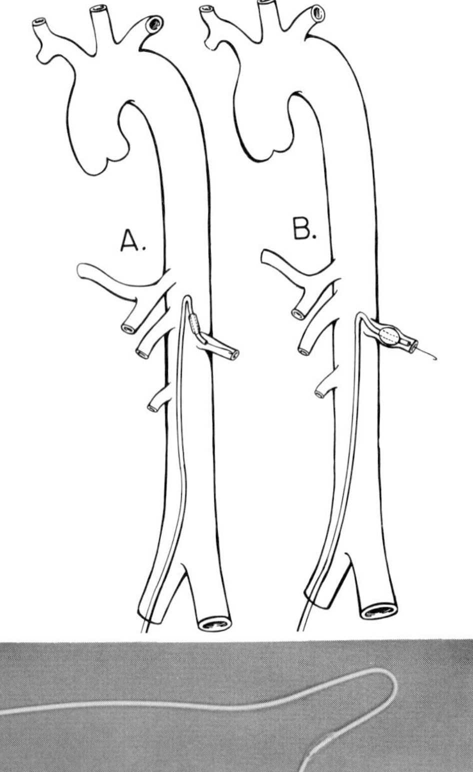

Fig. 20–2. *(A* and *B)* The transfemoral approach with a sidewinder catheter. *(Inset)* A sidewinder catheter.

INDICATIONS

There are three groups of patients in whom renal-artery angioplasty may be appropriate:

(1) Patients with renal-artery stenosis demonstrated angiographically and with unilateral renin hyperactivity. This group can be divided according to the cause of the stenosis: fibromuscular dysplasia; atherosclerosis; and vasculitis (Takayasu's arteritis, neurofibromatosis).

(2) Patients with renal-artery stenosis demonstrated angiographically but without renin lateralization. In this group, the long-term patency rate after angioplasty is similar to that in the previous group, but control of

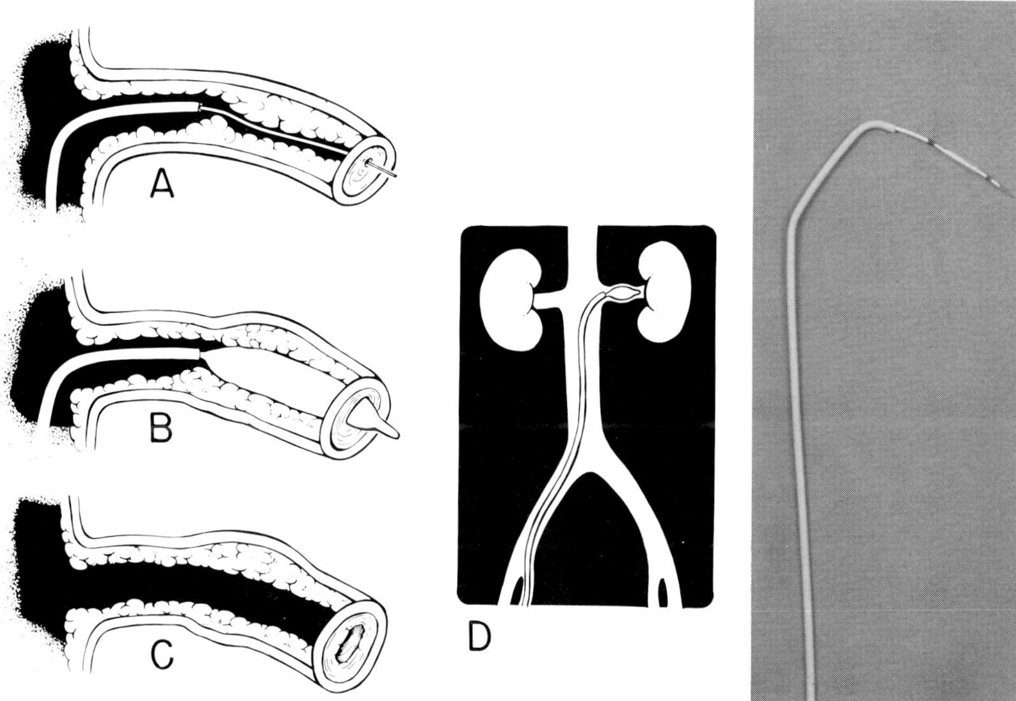

Fig. 20–3. Transfemoral approach with a coaxial system. *(A)* The guiding catheter has been placed in the renal artery proximal to the stenosis. *(B)* The balloon catheter has been passed through the guiding catheter and inflated. *(C)* Increase in lumen size after the procedure. *(D)* Overview of the coaxial technique. *(Inset)* The coaxial system with the balloon catheter protruding from the guiding catheter.

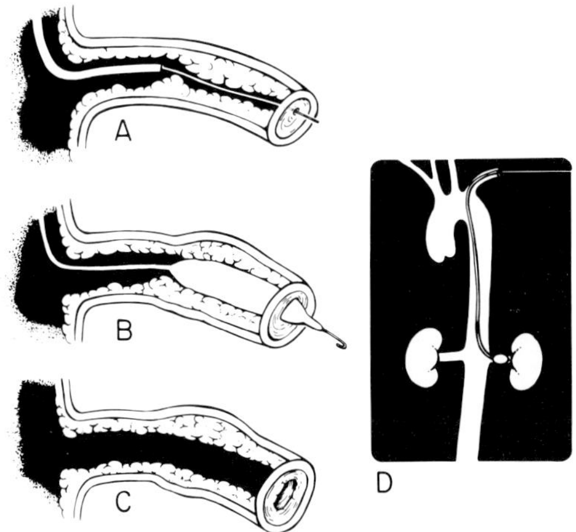

Fig. 20–4. *(A through D)* Transaxillary approach with a balloon catheter.

hypertension is less frequent. However, dilatation commonly allows a reduction in the doses of antihypertensive drugs.

(3) Patients with chronic renal failure with severe renal-artery stenosis; in these cases, angioplasty may be done to improve renal function.

PROCEDURE

Precautions

A vascular surgeon should be readily available, because major complications, such as rupture of the renal artery, require an immediate operation to save the patient's life. Also, a large venous cannula should be inserted before the procedure to allow rapid administration of fluid or blood. Finally, any long-acting hypertensive drugs the patient may be taking should be discontinued before the procedure. If necessary, the blood pressure should be controlled with short-acting drugs, such as nitroprusside.

Technique

Renal-artery angioplasty can be performed four different ways: by the femoral approach, using conventional balloon catheters (Fig. 20–1), preshaped balloon catheters (Fig. 20–2), or coaxial catheters (Fig. 20–3); or by the transaxillary or transbrachial approach, using conventional balloon catheters (Fig. 20–4). Initially, all cases can be attempted via the femoral approach with standard or preshaped balloon catheters unless the renal arteries form a sharp angle with the aorta (Fig. 20–5), in which case a sidewinder balloon catheter should be used. In the uncommon cases in which the femoral approach fails, the transaxillary approach may succeed, because the catheter is easily introduced into the renal arteries from above. If the renal-artery angulation is steep, it may be advisable to start with the transaxillary approach.

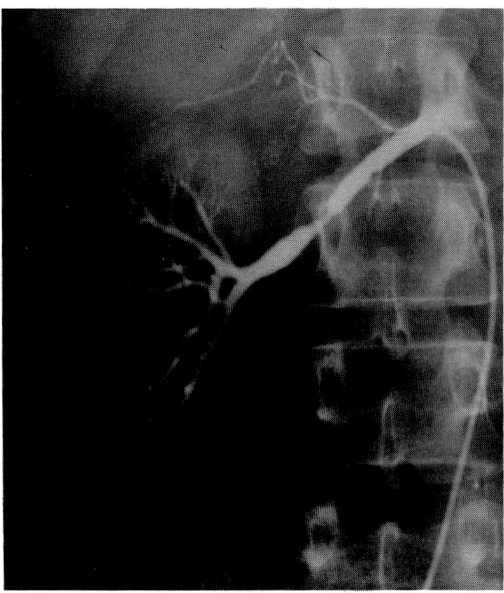

Fig. 20–5. A sharply angled renal artery narrowed by fibromuscular dysplasia. Sidewinder catheters are often useful in such cases.

The coaxial catheter system is not popular with radiologists because of its complexity and tendency to produce intimal dissections. However, there are cases in which balloon catheters do not follow the guide wire, necessitating the bracing possible with the coaxial technique.

An abdominal aortogram is performed to demonstrate the location of the stenosis, the contralateral renal artery, and the segmental arteries. The pressure in the abdominal aorta is recorded, and the catheter is replaced with a No. 5 or No. 6 preshaped renal curve or cobra catheter (Fig. 20–6) passed through a sheath introducer to prevent bleeding at the puncture site.

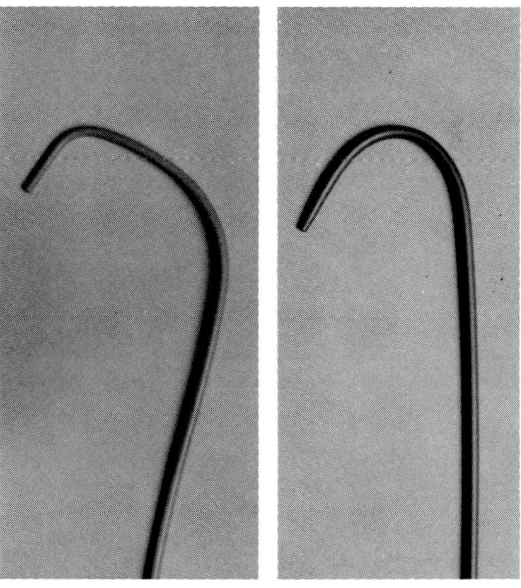

Fig. 20–6. Cobra *(left)* and renal curve *(right)* catheters.

Procedure for Using Unshaped Balloon Catheters. The stenotic renal artery is catheterized selectively if the catheter

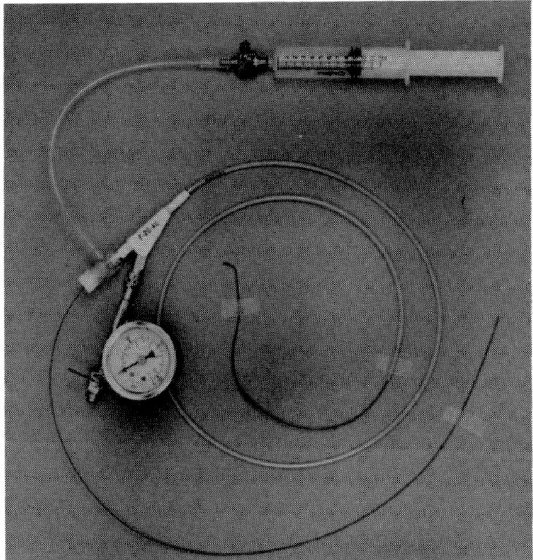

Fig. 20–7. Assembly of Grüntzig catheter, guide wire, Tuohy–Borst sidearm adaptor, and pressure gauge.

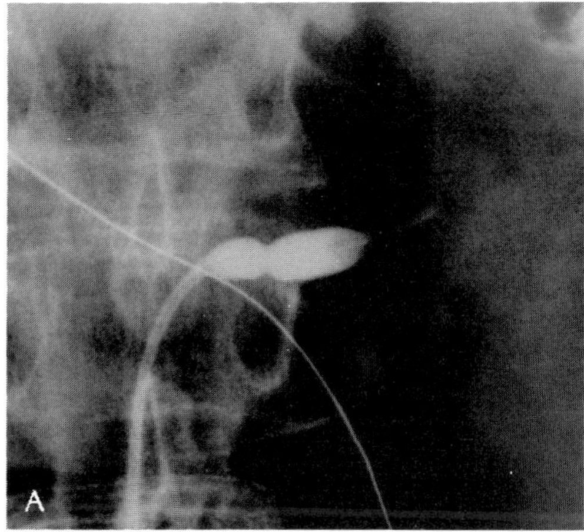

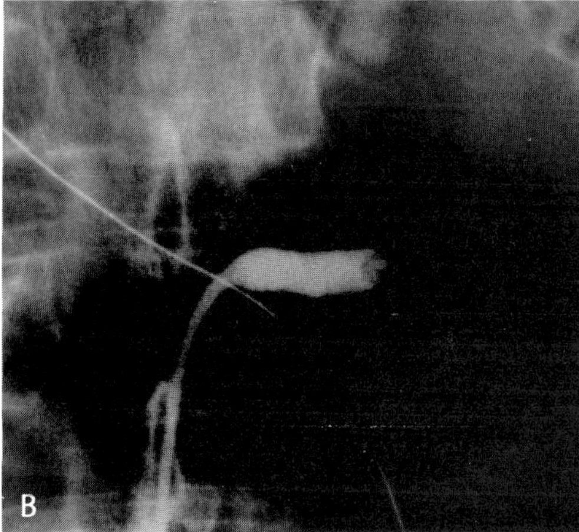

Fig. 20–8. Angioplasty of severely stenotic left renal artery. *(A)* Grüntzig balloon catheter inflated in stenosis; note hourglass deformity. *(B)* Disappearance of deformity after 30-second inflation.

can be passed beyond the stenosis. If the catheter does not pass by itself, the stenotic segment is carefully probed with either a floppy guide wire or a 3-mm J-tipped guide wire until the wire has passed across the stenosis and into one of the major branches of the renal artery. The catheter is then advanced over the wire until its tip lies beyond the narrowed area. Either at this time or just before the passage of the wire, systemic heparinization is established with 5,000–7,000 units of heparin.

The guide wire is drawn back, and the pressure is measured to determine the gradient across the stenosis. A stiffer guide wire is then passed through the catheter into one of the branches of the renal artery, and the catheter is withdrawn gently under fluoroscopic observation, keeping the tip of the wire in the same position. A Grüntzig catheter with a balloon size equal to the caliber of the unstenosed portion of the renal artery is advanced carefully over the guide wire until the balloon lies across the lesion; the guide wire remains in place with the use of the Tuohy–Borst sidearm adaptor (Fig. 20–7). The balloon is inflated several times to a pressure of 5 to 6 atmospheres, as determined by the pressure gauge. Several inflations of 30 to 120 seconds each usually erase the hourglass deformity in the balloon (Fig. 20–8), indicating the opening of the lesion; if this does not happen, the inflation pressure can be increased to 8 to 9 atmospheres, but in this range the balloon may rupture, particularly if it is made of polyvinyl chloride.

After the balloon deformity has disap-

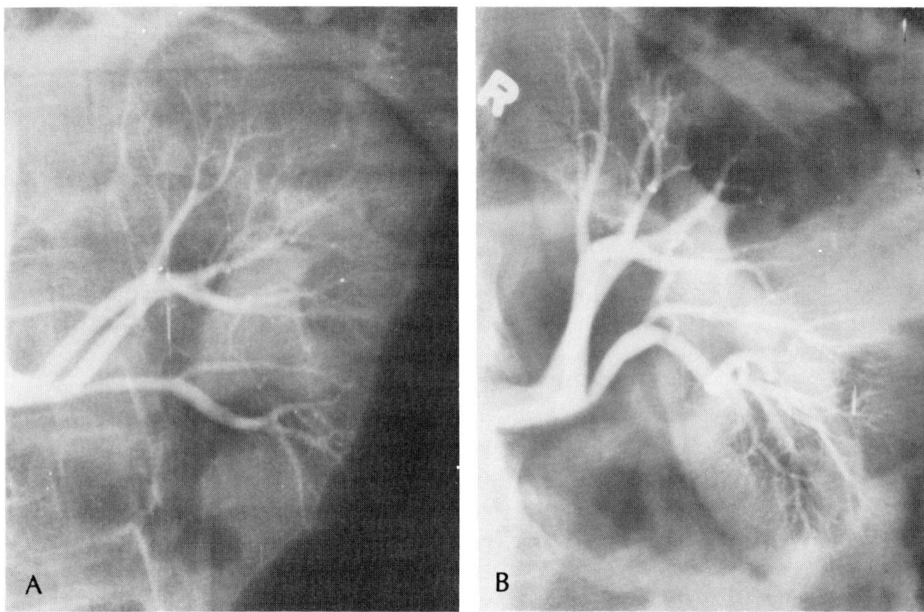

Fig. 20–9. *(A)* Severe fusiform narrowing. *(B)* Marked increase in lumen size after dilatation with a coaxial catheter.

peared, the guide wire is removed, and the pressure is measured through the balloon catheter (which may itself produce a gradient). If a small gradient is present, the guide wire is reintroduced, and the balloon catheter is replaced with a 5F catheter that is passed beyond the dilatation site. A more reliable pressure measurement is then obtained. If a pressure gradient of > 30 mm Hg is found, a larger balloon catheter can be introduced for further dilatation of the stenotic segment. It should be remembered, however, that a small residual pressure gradient does not preclude cure of the hypertension.

An abdominal aortogram or semiselective injection is then performed to document the status of the dilated renal artery angiographically.

Procedure for Using Preshaped Catheters. The balloon sidewinder is turned in the aortic arch and withdrawn with its tip pointed downstream and advanced into the ostium of the renal artery. The catheter should not be pulled across the area of stenosis, because a dissection can be produced. It is safer to advance a soft guide wire across the area first and then pull the catheter over the wire (see Fig. 20–2). The same technique is used with a balloon catheter having a renal curve.

With the coaxial technique, the guiding catheter is introduced into the ostium of the renal artery, and the balloon catheter is passed gently across the stenosis (see Fig. 20–4). This may be particularly useful for dilatation of severe narrowing and of branch stenoses, because the balloon catheters are smaller (Fig. 20–9).

COMPLICATIONS

Subintimal Dissections

If a small intimal flap is created by the guide wire or catheter, there is no significant impairment of blood flow. However, if the flap is large and flow is reduced, the procedure should be terminated and anticoagulants given. Redilatation should not be attempted for a minimum of four to six weeks. In the rare

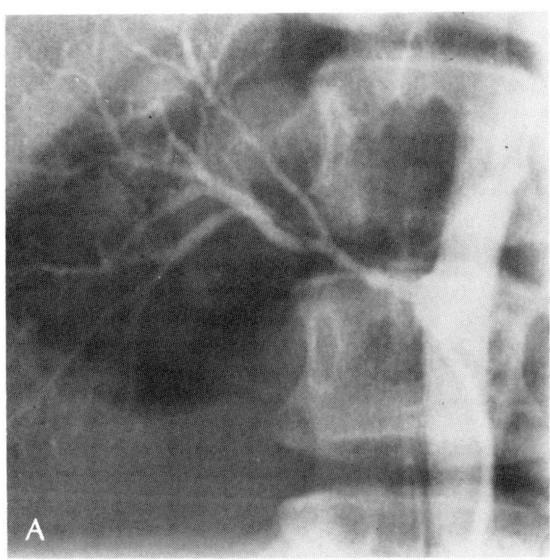

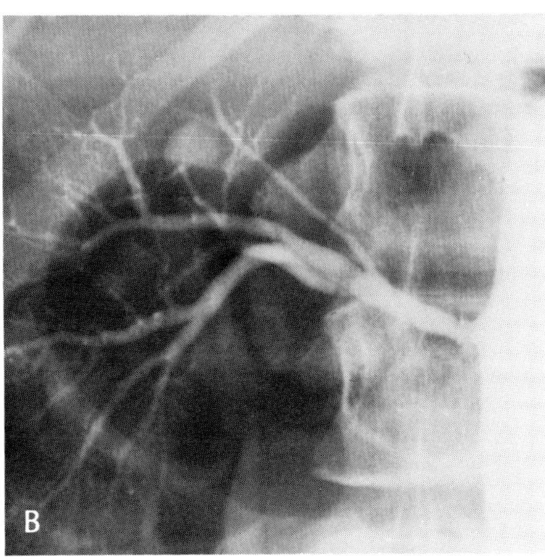

Fig. 20–10. *(A)* Severe spasm of renal artery and branches in an autotransplanted kidney in response to catheter balloon. *(B)* Angiogram after administration of vasodilators shows normal-caliber renal vessels.

case of complete renal-artery occlusion by an intimal dissection, an emergency bypass operation is required.

Plaque Detachment

The detachment of an atherosclerotic plaque with small segmental infarction requires no treatment and is usually of no clinical consequence. Anticoagulants may be given, but their value is not certain.

Arterial Rupture

Rupture of the renal artery is, fortunately, rare. If extravasation of contrast medium is seen, heparin should be reversed immediately with an adequate amount of protamine sulfate. If the balloon is in the renal artery it should be inflated to stop the bleeding, and the patient should undergo immediate surgical exploration.

Arterial Spasm

Spasm of the renal artery is usually secondary to catheter or guide wire manipulation and is particularly common in transplanted kidneys. It cannot be prevented, but if it occurs, a vasodilator, such as nitroglycerin or papaverine, may be injected. Occasionally these spasms can be severe, causing a marked pressure gradient (Fig. 20–10).

Puncture-Site Complications

Complications can occur at the puncture site, as in any other vascular catheterization procedure.

FOLLOWUP

After the procedure, the patient should be admitted to an intensive care unit or monitored closely for the first six to twelve hours, because profound hypotension may follow successful angioplasty. The patients are then discharged without anticoagulants, as the renal blood flow is sufficient to prevent occlusion by a thrombus. However, if there has been an intramural dissection with consequent partial renal-artery occlusion, anticoagulation should be carried out.

The patients are then followed on an outpatient basis. If hypertension recurs, renal angiography should be done to evaluate the dilatation site. If restenosis is seen, pressure measurements should be obtained and the lesion redilated in the same sitting.

In a few cases, patients may require

more than one angioplasty for permanent success.

CONCLUSIONS

Transluminal angioplasty is reducing the need for many open operations, including those on the renal arteries. It has been found especially useful for treating fibromuscular hyperplasia and has a somewhat lower success rate for atherosclerotic lesions. Even when it fails, little has been lost, because its use does not preclude surgery.

REFERENCES

1. Schwarten, D.E.: Percutaneous transluminal renal angioplasty. Urol. Radiol. (in press).
2. Brewster, D.C.: Surgical management of renovascular hypertension. AJR, *135*:963, 1980.
3. Grüntzig, A., and Hopff, H.: Perkutane Rekanalization chronischer arterieller Verschlusse mit einem neuen Dilatationskatheter: Modification der Dotter-Technik. Deutsch. Med. Wschr., *99*:2502, 1974.
4. Millan, V.G., Mast, W.E., and Madias, N.E.: Nonsurgical treatment of severe hypertension due to renal artery intimal fibroplasia by percutaneous transluminal angioplasty. N. Engl. J. Med., *300*:1371, 1979.
5. Grüntzig, A., et al.: Treatment of renovascular hypertension with percutaneous transluminal dilatation of a renal-artery stenosis. Lancet, *1*:801, 1978.
6. Grüntzig, A., Kuhlmann, U., and Vetter, W.: Percutaneous transluminal dilation of atherosclerotic renal artery stenosis. Circulation *58*(II):213, 1978.
7. Tegtmeyer, C.J., et al.: Percutaneous transluminal angioplasty in patients with renal artery stenosis: follow-up studies. Radiology, *140*:323, 1981.
8. Sos, T.: Late follow-up results of renal angioplasty. Presented at the Annual Meeting of the Society of Cardiovascular Radiology, Palm Springs, 1982.
9. Schwarten, D.E., and Gallant, T.E.: Transluminal renal angioplasty. *In* Transluminal Angioplasty. Edited by W.R. Castaneda-Zuniga. New York, Thieme-Stratton, Inc., 1983.
10. Pfeifer, J.R., et al.: Outpatient angiography as an adjunct to vascular surgery practice (abstract). *In* Ambulatory Surgery—Quo Vadis? Eighth Annual Meeting of the Freestanding Ambulatory Surgical Association, Washington, D.C., 1982.
11. Katzen, B.T.: Transluminal angioplasty for renal hypertension. Urol. Times, *10*:1, 1982.

21

Nonoperative Management of Vasculogenic Impotence

WILFRIDO R. CASTAÑEDA-ZUÑIGA, M.D., KEITH W. KAYE, M.D., F.C.S. (S.A.)., F.R.C.S. and KURT AMPLATZ, M.D.

The recent proof of the vascular origin of many cases of impotence[1] has led to the rapid development of various vascular reconstructive procedures to correct the condition, including aortoiliac endarterectomy, hypogastric endarterectomy, and implantation of small vessels directly into the corpora cavernosa.[2-4] Unfortunately, the results are often poor.

One of the most important recent advances in the management of impotence was the development of noninvasive techniques to measure penile blood pressures. Of these, plethysmography and Doppler ultrasound are the most widely used.[5,6] The latter, which measures the systolic blood pressure in the penis, appears to be simpler and more reliable and can produce separate values for the right and left sides of the penis.[7] Normally, the systolic blood pressure in the penis is slightly (< 20 mm Hg) below that in the brachial artery; the normal penile:brachial systolic pressure index (PBI) is 0.961 ± 0.053.[7,8]

Because of the high failure rate of reconstructive vascular procedures, the new techniques of percutaneous transluminal angioplasty have been evaluated for the management of vasculogenic impotence.[9] This procedure can be carried out safely under local anesthesia, and the results can be assessed immediately by measuring the penile blood pressure by Doppler ultrasound. It is most useful in the management of patients with aortoiliac occlusions and has less value in the management of occlusions of the pudendal artery. It probably will not be applicable to the management of penile-artery lesions.

EVALUATION

Outpatient Studies

The workup of a patient suspected of having vasculogenic impotence includes the taking of a sexual and medical history, a physical examination, psychologic testing (e.g., the Minnesota Multiphasic Personality Inventory), nocturnal penile tumescence monitoring, and laboratory analysis (glucose-tolerance test, serum testosterone measurements, and coagultion profile). Noninvasive vascular studies are then performed to identify those patients likely to have abnormal pelvic and internal pudendal arteries. Commonly, men with vasculogenic impotence have penile systolic blood pressures considerably lower than their brachial systolic pressures, often $\geq$ 50 mm Hg.[7] A PBI $\leq$ 0.8 suggests that the impotence is vasculogenic,[8] and these patients are candidates for iliac and pudendal arteriography. Conversely, patients with a PBI > 0.8 are not candidates. Such pressure studies are important even when one is reasonably certain that the impotence is vasculogenic, because it is difficult to determine the hemodynamic significance of obstructive lesions by angiography and because they provide a baseline against which to assess postprocedure results.

Inpatient Studies

The patient is admitted to the hospital early in the morning and seen by a cardiovascular radiologist, who explains that the angiogram will be performed under local anesthesia and mild sedation through the left axillary artery to show the pelvic vascular anatomy. If major vessels (common iliac, hypogastric, or proximal pudendal arteries) are obstructed, angioplasty can be carried out in the same sitting. If small-vessel obstruction is found, the patient will be referred for possible microsurgical revascularization.

Technique. In patients suspected of having aortoiliac obstruction, a left axillary approach should be used, since it facilitates selective catheterization of both iliac and hypogastric arteries. With the femoral approach, only the contralateral hypogastric artery can be entered with the balloon catheters currently available.

Although conventional arteriographic techniques may disclose obstruction in the aortoiliac region, more selective techniques may be needed to demonstrate obstructions of the pudendal or penile arteries. In 1978, Michal and Pospichal described a technique for retrograde phal-

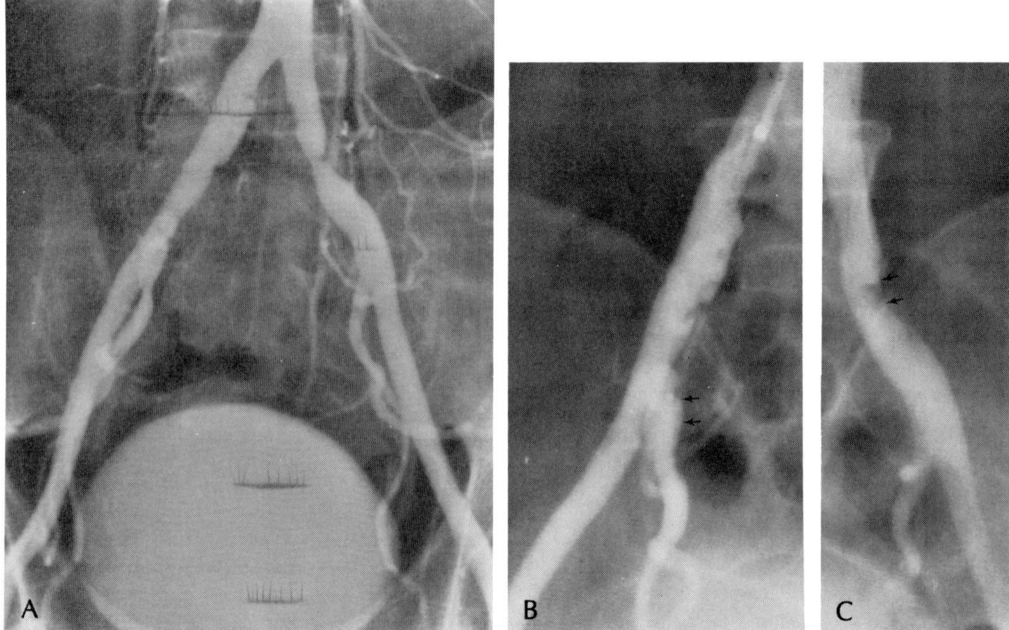

Fig. 21–1. *(A)* Pelvic arteriogram shows severe narrowing of the left common iliac artery, slight narrowing of the right common iliac artery, and a localized stenosis of the right internal iliac artery. *(B)* Iliac arteriogram after angioplasty shows increase in caliber of right common and internal iliac arteries *(arrows)*. *(C)* The caliber of the left common iliac artery also has been increased by angioplasty *(arrows)*.

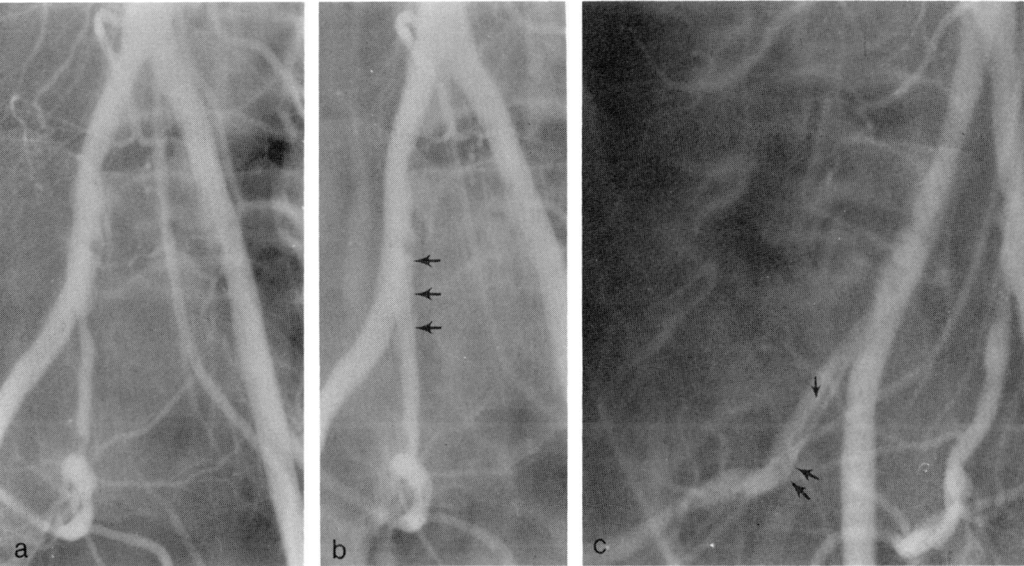

Fig. 21–2. *(A)* Pelvic arteriogram shows atherosclerotic narrowing of right common iliac artery and two narrow areas in right internal iliac artery; the left internal iliac artery is not well demonstrated. *(B)* Right posterior oblique arteriogram after angioplasty shows increased caliber of dilated areas in right common and internal iliac arteries *(arrows)*. *(C)* Left posterior oblique arteriogram after angioplasty shows an intimal flap *(small arrow)* and increased caliber of the distal lesion in the right internal iliac artery *(large arrows)*. Note severe narrowing of the origin of the left internal iliac artery at right of radiograph.

loarteriography that also allows determination of the amount of flow needed for erection.[10]

After systemic heparinization, pullback pressures are measured across the angiographically demonstrated lesion with a 5F catheter to document the pressure gradient. For transluminal angioplasty, the small catheter is then removed, and, over an exchange guide wire, a Grüntzig balloon catheter of the caliber of the normal artery proximal to the stenosis is introduced. Once across the area of stenosis, it is inflated to 4 to 6 atmospheres for 1 to 3 minutes until the hourglass deformity of the balloon disappears. If both the hypogastric and common iliac arteries are narrowed, the hypogastric artery should be dilated first, since it requires a smaller balloon catheter (Figs. 21–1 and 21–2). The balloon catheter is then removed, and penile pressures are recorded by Doppler ultrasound. If there is no gradient, a postangioplasty angiogram is performed; and if its appearance is satisfactory, the procedure is terminated. If there is a residual pressure gradient, the balloon catheter is reintroduced and reinflated until the gradient disappears or diminishes significantly. However, manipulation of catheters and guide wires through a recently dilated segment should be avoided, because embolic complications or local dissections may result. No postprocedure anticoagulants are needed routinely.

RESULTS

In our series of three cases, two patients had adequate documentation of vascular obstruction by ultrasound before transluminal angioplasty. Both patients reported return of normal sexual function for at least 18 months afterward. In the one case in which penile pressure had not been measured, there was only partial improvement in sexual function.[9]

Although only a few patients have been treated by transluminal angioplasty for the relief of impotence at our institution and elsewhere, the available long-term results are encouraging. It may be postulated that normal sexual function will be permanently restored in patients so treated for vasculogenic impotence provided the obstructive disease does not involve the pudendal or penile arteries, which are not readily accessible. As technical skills and technology improve, it may become possible to treat lesions in small arteries as well.

Fewer than 5% of patients suffered complications, and these were usually minor, such as hematoma formation at the puncture site. Major complications that may necessitate emergency surgery, such as rupture of a vessel, occur in fewer than 0.5% of patients.

CONCLUSIONS

Transluminal angioplasty is a new approach to vascular lesions, and the indications, contraindications, and risks of complications are still evolving. Application of the technique to the treatment of vasculogenic impotence is in its preliminary stages, and thus we have been admitting the patient early in the morning for the procedure and discharging him from the hospital the next day. Some medical centers are now performing angiography on an outpatient basis,[11] and with further experience we think it may be possible to perform angiography and angioplasty for vasculogenic impotence in hospital-based outpatient units, with the patient being released after 8 to 12 hours of observation.

REFERENCES

1. Zorgniotti, A.W. (ed.): Vasculogenic Impotence. 2nd Ed. Springfield, Charles C Thomas, 1980.
2. Michal, V., Kramer, R., and Pospichal, J.: Femoropudendal bypass, internal iliac thrombo-endarterectomy and direct arterial anastomosis to the cavernous body in the treatment of erectile impotence. Bull. Soc. Int. Chir., *33*:343, 1974.
3. Waterhouse, R.K., and Laungani, G.: Results of corpus cavernosum revascularization in vasculogenic impotence. *In* Vasculogenic Impotence. 2nd Ed. Edited by A.W. Zorgniotti. Springfield, Charles C Thomas, 1980.
4. Leeven, H.H.: Experience with techniques utilized to revascularize the penis in vasculogenic impotence. *In* Vasculogenic Impotence. 2nd Ed. Edited by A.W. Zorgniotti. Springfield, Charles C Thomas, 1980.
5. Britt, D.B., Kemmerer, W.T., and Robison, J.R.: Penile blood flow determination by mercury strain-gauge plethysmography. Invest. Urol., *8*:673, 1971.
6. Abelson, D.: Diagnostic value of the penile pulse and blood pressure: a Doppler study of impotence in diabetics. J. Urol., *113*:636, 1975.
7. Montague, D.K., James, R., and DeWolfe, V.: Diagnostic screening for vasculogenic impotence. *In* Vasculogenic Impotence. Edited by A.W. Zorgniotti and G. Rossi. Springfield, Charles C Thomas, 1978.
8. Engel, G., Burnham, S.J., and Carter, M.F.: Penile blood pressure in the evaluation of erectile impotence. Fertil. Steril. *30*:682, 1978.
9. Castaneda-Zuniga, W.R., et al.: Transluminal angioplasty for the treatment of vasculogenic impotence. AJR, *139*:371, 1982.
10. Michal, V., and Pospichal, J.: Phalloarteriography in the diagnosis of erectile impotence. World J. Surg., *2*:239, 1978.
11. Pfeifer, J.R., et al.: Outpatient angiography as an adjunct to vascular surgery practice. Presented at the 8th Annual Meeting of the Freestanding Ambulatory Surgical Association, Washington, D.C., 1982.

Section VII

Surgical Procedures

22

Percutaneous Renal Biopsy: Indications, Techniques, and Considerations of the Risk:Benefit Ratio in the Ambulatory Setting

ALFONSO CAMPOS, M.D., and ROBERT L. VERNIER, M.D.

Percutaneous renal biopsy was introduced in 1944 by Alwall[1] and first used systematically in the study of kidney disease by Iversen and Brun.[2] Modification of the original technique and introduction of the modified Franklin–Silverman needle[3] led to application of the method throughout the world, and renal biopsy is now a safe and essential part of the management of patients with renal disease. The technique offers invaluable aid in the diagnosis, and has contributed to the understanding of the causes, pathogenesis, natural history, and forms of treatment of many kidney diseases. Its value depends on the type of disease, the adequacy and quality of preparation of the sample, and the availability of a competent and experienced pathologist.

Traditionally, percutaneous renal biopsy has been an inpatient procedure because it carries a risk of renal bleeding. However, we have performed renal biopsy in older children in the ambulatory surgical unit of our hospital, observed the patients for 8 hours, and then discharged them home for an additional 24 hours of bed rest. The cost-effectiveness of such an approach must be weighed against the potential additional risks, and only low-risk patients should be selected. Typical patients in this category include cooperative older children and young adults who do not have bleeding disorders, vascular disease, or hypertension. The quality of supervision provided by the family and their reliability as observers are also important factors.

INDICATIONS

There are differences of opinion regarding the indications for a renal biopsy, but in every case the potential benefits to the patient must outweigh the risks involved.

Hematuria

Microscopic hematuria is a common isolated finding in otherwise asymptomatic patients, and in many instances, it is transient. Because acute poststreptococcal glomerulonephritis is still one of the most common causes of transient microscopic hematuria, it remains an important differential consideration, especially in children. Evidence of streptococcal infection (elevated anti-DNAase B titer or streptozyme test) and transient hypocomplementemia strongly suggest the diagnosis. Idiopathic hypercalciuria should also be considered in the differential diagnosis; an elevated urinary calcium:creatinine ratio will give a clue to the correct diagnosis.[4]

Other studies of persistent hematuria should also be selected to rule out urinary-tract infection, glomerulonephritis, renal cystic disease, anatomic abnormalities, familial nephritis, lithiasis, hematologic disorders, and bleeding diatheses. Cystoscopy should not be part of the routine evaluation of microscopic hematuria in children, because tumors are an exceedingly rare cause of hematuria in this population; but obviously malignancy of the bladder must be excluded in older patients. If, after the proper studies, the cause of hematuria is still uncertain, regular followup is all that is indicated provided that proteinuria is absent and the renal function and blood pressure are normal.

Should the isolated microscopic hematuria persist for more than a year, it may be important to know, for reasons of insurability, military service, parental anxiety, etc., whether the patient has a potentially serious disease. Under these circumstances, examination of a kidney biopsy specimen may allow definitive diagnosis of important diseases such as IgA nephropathy or hereditary nephritis and provide important prognostic information. In these circumstances, the finding of a "normal" kidney, after thorough study, may also have important implications for the patient.

Microscopic hematuria associated with proteinuria almost invariably signals glomerulonephritis, in which case renal biopsy is usually indicated.

Macroscopic hematuria in the adult patient usually suggests urinary-tract malignancy, lithiasis, or infection. In children and young adults, however, IgA–IgG nephropathy is the single most common cause of intermittent gross hematuria. In this syndrome, gross hematuria is usually preceded by an upper-respiratory infection or vigorous physical activity. The finding of segmental and focal glomerulonephritis with diffuse mesangial deposits of IgA in a biopsy specimen by immunofluorescence microscopy establishes the diagnosis. Alport's syndrome of hereditary nephritis with deafness also commonly presents as recurrent macroscopic hematuria and, in most instances, hematuria is also present in other members of the family. Again, the diagnosis is made by renal biopsy.

Proteinuria

In the older child and the young adult, the most frequent cause of asymptomatic proteinuria is orthostatic proteinuria, a normal variant that should be ruled out in the initial evaluation. Persistent asymptomatic proteinuria is often the first sign of many diseases such as membranoproliferative glomerulonephritis, membranous nephropathy, congenital anomalies, chronic pyelonephritis, hereditary nephritis, and polycystic disease. The initial evaluation should include urine cultures, creatinine clearances, 24-hour urinary protein excretion, complement levels, and radiographic studies. Persistent significant proteinuria in a child may be the prodrome of nil-lesion nephrotic syndrome.

Nephrotic syndrome is a clinical state rather than a single entity and is associated with a wide spectrum of pathologic changes, ranging from nil lesion, focal sclerosis, and membranous nephropathy, to membranoproliferative glomerulonephritis. It may be primary or idiopathic, or secondary to systemic diseases such as systemic lupus erythematosus, anaphylactoid purpura, malignancy, diabetes, and amyloidosis. There are several indications for a kidney biopsy in these patients. In children younger than 6 years, nil lesion is the most common pathologic finding (90%), and biopsy is not necessary if the patient responds to a trial of adrenocorticosteroids. If the patient has low complement levels or has unusual manifestations, biopsy is indicated to establish the pathologic diagnosis. In adults, renal biopsy is indicated in almost every instance unless the cause is apparent from the extrarenal manifestation, such as in diabetes mellitus.

Other Indications

In patients with renal insufficiency, it is often difficult to determine whether the renal disease is acute or chronic. Normal-sized or enlarged kidneys suggest an acute cause of renal failure. If, by clinical and laboratory evaluation, the cause of the renal insufficiency is not clear and obstruction is excluded, renal biopsy may be useful in the diagnosis, prognosis, and management of conditions such as glomerulonephritis, tubulointerstitial nephritis, Goodpasture's syndrome, Wegener's granulomatosis, and polyarteritis nodosa. Renal biopsy may also be valuable as a guide to prognosis in acute renal failure, such as in acute tubular necrosis when the condition continues for more than three or four weeks and after recovery from oliguria in patients with an atypical course when the diagnosis remains doubtful.

Anaphylactoid purpura, a form of small-vessel vasculitis, characteristically presents with purpuric skin rash, arthritis, and abdominal pain. Approximately 60% of the patients have renal involvement that may range from microscopic hematuria or proteinuria to nephrotic syndrome and acute renal insufficiency. If only microscopic hematuria is present, with otherwise normal renal function, renal biopsy is not indicated. Should decreased renal function, gross hematuria, or proteinuria occur, biopsy is recommended to assess the severity and prognosis of the renal involvement. Similarly, renal biopsy may be valuable in confirming the diagnosis of large-vessel vasculitis in suspected polyarteritis, Wegener's granulomatosis, and other systemic diseases.

In systemic lupus erythematosus, approximately 85% of the patients present with involvement of several organs other than the kidneys, although approximately half have urinary abnormalities. Eventually, the majority of patients develop renal manifestations. Because nephritis is the major cause of death, examination of renal tissue is necessary to classify and quantitate the renal lesions as a guide to therapy.

EVALUATION AND PREPARATION

The indications and possible value of the renal biopsy in management must be discussed with the patient or the parents of the child. The possible complications should be discussed and informed consent obtained. A detailed explanation of the procedure usually relieves the anxiety of the patient. The older child should be given the opportunity to practice his or her role in the procedure before the biopsy. Younger children may need simple reassurance, and the presence of the parents during the procedure may ease the child's anxiety.

A detailed medical history should be obtained, with special attention to evidence of bleeding disorders. In the physical examination, skeletal abnormalities or local skin disorders that might preclude placing the patient in the prone position must be ruled out. The blood pressure should be normal. The necessary laboratory studies include a complete blood and platelet count, prothrombin and partial thromboplastin times, and serum creatinine measurement. A urinalysis is performed to obtain baseline information for the evaluation of postprocedure hematuria. The urine should be sterile. Study of the size, configuration, and location of the kidneys is mandatory.

Patients are given nothing by mouth for 4 to 8 hours before the procedure. Sedation is given 30 to 60 minutes beforehand, but oversedation must be avoided because, except in the very young child, the patient's cooperation in suspending breathing is necessary. In children, we use meperidine hydrochloride (Demerol) 1–2 mg per kilogram and promethazine hydrochloride (Phenergan) 1 mg per kilogram or pentobarbital sodium (Nembutal) intramuscularly. In adults, meperidine and local anesthesia are usually adequate.

CONTRAINDICATIONS

Absolute contraindications are a solitary kidney or a bleeding diathesis. Infection and a perinephric abscess are also contraindications because of the risk of causing septicemia. Percutaneous renal biopsy should not be considered for patients with mass lesions (see Chapter 19). The risk of bleeding is also increased in patients with polycystic kidney disease, and we believe that a surgical approach to biopsy is preferable in patients with questionable and uncorrectable clotting:bleeding indices.

Relative contraindications include severe azotemia and hypertension, because they increase the risk of postprocedure bleeding.[5,6] The uremic patient should be dialyzed before the biopsy. Good blood-pressure control is also mandatory. Although some authors recommend kidney biopsy in patients with end-stage renal failure,[7,8] we believe that small, fibrotic, and scarred kidneys are more likely to bleed after the procedure. In addition, the yield of information that might change the management of the patient is likely to be minimal.

IMAGING METHODS

Accurate location of the kidney is essential to the success of a renal biopsy. Several methods, such as radiography, fluoroscopy, radionuclide imaging, and ultrasound, have been used for this purpose,[3,9–12] with surprisingly similar rates of success and complications.[13] It is best that the operator be allowed to choose the method with which he or she feels most confident, although the added cost, radiation exposure, and inconvenience of some of the methods limit their value.

Ultrasound

Since its introduction in 1975, this noninvasive and highly accurate method has gained wide acceptance and is especially helpful because the visibility of the kidney does not depend on the extent of renal function.[11,12] Using a B-mode scanner, and with the patient prone with a renal bag under the abdomen, the lower pole of the kidney is delineated in both axes during deep inspiration and marked on the skin directly over the kidney. The depth of the kidney in relation to the skin is determined by lateral scanning. Ultrasound also permits determination of the optimal angle for the biopsy needle. Scanning may be continued during the puncture, although there are certain disadvantages.

Fluoroscopy

In this method, the kidneys are imaged after intravenous injection of contrast medium. The advantage of the method is real-time imaging. The disadvantages are the radiation exposure of the patient and operating room staff, the longer operating time and higher costs, and the possibility of significant allergic reactions. The method should not be used in patients with renal failure (serum creatinine level $>$ 2 mg per deciliter), because opacification will be poor and because there is a significantly increased risk of acute renal failure after injection of contrast medium in patients whose renal function is already compromised.

With the patient prone, the skin is cleaned, and, using an aseptic technique, a radiopaque marker is placed on the patient's back and moved, under fluoroscopic observation, until it is over the desired puncture site. The biopsy needle is then inserted and advanced toward the kidney during fluoroscopic monitoring. Once the needle has reached the renal cortex, it and the kidney will move together.

Radiography

Since 1955, we have used either an intravenous pyelogram (IVP) or a tomogram for locating the kidneys and have had very little operative morbidity.[14] The patient is placed prone with a sandbag or a tight roll of blankets beneath the umbilicus between the rib cage and pelvic bones; this eliminates lordosis and creates radiologic topography that can be transferred accurately to the patient's back by palpation of bones and by measurement. The roll also may support the kidney and prevent its movement away from the biopsy needle. The radiographic studies are done at the end of inspiration.

PUNCTURE METHOD

We usually prefer to biopsy the left kidney unless splenomegaly is present. The lower pole is the target area. With the patient prone as described, the lumbar spinous processes, twelfth rib, posterior iliac crest, and sacrospinalis muscles are outlined on the skin with a marker pen (Fig. 22–1). Then, using the IVP films, the distance from the lower pole of the kidney to the lumbar spinous processes and posterior iliac crest is measured and transferred to the patient's back. Usually, the biopsy site falls at the angle formed by the intersection of the twelfth rib and the lateral border of the sacrospinalis muscle.

Using an aseptic technique, the skin is cleaned and draped, and the site selected for the biopsy is infiltrated with intradermal, subcutaneous, and intramuscular injection of procaine. A small incision is made in the skin with the point of a scalpel blade. The location and depth of the kidney are then determined using an exploring needle; we recommend a long No. 22 spinal needle, which is introduced at the biopsy site, parallel to the spine and in a slightly cephalad direction, at an angle of 15–20° (Fig. 22–2*A*). Once the needle is in the subcutaneous tissues, it should be advanced a few millimeters with each breath, as the patient holds his breath on inspiration, to avoid renal laceration. The subcutaneous and muscle layers can be felt independently by the experienced operator, and the distinct renal mass is recognizable on contact. Occasionally, one can feel a "pop" as the needle goes through the renal capsule. More characteristically, the arc or swinging of the exploring needle with each breath (Fig. 22–2*B*) and the vibration of the needle with the pulsation of the kidney are useful indications that the needle has reached the kidney.[3] These motions of the needle should cease if it is withdrawn a few millimeters. The probing needle is then removed while procaine is injected along the track, and the depth of the kidney is measured. It is important not to insert the biopsy needle until the kidney has been identified with reasonable certainty with the probe.

We prefer the Vim–Silverman biopsy needle as modified by Franklin. The 11.4-cm needle is used for the average adult patient; for obese patients, the 15.8-cm needle is recommended. For older children, the 7.8-cm needle is used. The Tru-Cut disposable needle (Travenol), available in different sizes, may also be used.

The biopsy needle is inserted along the same track, and to the same depth, as the probing needle. The needle and its stylet

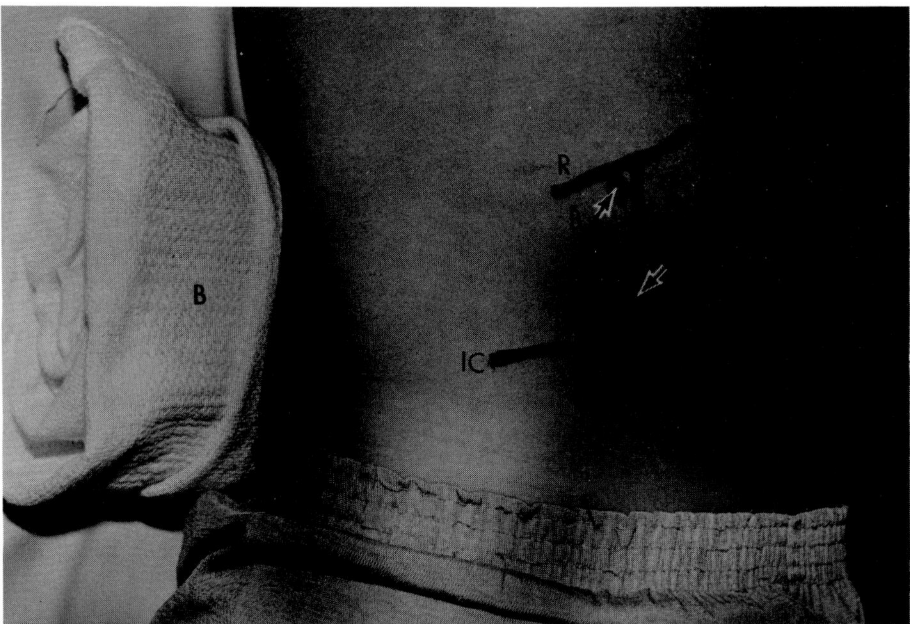

Fig. 22–1. Lateral view of patient, with lines indicating position of twelfth rib (R), iliac crest (IC), paraspinus muscle bundle (PS), vertebral processes (V), and biopsy site (Bx). These markings were developed from the intravenous pyelogram (IVP). Note blanket roll (B) protruding from under flank.

are slowly advanced (Fig. 22–3*A*) as described until the tip penetrates the renal capsule, as determined by the characteristic movements. Then the needle is embedded just 1 to 2 mm within the kidney, the stylet is removed, and the cutting needle is inserted until a characteristic resistance is met. If resistance is not found, it means that the outer needle has not penetrated the kidney; the stylet should be replaced and the needle redirected. At the time of the actual procedure, the patient is asked to hold his breath at the end of inspiration. Then, in rapid sequence, with the outer needle being held with the left hand at the skin level, the cutting needle is pushed with the right hand into the kidney with a sharp, rapid movement (Fig. 22–3*B*). The inner needle is then held steady while the outer needle is advanced 1 to 2 cm, cutting off the tissue sample (Fig. 22–3*C*). The whole needle is removed, with the outer needle covering the cutting prongs.

In the child who is unable to cooperate, each movement of the needle should be made during the expiratory phase. If the child is sleeping, the respiration movements are usually shallow; and if the biopsy is done rapidly and skillfully, the risk of capsular tear is small.[14,15]

We recommend that two biopsy cores be obtained to provide enough tissue for the different microscopic studies. Multiple attempts to puncture the kidney should be avoided, since the risk of injury probably increases with frustration. It is usually wise to allow the patient to be observed for 24 hours and then to try again the next day.

HANDLING OF TISSUE

The biopsy sample should be inspected for adequacy. With a hand lens or a dissecting microscope, glomeruli can be identified as red, flower-like blushes on the surface of the biopsy core (Fig.

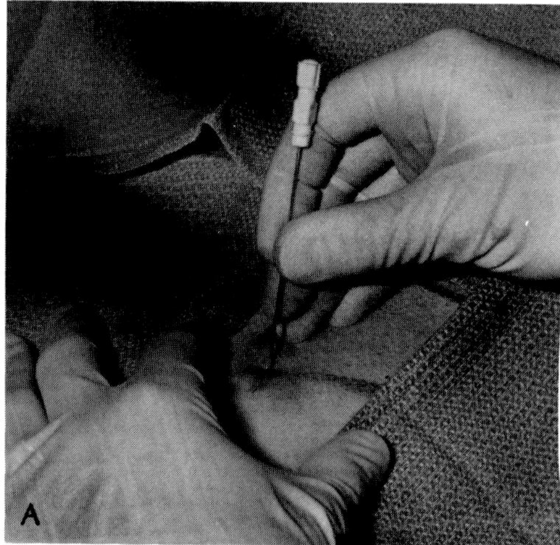

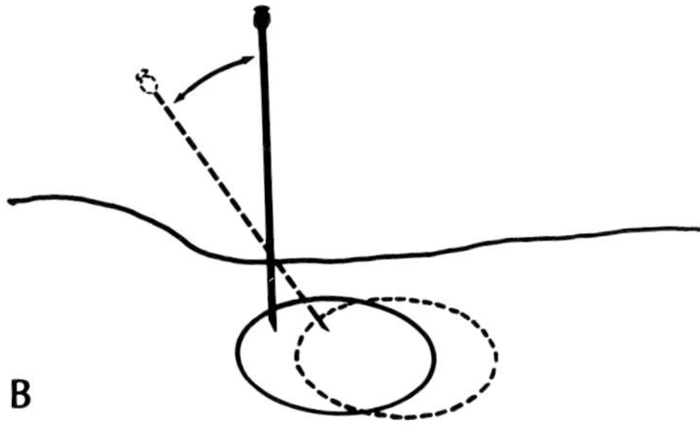

Fig. 22–2. Determining position and depth of kidney. *(A)* Introduction of No. 22 spinal exploring needle. *(B)* Diagram of cephalad motion of exploratory needle *(dotted line)* as the kidney moves with inspiration.

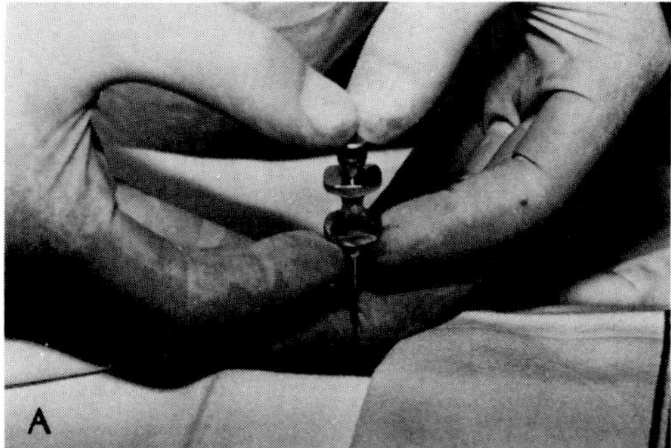

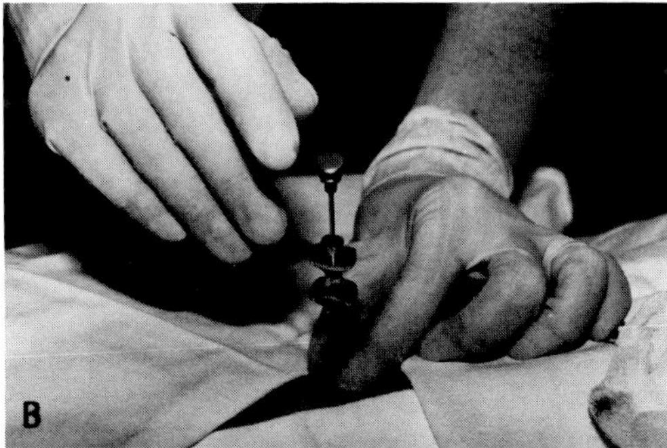

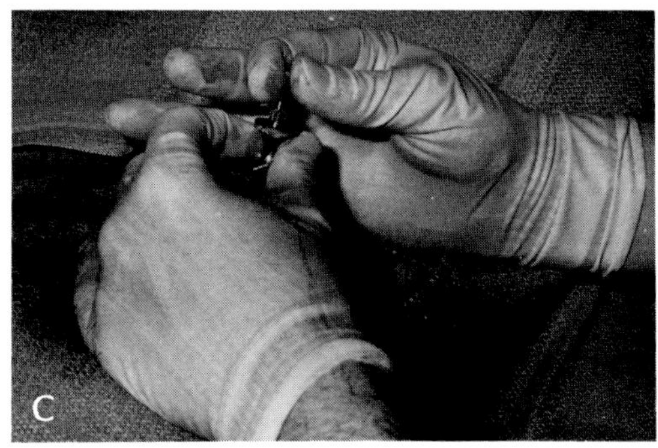

Fig. 22–3. Steps in insertion of biopsy needle and cutting specimen. *(A)* Biopsy needle and stylet are introduced through same track and to the same depth as exploratory needle. *(B)* Cutting needle is about to be advanced into renal parenchyma. *(C)* While cutting needle is held steady, outer needle is advanced over biopsy needle to cut off tissue specimen.

22–4).[16] At least 10 glomeruli must be present to minimize sampling error.

It is no longer reasonable to study the renal biopsy specimen by light microscopy alone; arrangements must be made in advance with the pathologist and the tissue divided into portions for light, immunofluorescence, and electron microscopy. Using a sharp razor blade on a wax board, 0.5–1-mm samples are taken from each end of the core for electron microscopy. The central core is then either divided longitudinally for immunofluorescence and light microscopy or a second biopsy core is obtained and the two samples divided appropriately. If little tissue is obtained, the nephrologist must decide which techniques are most likely to provide the needed information.

POSTPROCEDURE MANAGEMENT

Vital signs are monitored every 15 minutes for 1 hour, every 30 minutes for 2 hours if stable, and every hour for 4

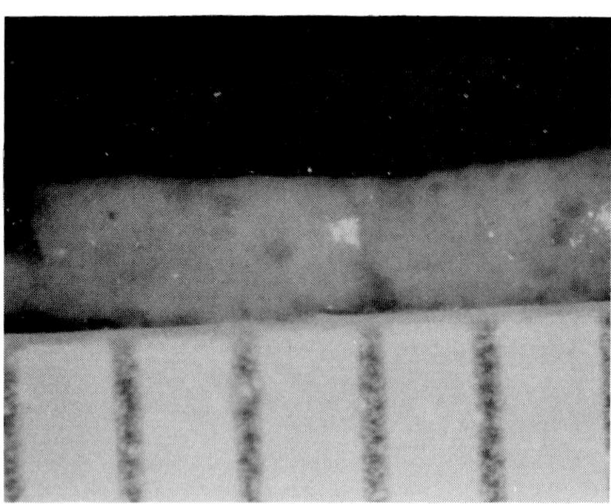

Fig. 22–4. Biopsy specimen as viewed with dissecting microscope. Note surface glomeruli distributed over specimen as small circular profiles. Ruler lines at bottom are 1 mm apart. (From Shapiro, R.S., et al.: Dial. Transplant., 6:46, 1977.)

hours. Patients should be kept supine for 12 to 24 hours but may be discharged to their homes 8 hours after the procedure if stable for further bed rest. All voided urine should be collected and portions kept for measurement of hematuria. Diuresis with oral fluids should be encouraged, and analgesics should be avoided, as they may mask a complication. The abdomen should be examined frequently for the first several hours, with auscultation of the flank and abdomen to detect any arteriovenous fistula. Pain, gross hematuria, fever, tachycardia, or hypotension should be reported immediately to the physician. The hemoglobin level and hematocrit should be obtained 6 hours after the procedure and before discharge. Body contact sports, diving, and other vigorous physical activity should be avoided for two weeks.

COMPLICATIONS

Microscopic hematuria and mild abdominal and flank pain that disappear within 24 hours are common and generally are not considered complications.[17–20] Bleeding manifested by gross hematuria or perinephric hematoma occurs in approximately 5% of cases.[5,6,14,15,17,21] Approximately 1 to 3% of patients undergoing percutaneous renal biopsy require a blood transfusion, and 0.3% require operation, often with nephrectomy. The frequency of hemorrhagic complications parallels the blood urea nitrogen level and the degree of hypertension.[5,6,17] Most of the time, the bleeding is apparent within 24 hours. Bleeding associated with a > 4% decrease in the hematocrit is likely to cause significant complications.

Gross hematuria usually responds to conservative management such as bed rest and transfusion as indicated and usually ceases within 24 hours. If it is accompanied by clots and renal colic, intravenous fluids and analgesics are recommended.

With followup by ultrasound or computed tomography, it has been found that perirenal hematoma is more common after biopsies than had been recognized.[21] Nevertheless, clinically significant hematomas occur in only 1.5 to 5% of cases.[5,17,21]

Arteriovenous fistulas occur in as many as 15% of patients according to the findings of angiography, but clinically significant fistulas occur in < 1% of cases.[17,22] Most are small and heal spontaneously within a few months. Those that persist may cause hypertension, hemorrhage, or heart failure and require surgical repair in most cases.

Other rare complications are renal and perirenal infections and punctures of other organs, such as the pancreas, liver, bowel, and spleen.

In large series, the mortality rate of renal biopsy is 0.1%.[17,18,23,24] When performed by experienced operators, the usefulness of the procedure clearly outweighs the risks.

CONCLUSIONS

Percutaneous renal biopsy is a safe diagnostic procedure with proven value through experience acquired over the past 30 years. The risks are minimal with carefully selected patients in the hands of an experienced operator. Given the extraordinary costs of hospitalization and the cost-effectiveness of the ambulatory setting, consideration should be given to performing percutaneous renal biopsy in selected patients in this setting.

ACKNOWLEDGMENTS

Supported in part by United States Public Health Service grants NIH #AI10704 and AM07087. The photographic talents of Mr. Marshall Hoff and the secretarial assistance of Ms. Cynthia Dawis are gratefully acknowledged.

REFERENCES

1. Alwall, N.: Aspiration biopsy of the kidney. Acta Med. Scand., *143*:430, 1952.
2. Iversen, P., and Brun, C.: Aspiration biopsy of the kidney. Am. J. Med., *11*:324, 1951.
3. Muehrcke, R.C., Kark, R.M., and Pirani, C.L.: Biopsy of the kidney in the diagnosis and management of renal disease. N. Engl. J. Med., *253*:537, 1955.
4. Moore, E.S., et al.: Idiopathic hypercalciuria in children: prevalence and metabolic characteristics. J. Pediatr., *92*:906, 1978.
5. Carvajal, H.F., et al.: Percutaneous renal biopsy in children: an analysis of complication in 890 consecutive biopsies. Texas Rep. Biol. Med., *29*:3, 1971.
6. Diaz-Buxo, J.A., and Donadio, J.V.: Complications of percutaneous renal biopsy: an analysis of 1000 consecutive biopsies. Clin. Nephrol., *4*:223, 1975.
7. Kropp, K.A., Shapiro, R.S., and Jhunjhunwala, J.S.: Role of renal biopsy in end stage renal failure. Urology, *12*:631, 1978.
8. Curtis, J.J., et al.: Evaluation of percutaneous renal biopsy in advanced renal failure. Nephron, *17*:259, 1976.
9. Mertz, J.H.O., Lang, E., and Klingerman, J.J.: Percutaneous renal biopsy utilizing unifluoroscopy monitoring. J. Urol., *95*:618, 1966.
10. Tully, R.J., et al.: Renal scan prior to renal biopsy—a method of renal localization. J. Nucl. Med., *13*:544, 1972.
11. Goldberg, B.B., Pollock, M.M., and Kellerman, E.: Ultrasonic localization for renal biopsy. Radiology, *115*:167, 1975.
12. Mailloux, L.U., et al.: Ultrasonic guidance for renal biopsy. Arch. Intern. Med., *138*:438, 1978.
13. Almkuist, R.D., and Buckalew, V.M.: Techniques of renal biopsy. Urol. Clin. North Am., *6*:503, 1979.
14. Vernier, R.L.: Kidney biopsy in the study of renal disease. Pediatr. Clin. North Am., *7*:353, 1960.
15. White, R.H.R.: Observations on percutaneous renal biopsy in children. Arch. Dis. Child., *38*:260, 1963.
16. Shapiro, R.S., Gunning, W.T., and Kropp, K.A.: Identification of adequate renal tissue at the time of biopsy. Dial. Transplant., *6*:46, 1977.
17. Wickre, L.C., and Golper, T.A.: Complications of percutaneous needle biopsy of the kidney. Am. J. Nephrol., *2*:173, 1982.
18. Dodge, W.F., et al.: Percutaneous renal biopsy in children. I. General considerations. Pediatrics, *30*:287, 1962.
19. Kark, R.M., et al.: An analysis of five hundred percutaneous renal biopsies. Arch. Intern. Med., *101*:439, 1958.
20. Muth, R.G.: The safety of percutaneous renal biopsy: an analysis of 500 consecutive cases. J. Urol., *94*:1, 1965.
21. Rosenbaum, R., et al.: Use of computerized tomography to diagnose complications of percutaneous renal biopsy. Kidney Int., *14*:87, 1978.
22. Ekelund, L., and Lindholm, T.: A-V fistula following percutaneous renal biopsy. Acta Radiol. [Diag.], *11*:38, 1971.
23. Karafin, L., Kendall, A.R., and Fleisher, D.S.: Urologic complications in percutaneous renal biopsy in children. J. Urol., *103*:332, 1970.
24. Slotkin, E.A., and Medren, P.O.: Complications of renal biopsy: incidence in 5000 reported cases. J. Urol., *87*:13, 1962.

23

Outpatient Orchidopexy in Children

RICARDO GONZALEZ, M.D.

Testicular maldescent occurs in 2.7% of full-term newborns; and at the age of one year, 0.8% of all males have persistent maldescent.[1] As a result, operations to correct this condition rank among those most frequently performed in children.

In a large proportion of patients, surgical correction of testicular maldescent can be accomplished in the ambulatory surgery unit without overnight hospitalization.[2] This approach has distinct advantages, not only in reducing cost but also in minimizing the psychological trauma to the child. Here, I review the indications and criteria used at the University of Minnesota for selecting patients for outpatient orchidopexy, as well as the surgical technique.

SELECTION OF PATIENTS

One must first determine whether the child has an absent, true undescended, or ectopic testis on one hand or a retractile testis on the other. This distinction is crucial, because in the latter group, an operation must not be performed.

The differential diagnosis of these conditions is based on repeated examinations under conditions conducive to the patient's relaxation and confidence in the examiner. If the gonad can then be palpated and manipulated to the bottom of the scrotum, the diagnosis of retractile testis is confirmed; and nothing else should be done, since after puberty the testis will remain in the scrotum and the fertility potential is normal.[3] It is helpful to remember that as many as 50% of children seen with suspected cryptorchidism in fact have retractile testes. Also, retractile testes are often bilateral, and the peak incidence occurs between the ages of five and six years.[4] If available, data from the neonatal examination are helpful, because true retractile testes must have been in the scrotum at that time, since the cremasteric reflex responsible for retractability is absent before the age of 6 months. In doubtful cases, administration of human chorionic gonadotropin (2,000 IU every other day for 5 doses for children over 2 years of age and 1,000 IU every other day for 5 doses for children between the ages of 1 and 2 years) will produce temporary or permanent descent of retractile testes. If this occurs, no further treatment is necessary. If descent does not occur, a corrective operation should follow shortly in order to take advantage of the temporary enlargement of the gonad and its blood vessels.

CRITERIA FOR OUTPATIENT OPERATION

Having excluded retractile testes, one must decide whether orchidopexy can be performed on an outpatient basis. The following factors must be evaluated:

(1) The location of the testes;
(2) The risk of anesthesia;
(3) The need for other surgical procedures at the same time; and
(4) The cooperation and understanding of the parents.

More than 70% of undescended testes are palpable. For example, Scorer and Farrington[4] reported that 44% of undescended testes are in the high scrotal position and 26% in Brown's pouch, and all these should be easily palpable except in the obese child. Most testes located in the inguinal canal, however, are difficult to palpate. Because many of these cases can be corrected on an outpatient basis, and because ultrasonography can detect approximately 65% of them,[5] this study should be done on all children with nonpalpable testes. Only children whose testes are known to be below the internal inguinal ring are considered for outpatient operations. When the testes cannot be located by ultrasonography, the child should be admitted to the hospital and laparoscopy performed before open exploration.

The second factor that determines whether the procedure can be done on an outpatient basis is the anesthetic risk, which is evaluated both by the surgeon during the initial examination and by the anesthesiologist the day the procedure is scheduled to be performed. The presence of congenital anomalies of the cardiovascular, respiratory, or central nervous system often precludes an outpatient procedure. Although rare, the need for endotracheal intubation does not mandate hospitalization. Less frequently, concomitant chronic or acquired illness must be taken into account. In a healthy child, the preoperative evaluation includes a thorough history, family history, and a physical examination. We confine the laboratory tests to a complete blood count and a urinalysis. If there is reason to suspect a bleeding tendency, coagulation studies should be performed.

A third factor determining the appropriateness of outpatient orchidopexy is the child's need for other major surgical procedures that require hospitalization. However, outpatient orchidopexies can be combined with less extensive surgical procedures, such as contralateral hydrocele repair, circumcision, minor hypospadias repair, etc. I do not hesitate to perform bilateral orchidopexies on an outpatient basis, provided that the location of both testes is known precisely preoperatively.

Finally, the parents should know what to expect in the postoperative period and should be prepared to handle the situation. Telephone consultation with a member of the surgical team should be available 24 hours a day. If the child lives far from the surgical unit, the referring physician should be consulted about his availability and willingness to provide emergency care if required. However, the incidence of serious complications from this operation and from general anesthesia is minute, and any problems can usually be detected by careful assessment before discharge of the child from the recovery area.

TIMING OF THE OPERATION

The objectives of the surgical correction of undescended testes are preservation of fertility, facilitation of early detection of testicular cancer (which is more prevalent in these patients), and prevention of the psychological consequences of an empty scrotum. It is clear that if fertility is to be preserved, the operation must be done before permanent changes occur in the testis; and these begin in the second year of life.[6] On the other hand, the operation should not be performed before the first birthday, since there is a decreasing incidence of maldescent during the first year of life and thus operation may be unnecessary. Consequently, the operation should be performed as soon as possible after the first birthday, and certainly before the age of 2 years. Whether such operations will decrease the chance of malignant transformation of the previously undescended testes remains to be seen.

OPERATIVE TECHNIQUE

The patient is examined by the surgeon or the referring pediatrician the day before the operation, and blood and urine samples are obtained. All fluids and solid food are withheld beginning at midnight for an early-morning procedure.

The objectives of an orchidopexy are to gain a sufficient length of spermatic cord to place the testis at the bottom of the scrotum, to fix the gonad in this position, and to correct the associated indirect hernia. The technique illustrated here is popular and has been reviewed by others.[7]

After induction of anesthesia, the patient is placed supine on the operating table with the legs spread. The surgical preparation should include the abdomen, genitalia, perineum, and upper thighs. The incision is made along the skin crease in the inguinal area beginning at the pubic tubercle and extending 5 cm laterally. The subcutaneous tissue is divided with diathermy.

If the testis is in Brown's pouch, it will be found after incising Scarpa's fascia. In this case, it is freed from its distal attachments, and the aponeurosis of the external oblique muscle is opened, beginning at the external ring, in a cephalad and lateral direction following the fibers, with care not to injure the ilioinguinal nerve. When the testis is not located subcutaneously, it will be exposed and freed after opening the aponeurosis (Fig. 23–1*A*,*B*,*C*, and *D*). After the cremasteric fascia has been opened, the peritoneal sac is separated from the spermatic vessels and vas deferens with gentle blunt dissection. The use of optical magnification greatly enhances the accuracy of this dissection. Once the sac is free, it is transected, and its distal end is left open. The proximal end is grasped with a hemostat and freed from the spermatic cord up to the point where the vas deferens and the spermatic vessels diverge, where it is suture-ligated with polyglycolic acid (Fig. 23–1*E*,*F*,*G*, and *H*). In the majority of cases of high scrotal and ectopic testes, a sufficient length of cord is obtained by this simple maneuver. When more length is needed, the epigastric vessels, which can be found medial to the internal ring, can be ligated and divided or dissected so that the spermatic cord can be redirected medial to them. I prefer to avoid skeletonizing the cord, because this maneuver carries a high risk of vascular injury. When still more length is required, the spermatic vessels are dissected off the posterior peritoneal surface in a cephalad direction. (When such extensive retroperitoneal dissection has been required, it is advisable to admit the patient to the hospital, since intravenous fluids may be required.) If it was necessary to disrupt the fascia transversalis and the posterior inguinal wall, these are repaired with interrupted sutures of polyglycolic acid lateral to the spermatic vessels and vas deferens (Fig. 23–1*I* and *J*).

The hemiscrotum is distended with a gauze sponge, and a transverse incision is made in the anterior aspect of the lower half. A pocket is created by dissecting between the skin and the dartos (Fig. 23–1*K*). The testis is brought down through a small incision in the dartos muscle, and the tunica vaginalis is opened and attached to the dartos fascia with interrupted sutures of 6–0 Vicryl. The testis is placed in the subcutaneous pouch, and the skin is closed with interrupted sutures of 6–0 chromic catgut. An external suture of 4–0 nylon tied over a cotton brace can be used for further fixation of the testis but is generally unnecessary (Fig. 23–1*L*,*M*,*N*, and *O*). If this

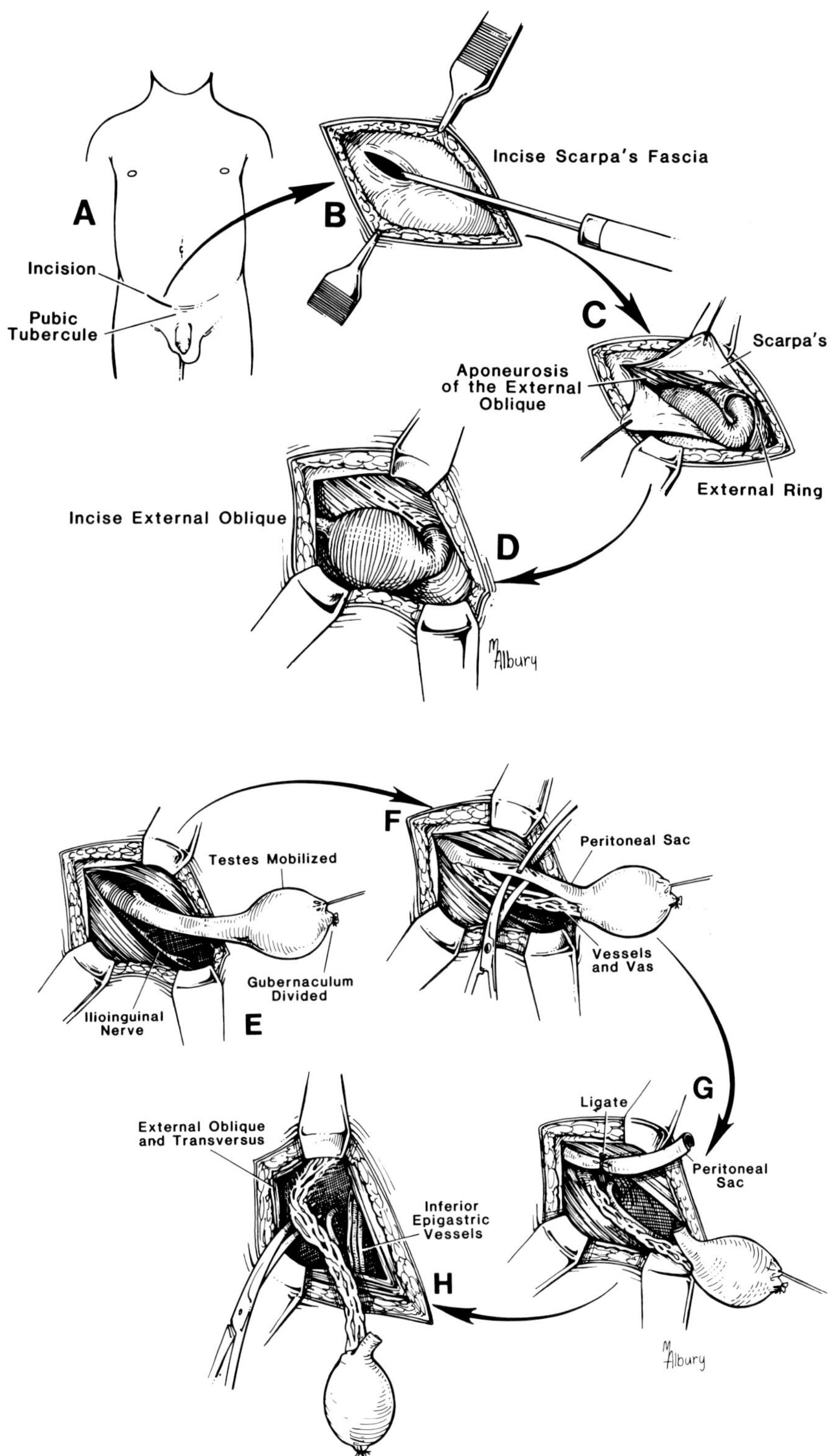

Fig. 23–1. *(A* through *R)* Technique of outpatient orchidopexy.

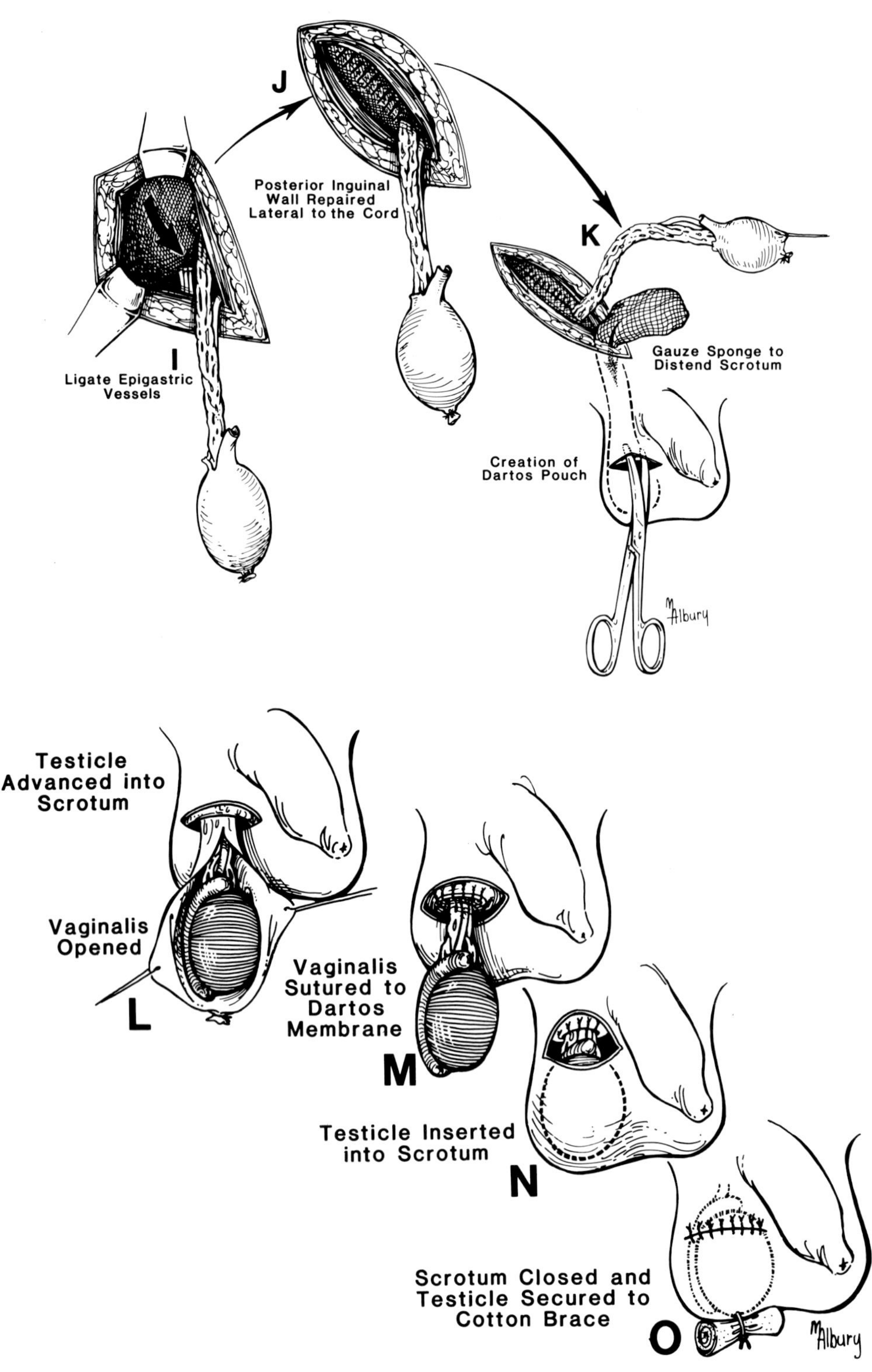

Fig. 23–1. ***(Continued)***

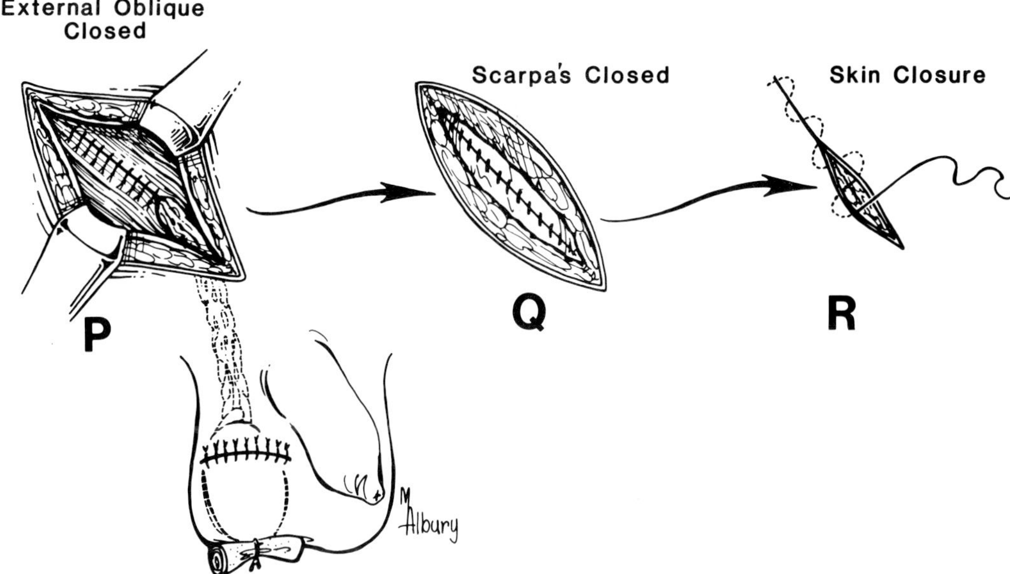

Fig. 23–1. *(Continued)*

suture is used, care should be taken to pass it through the tunica albuginea or the vaginalis and not to injure the epididymis or the vas deferens. The incision and vicinity of the ilioinguinal nerve are infiltrated with 0.25% bupivacaine. The aponeurosis of the external oblique muscle is closed with a running suture of polyglycolic acid, making sure that it is not closed too tightly around the spermatic cord. Scarpa's fascia is closed with a running suture of fine polyglycolic acid. I use an intradermic suture of polyglycolic acid in the skin. The closure is then reinforced with sterile strips (Fig. 23–1*P*,*Q* and *R*).

POSTOPERATIVE CARE

The patient is sent to the recovery room. The parents are allowed to be with the child from this time on.

The parents are instructed to place an antibiotic ointment over the scrotal incision four times a day. No attempt is made to keep the incision or the scrotum dry. If the child is still wearing diapers, a clear plastic adhesive dressing is applied and the parents are advised to change the diapers at approximately 3-hour intervals. This allows the incisions to be exposed to the air for long periods of time during the day. Immersion baths are avoided for one week.

I routinely prescribe acetaminophen for pain, but it is seldom required after the first postoperative day. The child is seen in the clinic one week later and again after three months to confirm the position of the testis. He is examined at yearly intervals thereafter.

RESULTS

Caldamone and Rabinowitz compared 77 outpatient orchidopexies with 459 done in hospitalized children and found no difference in the rates of complications in the two groups.[2] Five per cent of the children undergoing outpatient orchidopexy required overnight hospitalization because of complications that may have been caused by the length of the anesthesia or the extent of the dissection. (Fourteen per cent of the outpatients had either an intra-abdominal or an absent testis, conditions that necessitate considerable dissection.) With the method of patient selection outlined here, we have had no unplanned admissions to the hospital in our smaller series. Nevertheless, even a 5% rate of unexpected admissions is acceptable and certainly does not detract from the merits of outpatient orchidopexy.

CONCLUSIONS

An outpatient operation is possible in approximately 70% of boys with undescended testes. The main advantages of outpatient orchidopexy are a significant reduction in the cost of the operation, as well as minimal psychological trauma for the child.

REFERENCES

1. Scorer, C.G.: The descent of the testes. Arch. Dis. Child., *39*:605, 1964.
2. Caldamone, A.A., and Rabinowitz, R.: Outpatient orchidopexy. J. Urol., *127*:286, 1982.
3. Pari, P., and Nixon, H.H.: Bilateral retractile testes: subsequent effects on fertility. J. Pediatr. Surg., *12*:563, 1977.
4. Farrington, G.H.: The position and retractability of the normal testis in childhood with reference to the diagnosis and treatment of cryptorchidism. J. Pediatr. Surg., *3*:53, 1968.
5. Medrazo, B.L., et al.: Ultrasonographic demonstration of undescended testes. Radiology, *133*:181, 1979.
6. Hedinger, C.H.: Histopathology of undescended testes. Eur. J. Pediatr., *139*:266, 1982.
7. Fonkalsrud, E.W.: Technique for orchiopexy. *In* The Undescended Testis. Edited by E.W. Fonkalsrud and W. Menzel. Chicago, Yearbook Medical Publishers, 1981, p. 195.

24

Percutaneous Suprapubic Cystostomy

DAVID M. CUMES, M.D., and THOMAS A. STAMEY, M.D.

There are two methods of performing suprapubic cystostomy, the percutaneous and the open. The former method is becoming increasingly popular and is superseding the more traditional open method. Percutaneous cystostomy is a relatively minor procedure that can be performed in the urologist's office, emergency room, outpatient surgical suite, or hospital bed to allow temporary urine drainage until more definitive therapy is instituted. In most instances, patients are in urinary retention, which greatly facilitates the procedure.

INDICATIONS

Acute or Chronic Urinary Retention

Percutaneous cystostomy is a safe, effective alternative to urethral Foley catheter drainage, with several advantages. For example, it is usually more comfortable for the male patient and avoids the problems of urethral trauma, urethritis, urethral stricture, prostatitis, and epididymitis. For some patients with long-term urethral drainage, periurethral abscess, diverticulum, and fistula can be added to this list of complications. There are certain instances, moreover, in which suprapubic drainage is clearly preferable to urethral drainage. For example, in some patients, such as those with urethral stricture or bladder-neck contracture, one may be unable to pass a urethral catheter. Here, the definitive treatment of the underlying problem can be deferred until further diagnostic urethrography or endoscopy has been done. With the increasing use of visual urethrotomy, there is merit in deferring urethral dilation and substituting formal urethrotomy of the stricture in its undilated state. Certainly, for the nonurologist, urethral dilation is fraught with hazard, and percutaneous cystostomy is a safer technique that is easily learned by the emergency-room staff. Another example is patients in whom instrumentation of the urethra is undesirable, such as those with acute bacterial prostatitis, urethral trauma and disruption, urethritis, periurethral abscess, or urethral fistula.

Undesirability of Voiding through the Urethra

This is pertinent in patients who have undergone hypospadias repair or urethroplasty, in whom suprapubic diversion is advantageous to facilitate healing.

Monitoring of Residual Urine

This is useful in female patients after urethropexy for stress incontinence and in patients with neurogenic bladders on voiding trials. It is mainly in this group that percutaneous cystostomy is indicated in a female, since in other instances it has no advantage over urethral drainage, which is seldom contraindicated in the female.

Miscellaneous

There are numerous occasions when percutaneous cystostomy could be advantageous. For example, one may wish to use it in boys who are especially prone to urethral trauma because of a small urethral caliber; in patients who are undergoing bladder training before undiversion of a urinary conduit; as part of a urodynamic evaluation to monitor the intravesical pressure; to delay or prevent the bacteriuria that invariably follows the placement of a urethral Foley catheter, especially in the female; or in patients with postprostatectomy bleeding to allow continuous irrigation through the cystostomy and out through the urethral catheter in order to prevent clot retention.

SPECIFIC INDICATIONS FOR OPEN CYSTOSTOMY

There are instances where open cystostomy is preferable to the percutaneous method, such as when percutaneous placement is hazardous because of the risk of bowel perforation and when a large tube is necessary for management of gross hematuria with clots. (The caliber of the Stamey percutaneous tube, especially the 14F tube, will accommodate some bleeding and small clots, but it is inadequate for large clots.) An open procedure is also indicated when long-term suprapubic drainage is envisaged, although even in these patients it is possible to perform a percutaneous cystostomy initially, allow the tract to mature, and then insert a larger catheter after dilation of the tract. An open cystostomy is also indicated when optimal drainage is essential and blockage of a narrow tube could lead to complications.

Open cystostomy, in spite of being more invasive than the percutaneous method, is readily performed on an outpatient basis under local anesthesia and so should not be excluded from the armamentarium of the outpatient surgical suite.

CONTRAINDICATIONS TO PERCUTANEOUS CYSTOSTOMY

The percutaneous approach is contraindicated if it is likely to fail or to be associated with unacceptable morbidity. Thus, it should not be attempted when the bladder cannot be distended to a capacity at which it can be safely located above the pubis by an obturator needle, such as in patients with a contracted bladder secondary to tuberculosis, radiation, or interstitial cystitis. It also should not be done if there is likelihood of bowel adhesions in the lower abdomen that would prevent bowel displacement by distending the bladder or in patients with bladder cancer, in whom malignant cells could spread along the catheter tract. Percutaneous cystostomy is also contraindicated in the patient with a large intravesical prostate, in whom the insertion of the needle could impale the prostate, or in those who have bleeding diatheses or are receiving anticoagulants.

PERCUTANEOUS CYSTOSTOMY TUBES

There are several varieties of tubes available, including the Bonnano, Dow-Corning Cystocath, Argyle-Dover and Stamey suprapubic tubes (Table 24–1). The basic technique of placement is similar for all. Both the Stamey and the Bonnano tubes have a needle obturator that is withdrawn after placement. The Cystocath tube is based on the trocar and cannula principle, with the Silastic Cystocath tube being placed through the trocar once the cannula is removed. If a more generous punch cystostomy is required, the Campbell suprapubic cystostomy punch (Bard) can be used. The trocar will accommodate a 20F Foley catheter.

TABLE 24–1. Suprapubic Cystostomy Tubes

	Stamey	Bonnano	Cystocath	Argyle-Dover
Manufacturer	Cook Urological	Becton-Dickinson	Dow-Corning	Sherwood Medical Industries
Material	Polyethylene	Teflon	Silastic	Polyvinyl chloride
Catheter size	10F, 12F, 14F	8F	8F	12F, 14F, 16F
Introducer	18-, 16-, 15-gauge needle	18-gauge needle	10-gauge trocar and cannula	Trocar and cannula
Design	Malecot with 3 side holes (except 10F)	Pigtail with end hole and 3 side holes	End hole and 2 side holes	End hole and 3 side holes with 5-ml retention balloon and irrigation port
Connector	14F connecting tubing and 2-way stopcock	Rubber tubing and pinch clamp	3-way connector	Funnel integral connector

MATERIALS NEEDED

The technique of inserting the Stamey suprapubic catheter (Fig. 24–1) will be described. The materials required are:

(1) Razor
(2) Sterile gloves
(3) Sterile barrier drapes
(4) Syringes
(5) Needles
(6) 20-gauge spinal needle
(7) 1% lidocaine
(8) No. 15 or No. 11 scalpel blade
(9) Sterile gauze, 2 × 2 and 4 × 4 inches
(10) Needle holder

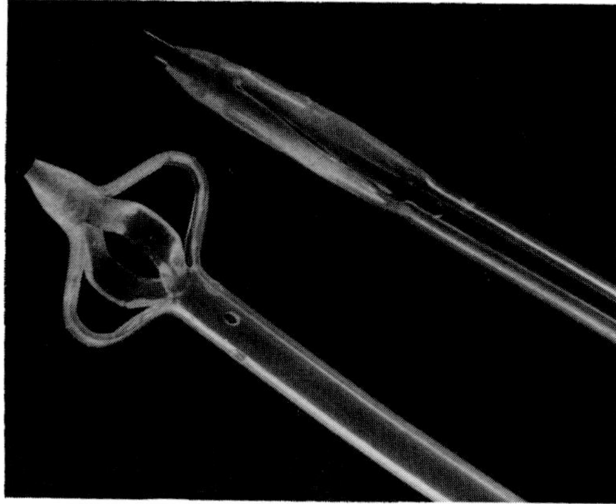

Fig. 24–1. Suprapubic Stamey catheter. *(Above)* Luer-Lok holds wings of Malecot catheter flat during insertion.

(11) Scissors
(12) Urine drainage bag

TECHNIQUE

Patient Position

The patient lies supine, preferably in the Trendelenburg position to displace the bowel loops from the suprapubic region.

Bladder Distention

Often, the patient is already in urinary retention, with the bladder distended above the symphysis pubis. If not, it can be filled in one of two ways.

Retrograde Filling. Usually, it is possible to pass a catheter through the urethra into the bladder and fill the bladder under gravity. If a catheter will not pass because of a urethral stricture or bladder-neck contracture, the catheter tip can be placed just distal to the obstruction and the bladder filled across the stricture by gravity. (This should not be done if there has been any recent urethral trauma or if there is a danger of sepsis from urethral bacteria.) In order to facilitate this maneuver, a Foley catheter with the tip cut off is used. The catheter is inserted until it is just distal to the obstruction. The Foley balloon is inflated gently in the urethra to facilitate one-way flow into the bladder, much the same way as a retrograde urethrogram is performed. If this technique is used, 80 mg of gentamycin should be given intravenously beforehand.

Antegrade Filling. In some instances, it is possible to pass an 18-gauge spinal needle suprapubically into the bladder. The incompletely distended bladder then can be filled by gravity from above.

Insertion of the Cystostomy Tube

The lower abdomen and suprapubic area are shaved and scrubbed. The skin is infiltrated 1 to 2 fingerbreadths above the symphysis pubis with 1% lidocaine. The position and depth of the bladder are ascertained by passing a 20-gauge spinal needle posteriorly through the anesthetized area; if urine does not flow after removal of the obturator, it can be aspirated with the syringe, or the needle can be repositioned. Under no circumstances should an attempt be made to pass the suprapubic tube unless aspiration with the spinal needle has been successful. Once the bladder is known to be immediately beneath the skin, 10 to 20 ml of 1% lidocaine (depending on the size of the patient) should be infiltrated between the skin and the mucosa of the bladder. With adequate anesthesia, the patient feels only pressure during the introduction of the 14F Stamey tube.

The suprapubic Stamey catheter is assembled (see Fig. 24–1). A small skin incision is made 1 to 2 fingerbreadths above the symphysis pubis with the tip of the scalpel, and the catheter assembly is inserted through it using firm pressure and aiming posteriorly and slightly inferiorly. The catheter should be controlled with a hand at skin level, so that when the resistance of the rectus fascia is overcome, the catheter does not plunge uncontrollably into the pelvis (Fig. 24–2). If urine does not flow freely from the end of the tube, correct positioning can be confirmed by aspiration with a syringe. The catheter is advanced an additional 3 to 4 cm into the bladder before withdrawing the needle obturator and allowing reexpansion of the Malecot wings.

The connecting tubing with a Luer-Lok stopcock is attached (Fig. 24–3) and the tube taped in position. We recommend taping it as shown in Figure 24–4. First, the skin and the tube are painted with a tincture of benzoin. While an assistant holds the tube vertically, a 2-inch strip of strong adhesive tape is placed beside the catheter, beginning where the tube emerges from the skin. The tape is pressed around the tube to overlap on itself for approximately 1 cm; this permits catheter movement. The remaining tape is then laid down flat on the abdominal wall. A second piece of tape is attached just distal to the first in the same way.

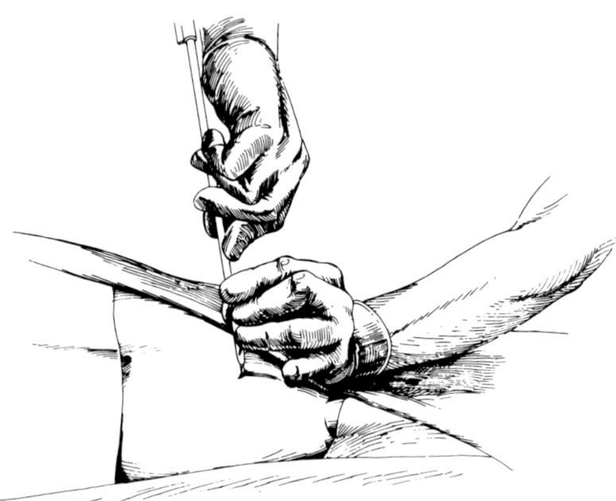

Fig. 24–2. Control of catheter at skin during insertion.

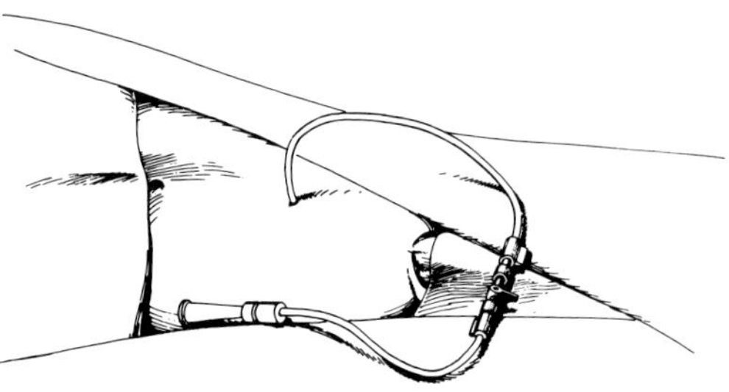

Fig. 24–3. Connecting tubing attached.

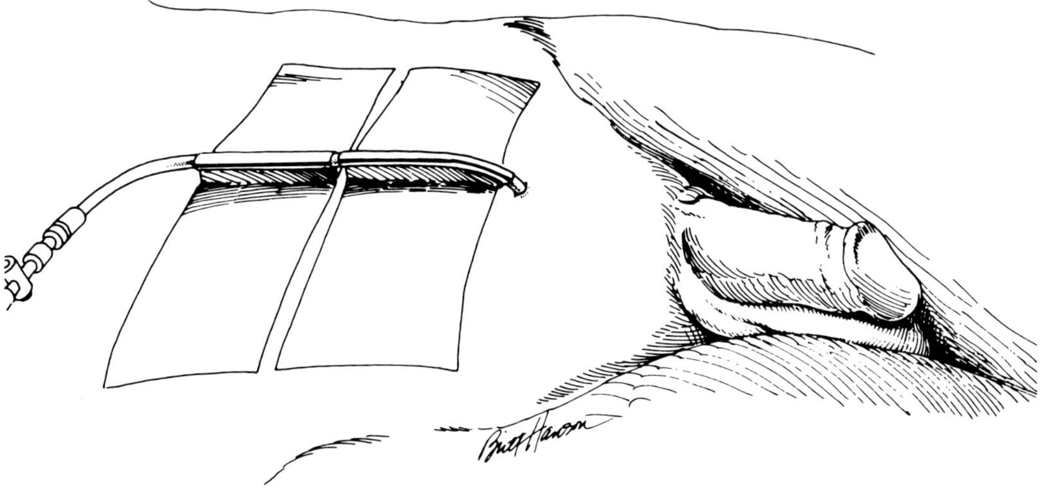

Fig. 24–4. Catheter taped to skin.

SPECIAL TECHNIQUES

If there is a history of lower-abdominal intraperitoneal surgery, it is crucial that the bladder be well distended for the cystostomy. In placing the catheter, it is safer to hug the symphysis pubis to stay away from the bowel.

Changing the Catheter or Replacing it with a Foley Catheter

If the catheter has been in place for several weeks and a good tract is established, a new catheter can usually be passed most simply through the old tract with minimal discomfort to the patient. An alternative is to use a guide wire, which is inserted through the lumen of the Stamey catheter into the bladder. The catheter is removed, leaving the guide wire in place, and a new Stamey catheter is assembled after the terminal end of the needle obturator has been broken off or removed.[1] The blunt end of the needle obturator, with its catheter, is threaded over the guide wire and pushed into the bladder. The guide wire and obturator are removed and the correct position of the catheter confirmed by irrigation.

If the catheter has been in place several weeks and a tract has formed, the tract can be dilated with Bard-Heyman followers over a guide wire or a Bard-Heyman filiform. A Foley catheter of suitable size is inserted in the usual fashion after an adequate tract has been established by dilation.

Miscellaneous Methods of Inserting a Suprapubic Tube Without Formal Open Exposure

The Campbell punch has already been mentioned as a method of inserting a larger catheter with a more adequate caliber. There are other techniques for doing the same thing that also can be done easily in the outpatient surgical suite, preferably under saddle anesthesia (see Chapter 10) with generous suprapubic local lidocaine.

The bladder is filled to capacity, and a Lowsley curved sound is inserted into it until it can be palpated through the abdominal wall above the symphysis pubis. A cutdown onto the sound is made with a scalpel and the sound delivered through the abdominal wall. The wings of the sound are opened so that a strong silk suture can be passed through it. The suture is anchored to the tip of a Foley catheter. The wings of the Lowsley sound are closed, and the catheter is pulled into the bladder and out of the external meatus.

The catheter is detached from the Lowsley sound and pulled back into the bladder, where the balloon is inflated. A similar technique is possible with a Van Buren sound, which has a hole through its terminal end to accommodate the suture.

COMPLICATIONS

If the contraindications and the technique are rigidly observed, the rate of complications such as bowel perforation or trauma to a large intravesical prostate should be negligible. The most common complication encountered is hematuria, which is usually self-limiting and of no consequence. If a large vessel is traumatized, however, especially with the trocar techniques, fulguration may be necessary; but we have never seen this complication with the Stamey or Bonnano catheters. Faulty placement and inadequate drainage is unusual if the bladder has been adequately distended.

As with all indwelling urinary catheters, bacteriuria is inevitable, but it is greatly delayed with suprapubic tubes in comparison with indwelling urethral catheters. With closed drainage systems in the hospital, the urine is usually sterile for at least a week with a percutaneous cystostomy.

CONCLUSIONS

There are several methods of performing suprapubic cystostomy in the outpatient urosurgical suite. The simplest and least traumatic is the percutaneous method using one of the commercially available suprapubic tubes. This is a safe, simple, and effective way of achieving bladder drainage and should not be associated with complications if the correct principles for safe placement are adhered to.

REFERENCES

1. Kauder, D.H., and Bucchiere, J.J., Jr.: Method for changing suprapubic Cystocath bladder drainage system. Urology, *18*:503, 1981.

25

Infrapubic Operations: Vasovasostomy and Bilateral Orchiectomy

KEITH W. KAYE, M.D., F.C.S.(S.A.)., F.R.C.S.

An incision that has proved particularly useful in the outpatient setting is the infrapubic. In 1978, Kelâmi advocated this approach for bilateral scrotal operations, such as placement of testicular prostheses, orchiectomy, orchiopexy, correction of testicular torsion, and vasovasostomy.[1] We have subsequently reported our experience with it for outpatient microsurgical vasovasostomy and vasoepididymostomy, bilateral orchiectomy for prostatic carcinoma, and placement of semirigid penile prostheses[2] (see Chapter 30). This incision is especially valuable for use in outpatients, as it is well suited to use with local anesthesia, is quick and easy, and has a low complication rate.

One of the principal concerns when performing surgery on an outpatient basis is that the patient may have some complication after discharge that would necessitate admission to a hospital, thus negating the advantage of the outpatient setting. Surgeons have been reluctant to discharge patients soon after any scrotal operation for fear of a hematoma, to which scrotal incisions are notoriously susceptible. In order to prevent this, numerous types of incisions and dressings, especially various pressure dressings, have been advocated;[3–7] one author even suggested encasing the scrotum postoperatively in plaster of paris! The infrapubic incision has largely overcome the problem of scrotal hematoma.

INCISION TECHNIQUE

The infrapubic incision is a short transverse incision approximately 5 cm long placed at the root of the penis. It must not be placed any higher on the abdominal wall, as this necessitates dissection through more fat, which may complicate the procedure.

After the skin and superficial layer of subcutaneous tissue have been incised, a Weitlander retractor is used to hold the wound open. Any branches of the superficial dorsal penile vein that may be visible at or near the midline are preserved. In order to facilitate this, and also to preserve the lymphatic channels, the subcutaneous tissue is left intact in the midline (Fig. 25–1); this prevents complications such as penile edema or thrombosis of the superficial dorsal penile vein. An Army–Navy retractor is placed in the lateral part of the wound, and the spermatic cord is palpated against the pubic bone with the forefinger. The subcutaneous fat is cut through and the external spermatic fascia incised. (Unless the fascia is cut, it can be frustrating

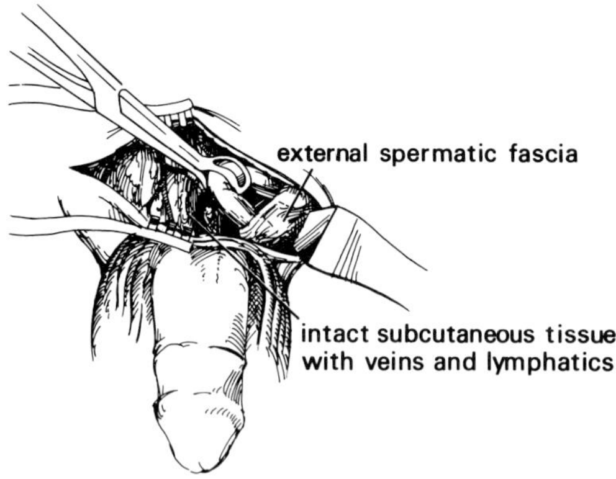

Fig. 25–1. Infrapubic incision and extraction of the spermatic cord. Note intact midline tissue. (From Kaye, K.W., et al.: J. Urol., *129*:992, 1983.)

trying to find the spermatic cord.) Once a small portion of the cord and overlying cremasteric muscle are visible, they may be grasped with Babcock's forceps and delivered easily into the wound.

After the surgical procedure has been performed, the wound is closed with a continuous 3–0 chromic suture to the subcutaneous layer and a 4–0 Vicryl subcuticular stitch. Thus, there are no sutures that require removal. A firm Elastoplast dressing is used that is bolstered laterally over the spermatic cord with gauze squares to provide slight pressure. No tight scrotal dressings are used; the patient is simply given a scrotal support.

Advantages and Complications

This incision is simple and safe and has the advantage of exposing both spermatic cords and testes, as well as the base of the penis if necessary, through a single incision. Early in our series, a few patients had mild postoperative penile edema, and in three cases there was thrombosis of the superficial dorsal penile vein, which was palpable as a firm cord in the penis. These minor complications were avoided in later cases by leaving a bridge of subcutaneous tissue intact in the midline. The superficial dorsal vein of the penis runs in the subcutaneous tissue to the symphysis pubis, where it divides into right and left branches that end in the superficial external pudendal veins.[8] Thus, at the site of the infrapubic incision, the vein is usually close to the midline, and, by leaving the subcutaneous tissues intact in this region, one spares the vein and the lymphatics.

The one contraindication to the use of this incision may be a previous lower midline incision such as that used for radical retropubic prostatectomy. In these patients, fibrosis may make the dissection difficult.

SPERMATIC-CORD BLOCK

Complementary to the infrapubic incision for scrotal surgery as an outpatient procedure is a technique for anesthetic nerve block of the spermatic cord. Many minor urologic procedures on the scrotum, spermatic cord, and testes are currently being performed under general anesthesia, either because it is expedient or because regional-block techniques are not sufficiently appreciated. We have found, however, that spermatic-cord block is simple to perform, safe, and highly cost effective in comparison with general anesthesia.[9]

Sensations from the testes, epididymides, their coverings, and the vasa deferentia are conveyed via the ilioinguinal nerve, sympathetic fibers surrounding the testicular vessels, and the genital branch of the genitofemoral nerve. The ilioinguinal nerve enters the scrotum along the anterolateral border of the spermatic cord, whereas the genital branch of the genitofemoral nerve is situated more posteriorly (Fig. 25–2). The scrotal skin receives sensory innervation from the pudendal nerve and the perineal branch of the posterior cutaneous nerve of the thigh. For this reason, in any operation involving a scrotal incision, the scrotal skin must be anesthetized separately before or after spermatic-cord block has been established.

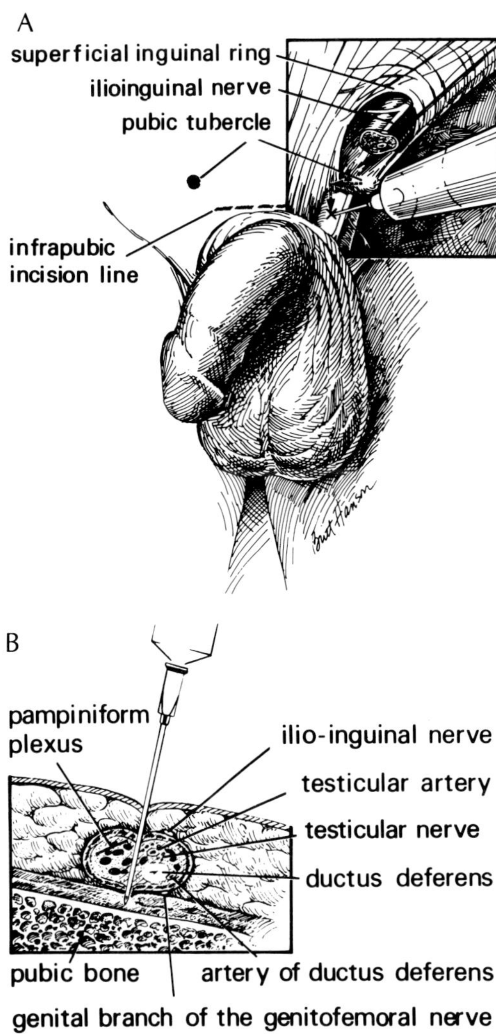

Fig. 25–2. Technique of spermatic-cord block. *(A)* Site of injection. *(B)* Path of needle. Anesthetic is injected as needle is withdrawn slowly. *(A)* From Kaye, K.W., et al.: J. Urol., *129*:992, 1983.) *(B)* From Kaye, K.W., et al.: J. Urol., *128*:720, 1982.)

Technique

The technique of spermatic-cord block is based on the fact that the cord, after emerging from the external inguinal ring, passes over the pubic tubercle then veers slightly medially on its course to the scrotum.

The anesthetic agent of choice is 0.5% bupivacaine hydrochloride without epinephrine, a long-acting local anesthetic that may be necessary for lengthy procedures such as microsurgical vasovasostomy and that also is desirable because it provides 4 to 6 hours of postoperative analgesia. It is injected before the full surgical preparation, to provide the 15 minutes of "soak time" necessary for full effectiveness. It is delivered with a 35-ml syringe with a 1.5-inch No. 25 needle.

The pubic tubercle is palpated, and the needle is passed from a point approximately 1 cm below and medial to the tubercle vertically down onto the anterior aspect of the pubic bone (see Fig. 25–2*B*). In its course, the needle thus passes through the spermatic cord and impales it against the bone. The plunger is pulled back slightly, to be certain the needle has not entered a blood vessel, and a total of 10–12 ml of anesthetic is injected slowly while the needle is being withdrawn. Injection must begin while the needle is at the bone to ensure blocking of the genital branch of the genitofemoral nerve. Usually, two or three passes are made through the cord at slightly different angles, injecting 3–4 ml each time, without withdrawing the needle completely through the skin. After the spermatic cord has been blocked, the skin and subcutaneous tissues at the site of the incision are infiltrated with the same anesthetic. If a bilateral operation is planned, the other side is then anesthetized the same way.

At times in thin patients, the spermatic cord can be palpated as it passes over the pubic tubercle. In these cases, it can be trapped between the surgeon's forefinger and middle finger and then injected.[10] In some patients, however, especially obese ones, it may be difficult even to palpate the tubercle. In such cases, an alternative is to grasp the cord between forefinger and thumb just above the scrotum and direct the needle into the cord with the other hand (Fig. 25–3).

With these techniques, no complications related to the anesthesia have oc-

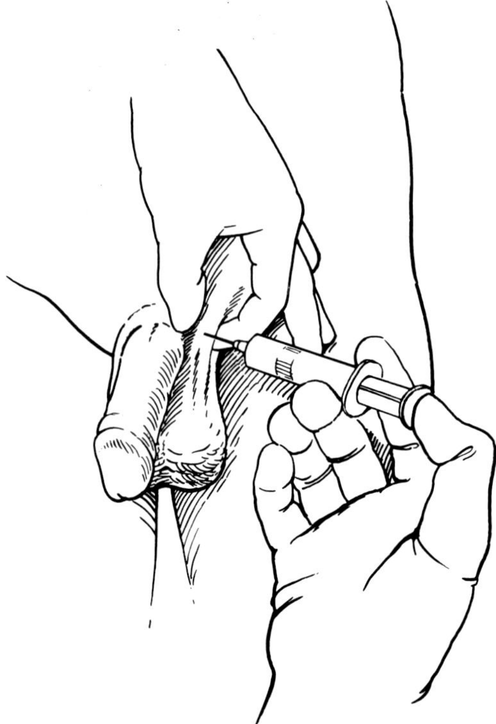

Fig. 25–3. Alternate method of spermatic-cord block appropriate for thin patients. (From Kaye, K.W., et al.: J. Urol., *129*:992, 1983.)

curred. In all patients, the testes, epididymides, and cord structures below the infiltration site could be manipulated with impunity, although in a few patients it was necessary to inject another 2–4 ml of bupivacaine directly into the cord after it had been exposed. Some patients complain of abdominal discomfort or nausea when there is heavy traction on the spermatic cord; however, this abates immediately when the traction is released.

Because 0.5% bupivacaine contains 5 mg of drug per milliliter and the maximum suggested single dose of this drug without epinephrine is 175 mg, a total of 35 ml of this agent may be used. This dose may be repeated after 3 hours, to a maximum of 400 mg in 24 hours. When 0.5% bupivacaine with epinephrine is used, the maximum single dose increases to 225 mg (45 ml). Reported adverse reactions are those characteristic of amide-type local anesthetics and usually result from excessive plasma levels, which may be due to overdosage, inadvertent intravascular injection, or slow metabolic clearance. These reactions and their treatment are outlined in Chapter 8.

MICROSURGICAL VASOVASOSTOMY

During the past decade, vasovasostomy has evolved from a rather crude macroscopic procedure, usually involving a stent, to a meticulous microsurgical operation, although controversy continues over which microsurgical technique is best. Certainly, the two-layer technique pioneered by Silber, in which the mucosa and muscularis are anastomosed in separate layers with a total of 14 to 18 interrupted sutures, has given excellent results.[11,12] However, this operation usually takes at least 3 to 3.5 hours and seems unsuitable for an outpatient setting.

Recently, it has been appreciated that a less laborious microsurgical technique, such as a 1½-layer anastomosis, can give results equivalent to those of the more difficult technique.[13–16] In these procedures, four full-thickness quadrant sutures are placed and reinforced by four or five interrupted seromuscular sutures. The great advantage of the 1½-layer technique is that it takes between 2 and 2.5 hours and thus is suitable for the outpatient setting. Sharlip found no difference between the 1½- and 2-layer techniques in the percentages of patients obtaining normal sperm counts and impregnation.[16] Thomas and associates, in an experimental study in dogs, likewise found no significant difference in the patency rates of one- and two-layer anastomoses.[17]

Preoperative Management

The patient is usually seen in the office the day before the operation, when a history is obtained and a physical examination performed. In particular, he is asked whether he has had any local anesthesia or has any allergies. Specific inquiries are made concerning recent aspirin ingestion, with its known antiplatelet action, and bleeding diatheses. Provided there is no evidence of abnormal bleeding, no routine laboratory studies are performed, and no radiologic studies are needed.

The nature of the procedure is outlined, and the patient is given the choice of local or general anesthesia. Almost invariably, patients elect to have their operations on an outpatient basis under local anesthesia, because in many regions, insurance companies will not pay for a vasovasostomy; and patients thus find the lower cost of the outpatient procedure and local anesthesia particularly attractive.

The patient is given a tube of Surgex* hair remover and instructed to apply it to his lower abdomen, scrotum, and inner thighs, taking care not to get any on the glans penis. We have found this far superior to shaving the incision site. The patient is permitted nothing by mouth beginning the evening before the operation.

After admission to the operating room, an intravenous line is inserted, and the patient is connected to a heart monitor. Spermatic-cord block is then performed. Preoperative and intraoperative sedation are rarely necessary. Throughout the procedure, the patient is reassured by the circulating nurse.

Technique

A short transverse infrapubic incision is made at the base of the penis, and the spermatic cord is delivered into the wound (see Fig. 25–1). The vasa deferentia are then mobilized above and below the vasectomy site and transected. If a prominent sperm granuloma is present, it is left in situ to reduce the chances of bleeding. When the vasectomy was performed low or near the convoluted part of the vasa, the testes are pulled up to make the sites accessible; when necessary, they are delivered into the wound. The luminal patency of the vasa is assessed distally by passing a 2–0 nylon suture and proximally by collecting the fluid with a micropipette and having it examined immediately for sperm.

A rubber dam is constructed for each side from the cuffs of surgical gloves to isolate the fields and keep them clear and blood free.[18] The cuffs are cut off and washed to remove the starch. The free ends of the vas are then brought through a pair of holes punched in a cuff approximately 2 cm apart with mosquito forceps. The dam is immobilized on the surgical drapes with Kelly hemostats. The distal lumen of each vas deferens is gently dilated with a microsurgical vessel dilator after the dam is in place.

Using a microclamp and Ethicon background material,* the 1½-layer anastomoses are made under direct vision with the operating microscope with 10–0 nylon† used for the four full-thickness quadrant sutures and 9–0 nylon‡ for the four or five interrupted seromuscular sutures (Fig. 25–4). The first suture placed is the most posterior full-thickness suture, and it is tied immediately (see Fig. 25–4, *center*). Great care is taken to ensure that this and the other full-thickness sutures are triangle sutures[14] (see Fig. 25–4, *top*). A large bite is taken of the serosa and muscle of the vas deferens, but the needle emerges from the mucosa immediately adjacent to the cut edge. This provides good muscle support yet perfect mucosal approximation. The posterior and uppermost full-thickness sutures are tied as they are placed, whereas

*Sparta Instrument Corp., 26602 Corporate Ave., Hayward, CA 94545.

*Ethicon Inc., Somerville, NJ 08876

†SSC DMIII, ⅜ circle needle; Societe Steril Catgut, Switzerland.

‡Supramed, ⅜ circle; S. Jackson, Inc., Washington, D.C.

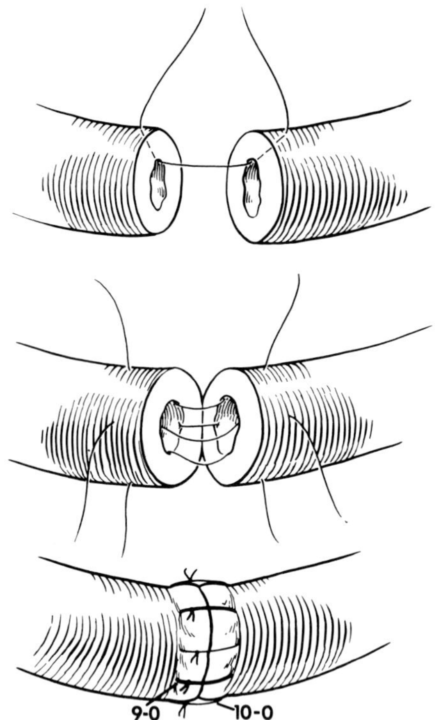

Fig. 25–4. The 1½-layer anastomosis technique. (From Kaye, K.W., et al.: J. Urol., *129*:992, 1983.)

both the anterior and the lower sutures are placed before they are tied. After the full-thickness quadrant sutures have been placed, the anastomoses are reinforced with one or two 9–0 nylon sutures between each of the original sutures (see Fig. 25–4, *bottom*).

After completion of the procedure on each side, the rubber dam is cut away with fine iris scissors under the operating microscope. The vasa deferentia are returned to the depths of the wound by gentle traction on the testes. The wound is closed as described.

Postoperative Management

Patients usually remain in the recovery room for less than an hour, as they have had no sedation. The wound is checked, and they are discharged home in the company of a responsible adult. They are given analgesic tablets and a typed list of instructions, which are:

(1) Telephoning the surgeon the next day to review the postdischarge course;
(2) An emergency telephone number where the surgeon can be reached;
(3) Return to work after one to two days, but no heavy lifting or vigorous exercise;
(4) Refrain from intercourse for one month;
(5) Return for postoperative check and first semen analysis at one month;
(6) Repeat semen analysis at two, three, and six months; and
(7) A basal body-temperature chart, with instructions, for the wife.

The couple is advised to attempt conception as soon as possible after the first month, in view of the occasional cases in which delayed scarring of the anastomoses blocks the vasa deferentia.

Results and Complications

This technique has been well accepted by patients and has given results similar to those of vasovasostomy performed on inpatients under general anesthesia. With experience, the operating time has been reduced to 2 hours. In more than 50 cases, there have been no serious complications, no patient has required admission to the hospital, and there have been no scrotal hematomas. Five patients have had minor problems, such as thrombosis of the superficial penile vein, slight penile edema, or small wound seromas; these all healed spontaneously within a few days, causing little discomfort.

At three months, more than 90% of patients have sperm counts > 20 million per milliliter. There have been two cases of delayed azoospermia, one detected 14 months after surgery (with a count of 48 million per milliliter at two months and the couple obtaining a pregnancy a month later) and another two years after vasovasostomy. The latter patient had a sperm count of 97.2 million per milliliter 16 months postoperatively and is believed to have the longest interval of good counts before scarring caused azoospermia.

Operating Costs

The cost of an outpatient vasovasostomy under local anesthesia averages $650 exclusive of the surgeon's fee (which is the same in any case). In comparison, the cost of an outpatient vasovasostomy under general anesthesia averages $1100 and that of an inpatient procedure under general anesthesia, $1650 (Table 25–1).

MICROSURGICAL VASOEPIDIDYMOSTOMY

At times, the surgeon may discover that a vasectomy was performed low on the convoluted part of the vas deferens or that there is a congenital obstruction in the tail of the epididymis. Either finding may necessitate low vasovasostomy or vasoepididymostomy, both of which require delivery of the testis into the wound. This is easily achieved under local anesthesia using the infrapubic incision simply by compressing the scrotum and having the testis slide up into the wound within the tunica vaginalis. At times, the incision may have to be extended laterally 1 to 2 cm to enable the testis to pass up easily. Once the testis is

TABLE 25–1. Comparison of Costs of Vasovasostomy Performed on Inpatient and Outpatient Basis Under Local or General Anesthesia

	Outpatient		Inpatient
	Local ($)	General ($)	General ($)
Preoperative tests (hemoglobin, urinalysis)	Not done	12.50	12.50
Hospital bed for 2 nights	—	—	432.00
Operating room (3 hours)	620.00	620.00	614.00
Intravenous access (500 ml of 5% dextrose; butterfly and syringe)	No charge	13.33	13.33
Anesthesia			
Gas and equipment (2.5 hours)	—	170.00	294.00
Bupivacaine (2 ampoules)	12.18	—	—
Anesthesiologist	No charge	200.00	200.00
Recovery room	25.00	90.00	102.00
TOTAL	$657.18	$1105.83	$1667.83
Saving with outpatient operation and local anesthesia (%)		448.65 (41)	1010.65 (61)

within the wound above the scrotum, the tunica is opened and the testis exposed (Fig. 25–5). It is not necessary to cut the gubernaculum, because pulling up the testis simply invaginates the scrotum, which then evaginates when the testis is returned.

Microsurgical vasoepididymostomy is then performed as outlined by Silber.[12] According to his technique, the epididymis is sectioned serially upward until sperm is obtained. At this level, eight to ten cut tubules can be seen under the microscope; however, careful examination will show fluid emerging from only one of these, and it is this one that is anastomosed to the vas deferens (Fig. 25–6*A*). Identifying this tubule may be difficult, as is the anastomosis, because the epididymal tubules are so delicate. Another, simpler, technique, suggested by A. J. Thomas, Jr.,[20] is not to transect the epididymis, but rather to cut a window from the visceral layer of the tunica vaginalis, thus exposing the epididymal tubules. A longitudinal incision is then made for a short distance along one tubule, and a connection is made between the end of the vas and the side of the tubule with interrupted microsutures (Fig. 25–6*B*).

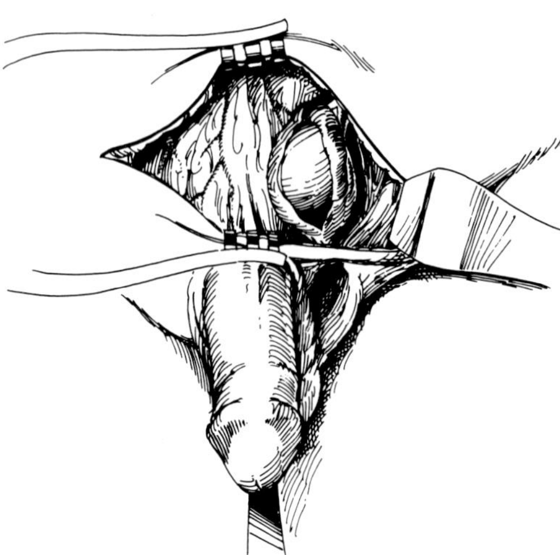

Fig. 25–5. Exposure of testis for vasoepididymostomy. Note invagination of the scrotum and intact gubernaculum.

BILATERAL ORCHIECTOMY

Bilateral orchiectomy is a common method of palliation for advanced carcinoma of the prostate. The majority of these patients are elderly, and many are substandard surgical risks, with cardiac and pulmonary disease. Estrogen therapy, which is the alternative to surgery, is, in many cases, poorly tolerated; and often there is poor compliance in taking the medication regularly. In other cases, the side effects, such as fluid retention, cardiac failure, venous thrombosis, and painful gynecomastia, may necessitate drug withdrawal. Bilateral orchiectomy under local anesthesia with early patient ambulation is a useful alternative to estrogen therapy and, in many instances, it is the method of choice.

Preoperative Evaluation

The patients have a history taken and a physical examination performed. The other studies are a complete blood count, a coagulation profile, blood urea nitrogen and electrolyte measurements, urinalysis, an electrocardiogram, and a chest radiograph. Any chemical abnormalities are corrected before surgery. The remaining perioperative instructions and management are as outlined for vasovasostomy.

Technique

The operation is performed with the patient in the standard supine position rather than the uncomfortable lithotomy position. No preoperative or intraoperative sedation is used in most cases. Bilateral spermatic-cord block is performed, and the infrapubic incision is made. The spermatic cords are exposed and mobilized, and the testes are delivered into the wound. The gubernaculum is transected and ligated with 2–0 chromic catgut, care being taken not to

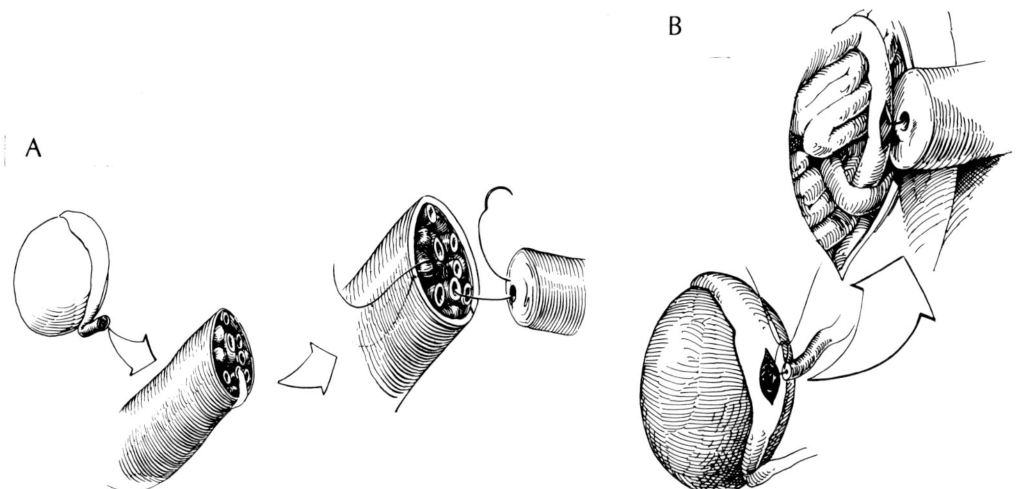

Fig. 25–6. Microsurgical vasoepididymostomy. *(A)* Anastomosis is made to the tubule from which the fluid is emerging. *(B)* End-to-side anastomosis of vas and epididymal tubule.

buttonhole the scrotal skin. Meticulous hemostasis is maintained. The spermatic cord is usually taken in two segments, each of which is ligated with a more-proximal suture of 2–0 silk and a distal 2–0 transfixion suture (Fig. 25–7). The wound is closed in standard fashion. A simple dressing is used, and the patient is given a scrotal support.

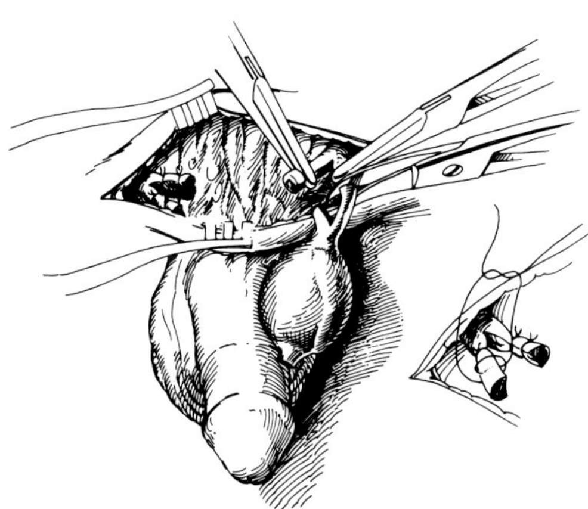

Fig. 25–7. Bilateral orchiectomy. Spermatic cord is cut and ligated in two parts.

Postoperative Management

The patient is given analgesic tablets and usually is discharged soon from the recovery room. He is instructed to walk around as soon as possible after his return home and to return for an office visit after one week. Many patients have little postoperative pain.

CONCLUSIONS

Use of the infrapubic incision and spermatic-cord block has facilitated the performance of several procedures on an outpatient basis. These have been well accepted by patients and are simple, reliable, and cost effective, with little morbidity. It has been suggested also that testicular torsion could be corrected in this way. Certainly, early spermatic-cord block could permit untwisting of the cord when no operating room is available; and in patients seen early, this could lead to the saving of some testes.[19]

REFERENCES

1. Kelâmi, A.: "Infrapubic" approach in operative andrology. Urology, *12*:580, 1978.
2. Kaye, K.W., Reddy, P., and Suryanarayanan, V.: Infrapubic incision in operative andrology. Urology, *21*:524, 1983.

3. Human, L.: The problem of postoperative hematoma of the scrotum. S. Afr. Med. J., *34*:969, 1960.
4. Wright, J.E.: The midline scrotal incision and a simple scrotal dressing. Med. J. Aust., *2*:14, 1966.
5. Mandler, J.I.: An improved scrotal pressure dressing. J. Urol., *96*:235, 1966.
6. Straffon, W.G.E.: A useful scrotal dressing. Med. J. Aust., *1*:320, 1974.
7. Burkitt, D.P.: Primary hydrocele and its treatment: a review of 200 cases. Lancet, *1*:1341, 1951.
8. Romanes, G.J.: Cunningham's Textbook of Anatomy. 10th Ed. London, Oxford University Press, 1964.
9. Kaye, K.W., Lange, P.H., and Fraley, E.E.: Spermatic cord block in urologic surgery. J. Urol., *128*:720, 1982.
10. Fuchs, E.: Cord block anesthesia for scrotal surgery. J. Urol., *128*:718, 1982.
11. Silber, S.J.: Microscopic vasectomy reversal. Fertil. Steril., *28*:1191, 1977.
12. Silber, S.J.: Reversal of vasectomy and the treatment of male infertility. Urol. Clin. North Am., *8*:53, 1981.
13. Kaye, K.W., Gonzalez, R., and Fraley, E.E.: Microsurgical vasovasostomy: outpatient procedure under local anesthesia. J. Urol., *129*:992, 1983.
14. Schmidt, S.S.: Vasovasostomy. Urol. Clin. North Am., *5*:585, 1978.
15. Howards, S.S.: Vasovasostomy. Urol. Clin. North Am., *5*:165, 1981.
16. Sharlip, I.D.: Vasovasostomy: comparison of two microsurgical techniques. Urology, *17*:347, 1981.
17. Thomas, A.J., et al.: Vasovasostomy: evaluation of four surgical techniques. Fertil. Steril., *32*:324, 1979.
18. Fuchs, E.F.: Inexpensive readily available rubber dam for vasovasostomy. Urology, *17*:374, 1981.
19. Spark, J.P.: Torsion of the testis. Ann. Coll. Surg. Engl., *49*:77, 1971.
20. Thomas, A.J.: Personal communication, 1983.

26

Scrotal and Related Procedures

KEITH W. KAYE, M.D., F.C.S.(S.A.)., F.R.C.S.

Because hematomas are frequent after scrotal surgery, many surgeons have been reluctant to discharge patients soon after operation on the scrotal contents. For example, one of the most common scrotal operations—hydrocelectomy—is usually performed under general or spinal anesthesia, with an average hospital stay of two to six days.[1,2] However, it is now being realized that by using certain techniques and avoiding others, the surgeon can perform many scrotal procedures safely on an outpatient basis.

Peter Lord has described an operation for treatment of idiopathic hydrocele, which, through the years, has proved to give the best results.[1-5] Another operation described by Lord is for removal of large spermatoceles or epididymal cysts.[6] We have adapted both of these for performance under local anesthesia on an outpatient basis and had excellent results.[7]

Another consideration is the fact that insurance companies are now beginning to see the cost-benefit advantages of outpatient scrotal operations; indeed, in some regions, including Minnesota, Blue Cross/Blue Shield will no longer pay for hydrocele operations done on an inpatient basis. Also, at many academic and federal institutions, minor operations such as hydrocelectomy have such a low priority for beds and operating-room time that patients must wait many weeks for an inpatient operation, whereas time is available soon in the outpatient unit.

HYDROCELECTOMY

Preoperative Preparation

This is as outlined in Chapter 25. Young, fit patients need no laboratory investigations, whereas in older individuals appropriate tests are done. All patients are given Surgex hair remover, with instructions to apply it to the lower abdomen, scrotum, and inner thighs the evening before admission.

Operative Technique

With the patient supine, spermatic-cord block is performed using 0.5% bupivacaine hydrochloride without epinephrine (see Chapter 25).[8] Usually, no sedation is used. The patient is then scrubbed and draped. It is useful to transilluminate the scrotum with a sterile endoscopy cold light to define the position of the testis within the sac and to help determine whether there are any associated epididymal cysts.

The hydrocele is grasped so as to stretch the scrotal skin, and this grip is maintained during the early stages of the operation. Transverse scrotal vessels can then be seen; an incision site is chosen to run between them on the anterior wall opposite the testis (Fig. 26–1). Anesthetic is injected into the skin and sub-

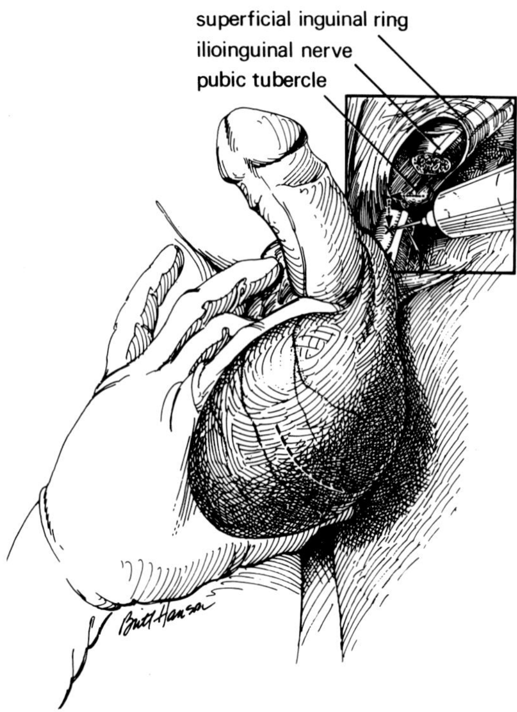

Fig. 26–1. Selection of incision site between scrotal vessels. Insert shows technique of spermatic-cord block. (From Kaye, K.W., et al.: J. Urol., *130*:269, 1983.)

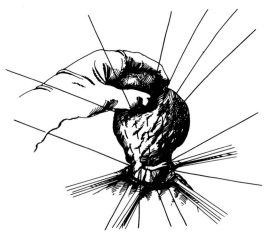

Fig. 26–2. Plication of the tunica vaginalis with chromic catgut. (From Kaye, K.W., et al.: J. Urol., *130*:269, 1983.)

cutaneous scrotal layers, the skin being kept taut to prevent displacement of the incision line; and, after the drug has taken effect, a 4- to 5-cm incision is made in the stretched skin. After the dartos layer has been incised, Allis forceps are placed on the subcutaneous tissues, and any small bleeding vessels are coagulated. The incision is deepened through the tunica vaginalis into the hydrocele sac, and the fluid is removed. To ensure hemostasis, cautery is used to open the sac further.

The testis is delivered through the incision. Starting at the cut edge, the tunica vaginalis is plicated with bites of 3–0 chromic catgut that contain only the layer of the tunica to prevent bleeding (Fig. 26–2). After eight to ten of these sutures have been placed, they are tied, thus gathering the tunica into a collar around the junction of the testis and epididymis. The testis is then returned to the scrotum. Allis forceps are placed on the subcutaneous tissues at either end of the wound, and the tissues are closed with a continuous 3–0 chromic catgut suture, which is run back as a subcuticular stitch and tied to its original free end (Fig. 26–3). This provides an excellent hemostatic suture and obviates suture removal.[9] However, the suture must not be pulled too tight, or it will cause ischemic necrosis.

No drains are used. Early in our experience, we applied a tight scrotal pressure dressing, but more recently, we have found a simple dressing to be satisfactory. The patient is given a scrotal support.

Postoperative Management

The patient remains in the recovery room for approximately 1 hour and then, after the wound has been checked, is discharged home. He is given analgesic tablets, advised to rest in bed for the remainder of the day, and told to telephone the surgeon the following morning. The dressing is removed by the patient after 48 hours, and thereafter he simply places

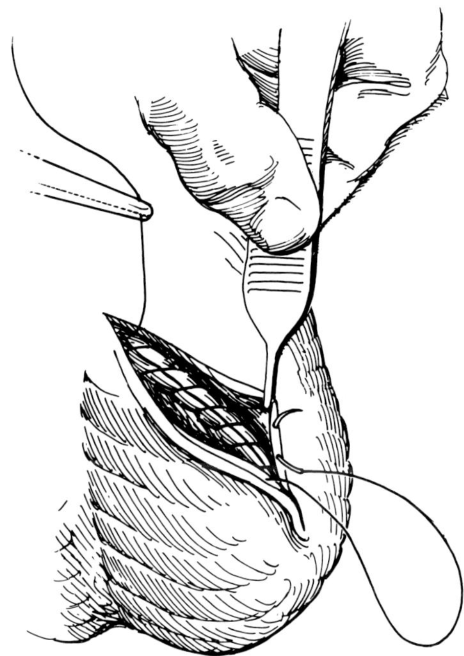

Fig. 26–3. Closing the wound. This technique makes suture removal unnecessary. (From Kaye, K.W., et al.: J. Urol., *130*:269, 1983.)

clean gauze within the scrotal support. He is examined in the office 10 to 12 days later.

Complications and Results

This technique has been used for more than 30 patients, and complications have been few and minor. The local anesthesia is well tolerated; and, despite the fact that at times considerable pressure is required to return the testis to the scrotum, the patients have had no discomfort or pain. Postoperatively, many patients have required only two or three analgesic tablets.

Early in our experience, in an effort to prevent scrotal hematomas, tight pressure dressings were used; and the skin sutures were pulled tight. These measures proved to delay wound healing. Now, care is taken not to pull the subcutaneous and subcuticular stitches too tight and not to bunch up the wound. Only simple scrotal dressings are used. These measures virtually eliminated wound-healing problems.

Only one patient in our recent experience was admitted to the hospital. He had a spermatocele as well as a thick-walled hydrocele that had been punctured for aspiration several times; and we were concerned about possible hematoma. A Lord's procedure was performed, and he was discharged the next morning. At followup three months later, he was cured, with only a small intrascrotal mass remaining.

Cost-Benefit Analysis

Outpatient hydrocele repair under local anesthesia costs $250 exclusive of the surgeon's fee and laboratory investigations, in contrast to $966 for an inpatient procedure under general anesthesia (Table 26–1). The saving shown is probably a conservative estimate, as most surgeons hospitalize their patients for more than two days.[1,2]

Contraindications

The only contraindications to performing this procedure on an outpatient basis

TABLE 26–1. Comparison of Costs of Hydrocele Repair Performed on Outpatient Basis Under Local Anesthesia and Inpatient Basis Under General Anesthesia

	Outpatient Local ($)	Inpatient General ($)
Hospital bed (two nights)	—	432
Operating room (1 hour)	220	282
Anesthesia		
Gas and equipment (45 minutes)	—	75
Bupivacaine (1 ampoule)	6	—
Anesthesioloist	No charge	75
Recovery room	25	102
TOTAL	251	966
Saving (%)		714 (74)

under local anesthesia (aside from the standard medical contraindications) are allergy to local anesthetics, bleeding diatheses, previous scrotal surgery, or a thick-walled hydrocele that already has been aspirated several times.

SPERMATOCELECTOMY

At times, it is necessary to excise a large, uncomfortable spermatocele or epididymal cyst. It is also not uncommon to see patients who have both a hydrocele and a spermatocele, which can be treated at the same time through a single scrotal incision. The perioperative management and spermatic-cord block are performed as described.

Operative Technique

With one hand grasping the cyst to stretch the scrotal skin, bupivacaine is injected into the skin and subcutaneous tissues between visible vessels. A 1.5-cm incision is made through the skin, dartos, and areolar tissue. (A larger incision is needed for concurrent hydrocele repair.) At this stage, one Allis forceps is placed on the subcutaneous tissue on either side of the wound for hemostasis. Using either iris scissors or mosquito forceps, the areolar tissue is gradually dissected until the bluish wall of the cyst is reached.

The key to the success of this operation is getting into the correct tissue plane directly on the cyst wall, because surrounding the wall is an avascular plane that permits simple, bloodless extraction of the cyst. Initially, one may have some difficulty in deciding when one has reached this plane, but with experience one soon comes to recognize the characteristic bluish appearance of the cyst wall. Use of Adson's forceps to grasp tissue layers is helpful. Often, there is a thick tissue layer immediately outside the cyst that must be opened by sharp dissection.

After the cyst wall is exposed, an area the size of the incision is cleared of overlying areolar tissue. Then one either makes a small incision into the cyst wall or aspirates most of the fluid with a syringe, permitting the removal of a cyst of any size through a small incision (Fig. 26–4). However, a small volume of fluid should be left in the cyst to facilitate further dissection. Mosquito forceps are placed on the wall to close the hole and for use as a retractor. Usually, the entire cyst can be delivered intact from the scrotum by gentle retraction of the forceps, with blunt dissection required only occasionally to wipe away loose areolar tissue (Fig. 26–5). If there is any bleeding, or if many small vessels are encountered on the surface of the cyst, one is in the wrong tissue plane.

When the entire cyst has been exteriorized, remaining attached only at its site of origin from the epididymis, the surgeon will usually see one or two small blood vessels in the stalk connecting the epididymis and cyst. These are either fulgurated with a bovie or cross-clamped and ligated (Fig. 26–6). This separates the cyst, with its remaining fluid, from

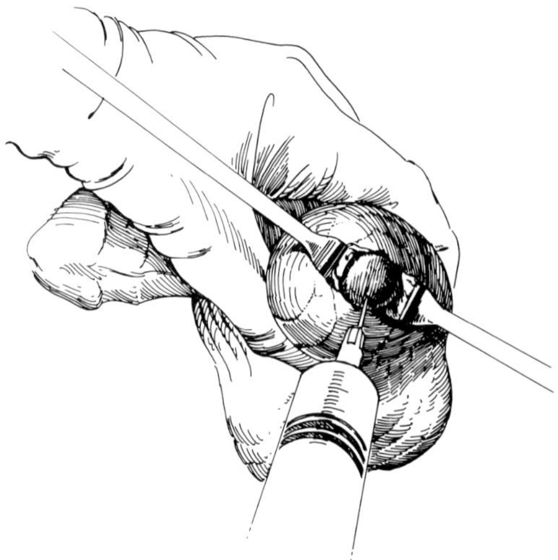

Fig. 26–4. Drainage of part of the fluid from a cyst. Some fluid should be left to facilitate further dissection. (From Kaye, K.W., et al.: J. Urol., *130*:269, 1983.)

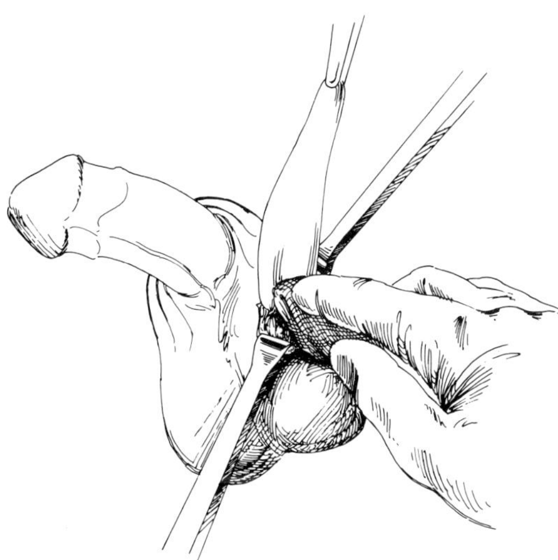

Fig. 26–5. Use of sponge to wipe away loose areolar tissue. (From Kaye, K.W., et al.: J. Urol., *130*:269, 1983.)

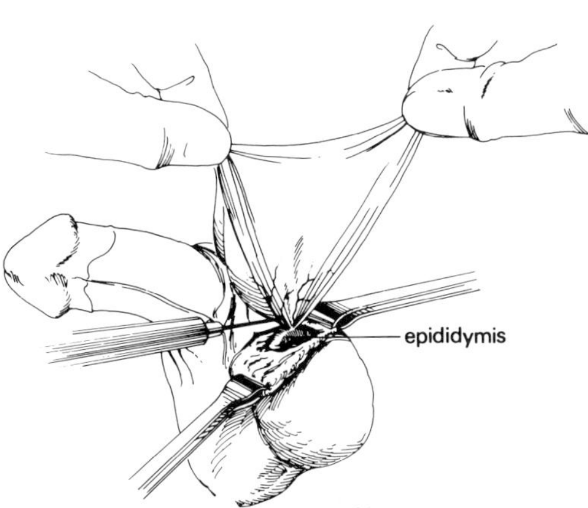

Fig. 26–6. Cyst connected to epididymis by stalk. The blood vessels are fulgurated or ligated. (From Kaye, K.W., et al.: J. Urol., *130*:269, 1983.)

the epididymis, usually intact. The wound is closed by placing skin hooks at either end and inserting a running 3–0 chromic catgut suture to close the dartos and subcutaneous tissue in one layer. The suture is then run back as a subcuticular stitch and tied to its original free end. No drains are used. The patient is given a simple scrotal support.

VASECTOMY

Vasectomy is the urologic surgical procedure most often performed on an outpatient basis; at present, approximately 250,000 vasectomies are performed annually in the United States. The other side of this, however, is the fact that about half of all malpractice claims against urologists involve vasectomies. For this reason, it is essential that the patient and his wife have a full understanding of the procedure, with all aspects of the technique, possible complications, followup, and the small chance of failure being made clear. Several companies now supply well-illustrated brochures* that can be sent to the couple by mail before the first office visit or along with the list of preoperative and postoperative instructions.

Legal Aspects

In order to avoid litigation, the following precautions are suggested.[10,11]

Informed Consent. Besides being given a brochure, the couple should be interviewed by the surgeon to answer further questions. In particular, they must be told to continue the usual contraceptive measures until at least 20 ejaculations have occurred *and* a semen analysis has proved the absence of sperm (usually eight to ten weeks after the procedure), with a second negative study two weeks later. The couple must realize that, despite all efforts, spontaneous recanalization occurs months or years after the operation in approximately one of every 1,000 cases; this fact should be included in the consent form. Other possible complications should be reiterated at this stage.

*Leader, Abel J.: Elective Vasectomy. Norwich-Eaton Pharmaceuticals, Norwich, NY 13815; The Facts about Vasectomy. Parke, Davis & Co., Morris Plains, NJ 07950; Miller, Norman G.: Vasectomy: Facts about Male Sterilization. Patient Information Library, 345 G. Serramonte Plaza, Daly City, CA 94015.

Be Selective. During the initial discussion, it may become apparent that the patient is not suitable for vasectomy. One may be justified in refusing surgery to a man who has persistent questions about loss of virility or potency after the matter has been discussed on several occasions.

Surgical Consent Form. In most states, special consent forms are required for sterilization in addition to, or instead of, the regular surgical consent form. This should be prepared by a lawyer in accordance with the law of your state and should include a statement about the risk of recanalization and the necessity for alternative contraceptive measures until sperm counts are negative (Fig. 26–7).

Operation Notes. These must be meticulous and should be made as soon after the operation as possible. It is advisable to have histologic proof in all cases that a segment of vas deferens was resected on both sides.

Followup. If the patient does not keep his followup appointment after eight to ten weeks for semen analysis, every effort should be made to contact him; and these efforts should be documented in the chart.

Preoperative Instructions

The following list of instructions was prepared by Leader from the Houston Vasectomy Clinic:

(1) Make every effort to keep your appointment, since the time required for this procedure has been reserved for you.

(2) Shave as much hair from around the testicles and penis, on the evening before or on the day the vasectomy is to be done, as you possibly can. (Do not use an electric razor.) [Our preference is that patients use a depilatory.]

(3) After shaving the area, wash the penis and scrotum thoroughly, then shower or bathe to remove all loose hairs.

(4) If you prefer, you may get someone to drive you to and from the office, although this is not essential.

(5) Before you come to the office, stop at a drugstore and buy either an athletic supporter ("jock strap") or a scrotal suspensory suitable to your size. Specify "no leg straps." If you buy a suspensory, get the large size.

(6) If you have not already done so, bring your signed operation consent form (which your wife must also sign) and the fee agreed upon with you. If you have insurance coverage that will reimburse you in whole or in part for this operation, bring your forms with you and we will gladly fill them in for you. You must, however, pay for this surgery at the time that it is done.[12]

Operative Technique

The vas deferens is palpated between forefinger and thumb through the scrotal skin, separated from the other cord contents, and then rolled toward the anterolateral aspect of the scrotum and immobilized between the forefinger and thumb. (One should avoid performing the vasectomy too close to the convoluted part of the vas deferens, as is often done, because this makes any later vasovasostomy more difficult.) Local anesthetic (2% lidocaine) is injected via a 25-gauge needle into the skin between the vas and the fingers (Fig. 26–8*A*). The vas deferens is secured with towel clips or Allis forceps (Fig. 26–8*B*), and more local anesthetic is injected into the skin overlying the vas and into the vas itself.

A short (< 1-cm) scrotal incision is made directly over the vas and deepened to expose the structure. The vas is grasped with another small Allis forceps, releasing the first one applied, and delivered into the wound. A short segment is

CONSENT FOR STERILIZATION OPERATION

WHEREAS, ..., physician, has been asked to perform an operation of sterilization on the undersigned husband, such an operation being known as a vasectomy (or vas section and ligation) and WHEREAS, said physician is willing to perform said operation only upon the written consent of the undersigned husband and wife, freely and fully given, and WHEREAS, the undersigned by execution of this agreement, hereby give their consent and agreement, individually and jointly, to the performance of a vasectomy upon the husband with the full understanding that said operation may forever and irrevocably deprive said husband of the ability to produce children or cause pregnancy in a female partner.

The undersigned further agree that ...., physician, shall not be responsible in any way for any deleterious consequences resulting from said operation, and hereby release and discharge him from any or all claims and demands whatsoever which they, their heirs, executors, administrators or assigns have or may have against said physician by reason of any matter relative or incident to such operation.

We further certify that we have read and fully understand all of the details of the brochure on Vasectomy which was given to us by said physician and of which this consent form was an intrinsic part. We certify further that having read this brochure we were asked by said physician whether any additional information was required, and we have answered to the contrary.

Signed this..................day of.................................., 19........

at...

....	....
(Husband)	WITNESSES:
....	....
(Address)	(Address)
....	....
(City, State)	(City, State)
....	....
(Wife)	
....	....
(Address)	(Address)
....	....
(City, State)	(City, State)

Fig. 26–7. Consent form for surgical sterilization. Note reference to permanency of procedure and to booklets providing information about need to continue contraceptive precautions (described in text).

freed from its fascial coverings (Fig. 26–9). Hemostasis must be secured.

Mosquito forceps are placed 1 cm apart on the vas, and the intervening segment is excised and sent for fixation (Fig. 26–10*A*). The lumen is coagulated for a short distance on both sides, and the vas is ligated with a permanent 3–0 suture such as Tevdek (Fig. 26–10*B*). It is important not to tie these ligatures too tight in order to avoid cutting through the vas, because if this happens, a sperm granuloma with subsequent recanalization may result.

The proximal side of the cut vas is returned to its fascial sheath, which is sutured over it with 3–0 chromic catgut (Fig. 26–10*C*) to get the two ends of the vas into different fascial compartments to help prevent spontaneous recanalization. The vas is returned to the scrotum. Skin sutures are not usually necessary; if they

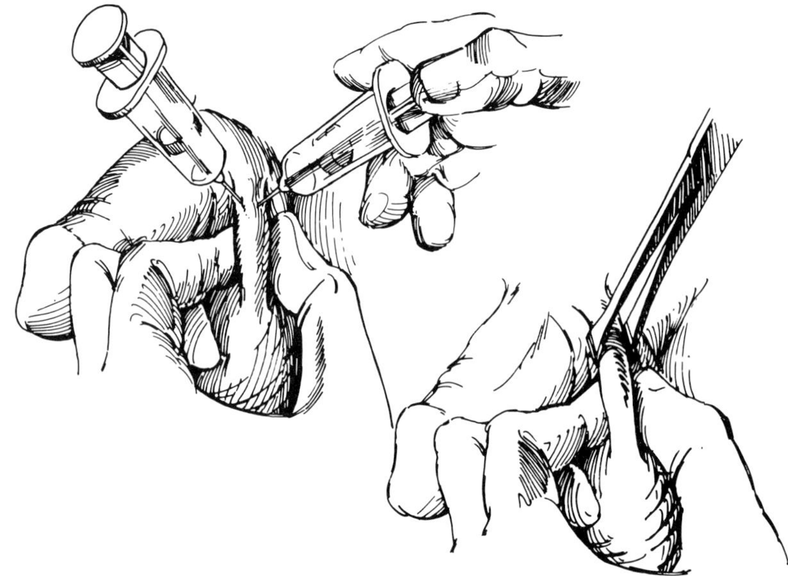

Fig. 26–8. Anesthesia for vas deferens. *(A)* Injection of the skin behind the vas. *(B)* Securing of the vas with clips or forceps.

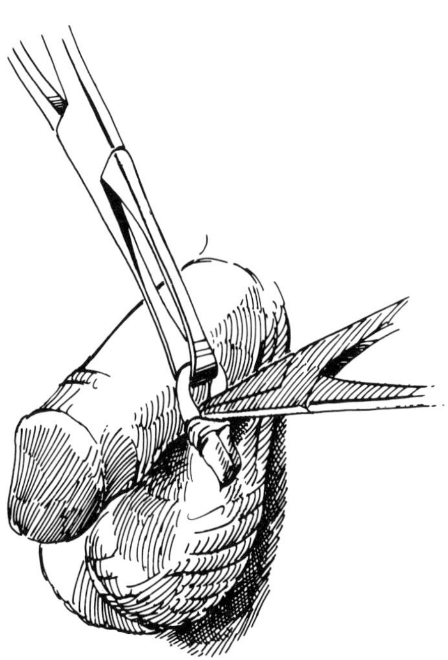

Fig. 26–9. A segment of vas freed from its fascial coverings.

are, one or two sutures of 3–0 chromic catgut will suffice. After the procedure has been repeated on the other side, a simple dressing and scrotal support are applied, and the patient is soon discharged home with a responsible adult.

Postoperative Instructions

The instructions should include the following points, as set forth by Leader:

(1) Wear the scrotal support for at least 24 hours. Thereafter, you may wear it as long as you are more comfortable with it on than without it.

(2) Avoid strenuous physical exercise for about five days. You may perform all other usual activities.

(3) You may shower or bathe on the day following vasectomy and thereafter.

(4) If stitches have been used to close the skin incision, they will dissolve by themselves and do not require removal. If a stitch comes away prematurely, the incision may open a little, and possibly there may be a slight discharge from the wound. Do not worry about this. Continue to

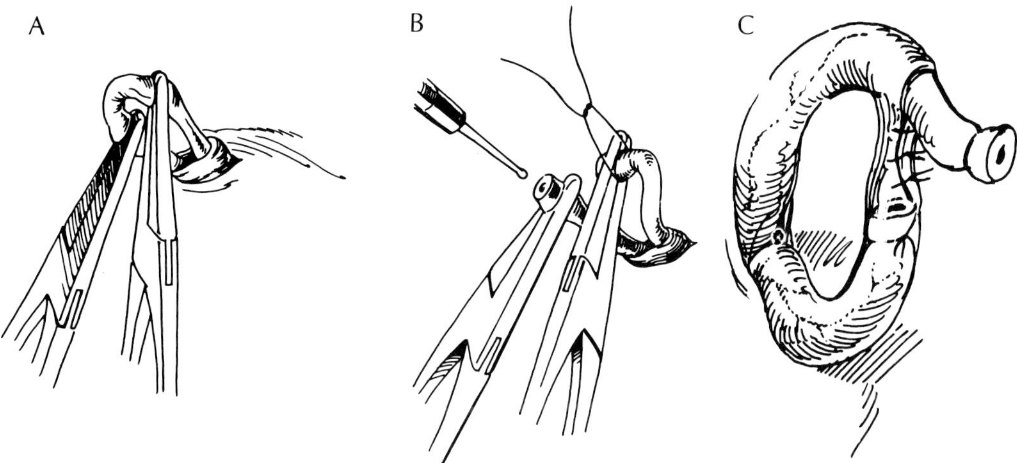

Fig. 26–10. Vasectomy. *(A)* Segment between mosquito forceps is excised and sent for fixation. *(B)* The lumen is coagulated and ligated on both sides. *(C)* Suturing of fascial sheath over proximal end of vas.

bathe as before and place a small gauze sponge inside the suspensory over the incision. You may purchase these small sponges at a drugstore. Continue to wear the scrotal suspensory with the sponge inside until the incision dries completely. Because of the small size of the incision, many physicians prefer not to use skin sutures or stitches, because the edges will heal more quickly without them.

(5) If you have pain or discomfort immediately after the operation, take two pain tablets at 4- to 6-hour intervals. An ice bag will provide additional comfort after the local anesthetic wears off if used for several hours. Attempt to lie flat for a number of hours after the operation in order to avoid the discomfort associated with movement.

(6) A slight oozing of blood (enough to stain the dressing), some tenderness, and mild swelling in the areas of the incisions are not unusual and should subside within 72 hours. These should cause no alarm. But if there is an unusual amount of pain, a large swelling of the scrotum, or continued free bleeding, do not hesitate to call your doctor at any time of the day or night. If for any reason you cannot reach him, go to the emergency room of the hospital that he has indicated.

(7) Maintain the usual contraceptive precautions for the time required for a minimum of 20 ejaculations. But, before proceeding to unprotected intercourse, bring a semen specimen to the office, produced by masturbation into a wide-mouth dry receptacle, for microscopic examination.[12]

MODIFIED HIGH APPROACH TO VARICOCELECTOMY USING LOCAL ANESTHESIA

Varicocelectomy is an accepted method of treatment for those infertile patients who have a low sperm count with reduced motility and a clinically evident varicocele, in whom no other cause for abnormal semen can be found. A significant improvement in semen quality is found in 75 to 80% of these patients, with pregnancy rates ranging from 45 to 55%.[13,14]

Most surgeons use the inguinal or the high (Ivanissevitch) approach with light general or with spinal anesthesia. However, Ross et al. reported a modification of the Ivanissevitch approach that can be done on an outpatient basis with local anesthesia.[15] Since then, we have used a similar procedure with a small change in the technique of anesthetic administration.

Criteria for Patient Selection

The patient should have a somewhat asthenic body, should have no allergies to the drugs used, and should accept having the procedure performed under local anesthesia. The preoperative management is as previously outlined.

Anesthetic Technique

The landmarks—the anterosuperior iliac spine, pubic tubercle, and deep inguinal ring (2 cm above the midpoint between the iliac spine and the tubercle)—are marked on the skin with a surgical marking pen. A point is chosen two fingerbreadths medial to the anterosuperior iliac spine to block the ilioinguinal and iliohypogastric nerves. A 1.5-inch 25-gauge needle on a 30-ml syringe is first advanced vertically downward through this point to penetrate the aponeurosis of the external oblique muscle (which can be felt as a resistance), and approximately 4 ml of 0.5% bupivacaine is injected into the muscles in the front of the pelvic bone as the needle is gradually withdrawn to the subcutaneous layer. The procedure is repeated, angling the needle first slightly medially, then laterally, and injecting about 4 ml on each occasion to a total of 12 ml (Fig. 26–11*A*). A spermatic-cord block may then be performed (see Chapter 25) with another 12 ml of the same anesthetic, although usually this is unnecessary. The line of incision is drawn from 2.5 cm above and below the deep inguinal ring parallel to the inguinal ligament. At this stage, it is safer to use 0.25% bupivacaine hydrochloride with epinephrine, which is injected along the line of incision. After the skin incision has been made, a further 2–4 ml of the 0.25% solution is injected under the external oblique fascia before it is incised. All injections except the last are made before full surgical preparation, to give time for the anesthetic to become fully effective without delaying the procedure.

Operative Technique

The 4- to 5-cm incision is made and deepened through the subcutaneous tissue and aponeurosis of the external oblique muscle. The arching fibers of the internal oblique and transverse abdominus muscles thus revealed are retracted cephalad (Fig. 26–11*B*). It is not necessary to incise any muscle. The transversalis fascia is bluntly dissected, exposing the one or two large spermatic veins, which lie preperitoneally above the vas deferens, which is passing down medially into the pelvis immediately before the veins curve around to lie retroperitoneally on the psoas major muscle. The veins are easily ligated at this point. Routinely, we use a sterile Doppler probe, both to ensure that all veins have been ligated and to be certain that the artery remains intact.[16] The wound is then closed in layers. The operating time averages 30 minutes.

Postoperative Management and Results

Patients are usually discharged from the recovery room within an hour when no sedation has been used. They are given analgesic tablets, although many will require none. The following day, a telephone check ensures that nothing untoward has occurred; and the patient is seen in the office one to two weeks later. Patients usually return to work after three or four days and return to the office after

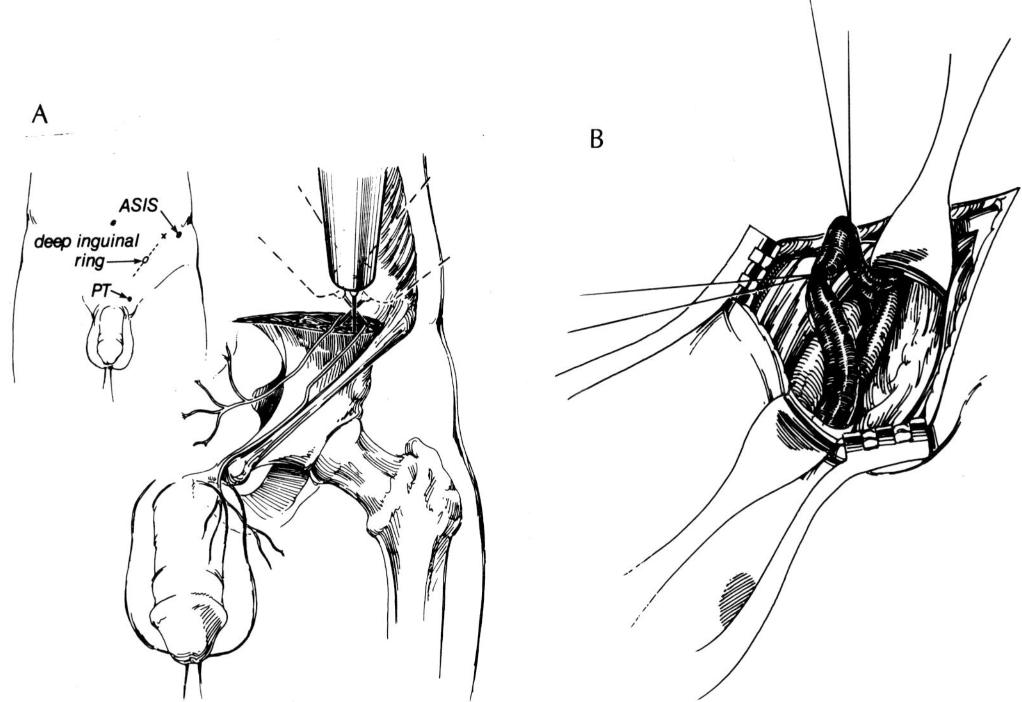

Fig. 26–11. Modified high approach to varicocelectomy. *(A)* Anesthetic technique. ASIS = anterior superior iliac spine; PT = pubic tubercle; X = injection site. *(B)* Exposure of vas, which is passing medially and curving down into pelvis. Note preperitoneal exposure of veins (in sutures) and intact testicular artery.

three months for their first semen analysis.

In both Ross's experience and ours, there have been no complications other than mild subcutaneous ecchymosis at the site of anesthetic injection. Early in our series, some patients had flank pain when undue traction was used in dissecting the spermatic veins from the cord; this was eliminated by avoiding hard pulling on the cord.

OPERATIVE MANAGEMENT OF ACUTE EPIDIDYMITIS

Acute epididymitis is generally treated conservatively until it becomes obvious that this has failed and an intrascrotal abscess, with or without testicular infarction, has appeared, necessitating epididymectomy or orchiectomy. Either of two operations will prevent this organ-destroying process, often with dramatic results.

Incision of the External Inguinal Ring

In 1973, Costas and van Blerk first reported noticing, at surgical exploration for nonresolving acute epididymitis, that the spermatic cord was markedly edematous and engorged up to the external inguinal ring.[17] The cord above the ring was not swollen, and upon incising the edge of the ring, the surgeons saw the edema and congestion abate dramatically. It thus appeared that the rigid external inguinal ring was obstructing venous and lymphatic return. Certainly, in advanced cases of severe, acute epididymitis, testicular infarction may occur. Half of Costas and van Blerk's patients were treated by incision of the ring alone, and half by concomitant epididymotomy, resulting in immediate testicular salvage in all but one patient, in whom testicular infarction had already occurred and orchiectomy was necessary.

I have used this simple operation on several occasions with the patients under local anesthesia, with dramatic relief of testicular pain, swelling, and fever. The key to its success, however, is not to delay: to act promptly when a patient who is being treated conservatively for epididymitis does not respond quickly.

Indications for External-Ring Release. Marked tenderness and thickening of the spermatic cord when acute epididymitis is diagnosed is probably in indication for either immediate operation or for no more than a short trial of conservative treatment. An operation is indicated if swelling and tenderness of the spermatic cord appear during conservative treatment, especially if there is increasing pain. Testicular pain that appears or increases suddenly in severity during conservative treatment may indicate impending infarction and is another indication. Finally, an immediate operation is indicated when there is a worsening of local symptoms and signs, with more severe pain, increased swelling, and loss of the ability to distinguish the testis from the epididymis, especially if this was previously possible.

Operative Technique. This simple procedure is performed using local anesthesia, 2% lidocaine injected into the skin and subcutaneous tissues over the external inguinal ring. (The midpoint of the external ring is 1 cm above the pubic tubercle.) A 3- to 4-cm incision is made obliquely in the lower inguinal region centering on the superficial inguinal ring and deepened to expose the spermatic cord emerging from the ring. Another 2 ml of lidocaine is injected into the fibers of the aponeurosis forming the external ring, which is then incised in a superolateral direction for 2 to 3 cm to open into the lowermost part of the inguinal canal (Fig. 26–12). The constrictive area on the spermatic cord may now be seen easily and the obstruction relieved. Subcutaneous tissue and skin are closed in standard fashion with no drains. Many patients have no pain except from the incision.

Epididymotomy

If the infection is more advanced, testicular exploration with possible epididymotomy should be performed in conjunction with the external-ring release. At exploration, a necrotic testis may be found, necessitating orchiectomy, although in many instances the testis and epididymis can be salvaged by epididymotomy.[18] This is usually performed under general or spinal anesthesia, because one would hesitate to perform spermatic-cord block on an already edematous and engorged structure and because at this stage the patient is invariably hospitalized.

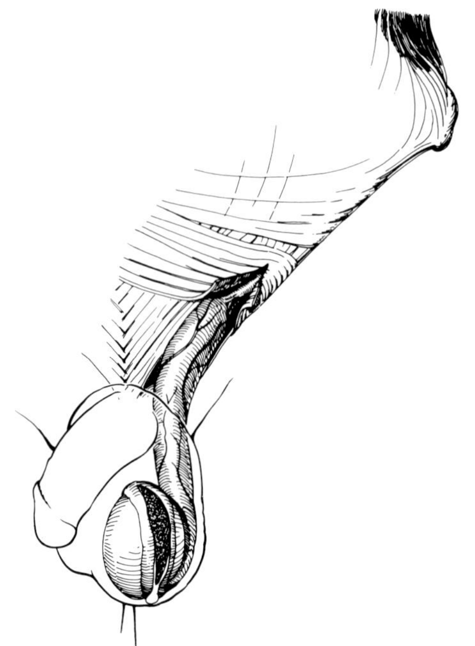

Fig. 26–12. External-ring release and epididymotomy.

Indications for Epididymotomy. This procedure is indicated when external-ring release alone fails to cure the condition. It also is indicated when the scrotal wall is fixed over the epididymis, as this indicates severe inflammation with potential suppuration. Persistent pyrexia, a raised leukocyte count, and severe testicular pain and scrotal edema also are indications. Careful judgment will be needed in deciding whether to attempt external-ring release alone under local anesthesia or to go ahead immediately with scrotal exploration, ring release, and epididymotomy under spinal or general anesthesia.

Operative Technique. An inguinoscrotal incision, extending only into the upper part of the scrotum, is preferred, as this, together with careful epididymotomy, has been found to prevent wound disruption with discharge of sloughing testicular tissue. The testis is exposed by opening the visceral layer of the tunica vaginalis, with great care not to incise the epididymal tubules (see Fig. 26–12). A shallow vertical incision is then made in the epididymis from the head to the tail. Pus will be seen in some cases, whereas in others only severe edema is found. A drain is placed at the epididymis and brought out through the scrotum inferiorly.

These techniques, together with regular evaluation of the patient, result in markedly reduced morbidity from acute epididymitis. It is suggested that this condition no longer be thought of as requiring either conservative treatment or ablative surgery but rather that organ-sparing operations be used more frequently.

CONCLUSIONS

Operations on the scrotum and its contents are ideal for the ambulatory surgery unit, particularly when one considers the low priority usually given to such procedures by hospital operating rooms. The financial savings are approximately 74%, a further inducement to outpatient care.

REFERENCES

1. Dahl, D.S., et al.: Lord's operation for hydrocele compared with conventional techniques. Arch. Surg., *104*:40, 1972.
2. Haas, J.A., et al.: Operative treatment of hydrocele: another look at Lord's procedure. Urology, *12*:578, 1978.
3. Lord, P.H.: A bloodless operation for the radical cure of idiopathic hydrocele. Br. J. Surg., *51*:914, 1964.
4. Efron, G., and Sharkey, G.G.: The Lord operation for hydrocele. Surg. Gynecol. Obstet., *125*:603, 1967.
5. Rodriguez, W.C., Rodriguez, D.D., and Fortuno, R.F.: The operative treatment of hydrocele: a comparison of four basic techniques. J. Urol., *125*:804, 1981.
6. Lord, P.H.: A bloodless operation for spermatocele or cyst of the epididymis. Br. J. Surg., *57*:641, 1970.
7. Kaye, K.W., Clayman, R.V., and Lange, P.H.: Outpatient hydrocele and spermatocele repair under local anesthesia. J. Urol., *130*:269, 1983.
8. Kaye, K.W., Lange, P.H., and Fraley, E.E.: Spermatic cord block in urologic surgery. J. Urol., *128*:720, 1982.
9. Blandy, J.: Surgery of the testicle. *In* Operative Urology. London, Blackwell Scientific Publications, 1978.
10. Beil, D.A.: Vasectomy and lowering surgeon's risk of liability. Urology, *12*:682, 1978.
11. West, P.J., and Bartelt, R.C.: Medicolegal aspects of urology. Urol. Clin. North Am., *7*:153, 1980.
12. Leader, A.J.: Elective Vasectomy. Norwich-Eaton Pharmaceuticals, Norwich, NY, 1982.
13. Dubin, L.J., and Amelar, R.D.: Varicocelectomy: 986 cases in a 12-year study. Urology, *10*:446, 1977.
14. Lome, L.G., and Ross, L.: Varicocelectomy and infertility. Urology, 9:416, 1977.
15. Ross, L.S., Lepson, S., and Dritz, S.: Surgical treatment of varicocele. Urology, *19*:179, 1982.
16. Gonzalez, R., et al.: Comparison of Doppler examination and retrograde spermatic venography in diagnosis of varicocele. Fertil. Steril., *40*:96, 1983.
17. Costas, S., and van Blerk, P.J.P.: Incision of the external inguinal ring in acute epididymitis. Br. J. Urol., *45*:555, 1973.
18. Witherington, R., and Harper, W.M., IV: The surgical management of acute bacterial epididymitis with emphasis on epididymotomy. J. Urol., *128*:722, 1982.

27

Evaluation and Treatment of Male Infertility

ROBERT M. WEISSMAN, M.D., and LARRY I. LIPSCHULTZ, M.D., F.A.C.S.

The evaluation and treatment of the subfertile couple are especially well suited to the outpatient setting. This chapter deals with several aspects of that evaluation and treatment, emphasizing the techniques. First, the most common therapeutic operation, varicocele ligation, will be discussed. Second, transscrotal testicular biopsy, with and without vasography, will be described. Finally, the appropriate techniques of artificial insemination will be reviewed. Other relevant material—on vasovasostomy and the nonoperative treatment of varicocele—will be found in Chapters 25 and 18, respectively.

VARICOCELE LIGATION

Incompetent valves of the internal spermatic vein occur in approximately 20% of males and appear to cause abnormal semen quality in some subfertile men.[1] Improvement in semen quality and increased pregnancy rates have been reported after varicocele ligation by numerous investigators.[2–4] There are three basic approaches to the surgical ligation of the internal spermatic vein: scrotal, retroperitoneal and inguinal.

Scrotal Approach

Although proponents of the scrotal approach contend that it allows a more complete ligation of the gonadal veins, including those that may not anastamose with the internal spermatic vein, we do not favor such a procedure for several reasons. First, because of the complexity of the dilated pampiniform plexus, the scrotal operation is more time consuming, and it is more difficult to be certain that all venous branches have been adequately ligated. In addition, it is much easier to injure the blood supply to the testis, including the internal spermatic, cremasteric, and deferential arteries. Finally, there is the potential for increased postoperative morbidity from intrascrotal hemorrhage and edema.

Our institutions are equipped with well-functioning outpatient surgical units, allowing the brief use of a general anesthetic and a short stay in the postoperative recovery room before discharge. Under these conditions, both the high retroperitoneal ligation (Palomo) procedure and the inguinal (Ivanissevitch) approach are performed.[5,6] In general, we favor the inguinal approach, especially if local anesthesia is contemplated. High ligation is reserved for those patients who have previously undergone an inguinal operation, such as a herniorrhaphy or an inadequate varicocele repair.

Retroperitoneal Approach

The retroperitoneal approach begins with the patient supine and in the reverse Trendelenburg position. A short transverse incision is made just medial to and below the anterosuperior iliac spine (Fig. 27–1); this should place the incision at the level of the internal inguinal ring. The skin incision is carried down to and through Scarpa's fascia, exposing the aponeurosis of the external oblique muscle. This fascia is sharply incised in the direction of its fibers, and the internal oblique muscle is encountered. At this point, an abdominal retractor is inserted such that the internal oblique muscle is retracted cranially (Fig. 27–2*A*). The dilated internal spermatic veins are now easily visible as they course through the internal ring (Fig. 27–2*B*). The veins are then freed from the artery by both blunt and sharp dissection. Care must be taken to ensure that no anastomosing collaterals are missed. The veins are ligated with nonabsorbable, 3–0 silk ligatures (Fig. 27–2*C*), and a short segment of each is removed (Fig. 27–2*D*). Inadvertent tearing of a vein by rough handling of the tissues may result in retraction of the vessel into the retroperitoneum, requiring a much more extensive surgical procedure. The vas deferens can sometimes be seen curving into the pelvis in the lower, medial aspect of the incision.

With the completion of the dissection, the internal oblique muscle is allowed to fall back into position. The external oblique fascia is closed with interrupted 2–0 Dexon sutures. Scarpa's fascia is closed with a 3–0 chromic suture, and the skin is reapproximated with a running 4–0 Dexon subcuticular stitch reinforced with Steri-strips.

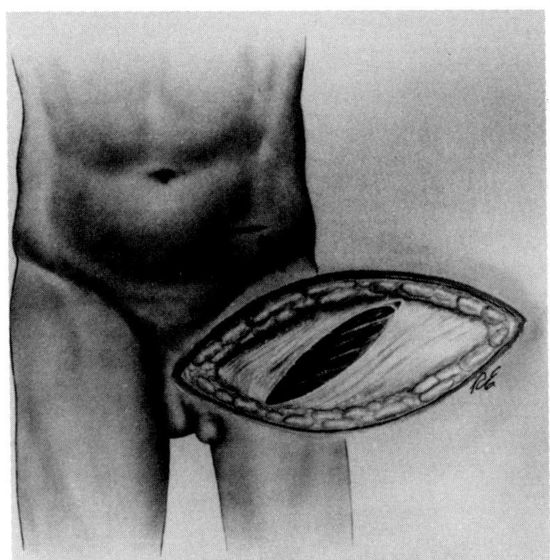

Fig. 27–1. Incision for retroperitoneal approach to varicocele ligation.

Inguinal Approach

The inguinal approach lends itself nicely to both general and local anesthesia. Again, the patient is placed supine in the reversed Trendelenburg position, to allow retrograde filling of the dilated veins within the spermatic cord. The medial aspect of the incision is begun two fingerbreadths above the symphysis pubis and perpendicular to the lateral border of the scrotum (Fig. 27–3*A*). The incision courses obliquely toward, but not to, the anterosuperior iliac spine. If local anesthesia is preferred, skin wheals are raised with 1% lidocaine without epinephrine along the line of the incision.

The incision is carried down through Scarpa's fascia to the external oblique fascia. Approximately 5 ml of 1% lidocaine is administered beneath this fascia before it is divided in the direction of its fibers. A Weitlander self-retaining retractor is inserted. The ilioinguinal nerve is identified and directed away from the operative site. Regardless of whether the procedure is performed under general anesthesia, approximately 5 ml of bupivacaine hydrochloride without epineph-

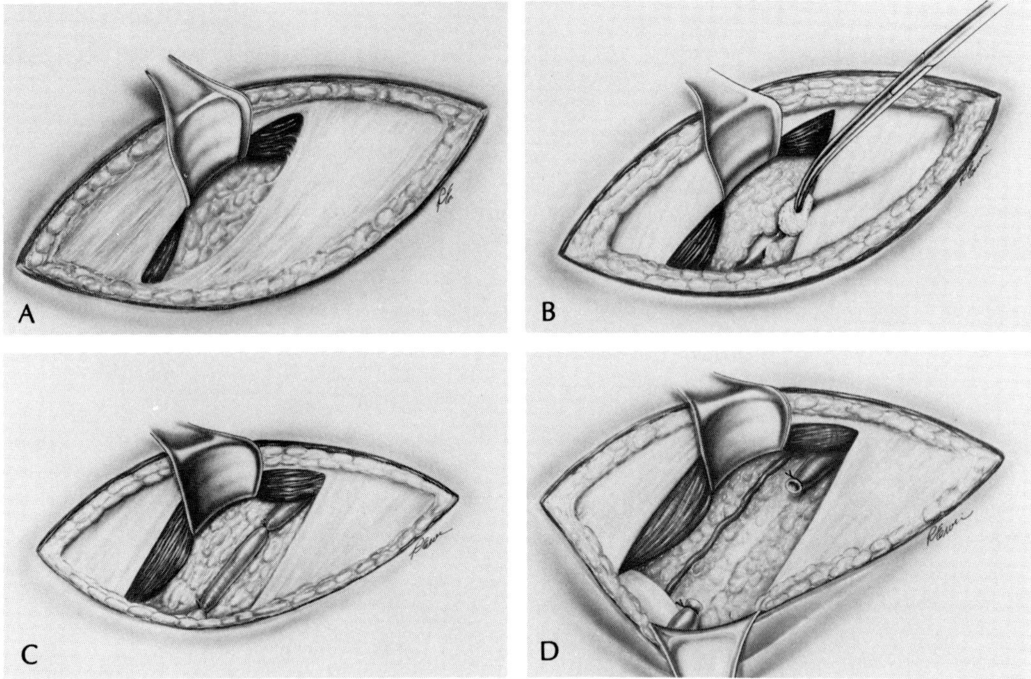

Fig. 27–2. Varicocele ligation via the retroperitoneal approach. *(A)* Abdominal retractor used to retract the internal oblique muscle cranially. *(B)* Exposure of the dilated spermatic veins. *(C)* Ligation of the veins with nonabsorbable sutures. *(D)* Removal of a short segment of each vein.

rine is injected around this nerve to decrease postoperative pain. If general anesthesia is not being used, 1% lidocaine is injected circumferentially around the spermatic cord and into the periosteum of the pubis. The cord is then mobilized and a Penrose drain placed beneath it for retraction (Fig. 27–3*B*). The spermatic fascia is incised (Fig. 27–3*C*), and usually two or three vessels are easily identified. These are dissected free (Fig. 27–3*D*), ligated with 2–0 silk, and incised (Fig. 27–3*E*). Care must be taken not to dissect around the vas deferens in order to preserve the deferential artery and thus maintain the testicular blood supply should the other arteries of the testis be injured. Before closing, it is also important to look for a dilated cremasteric vein at the external inguinal ring. In some patients, this is an important collateral contributor to the varicocele, and it should be ligated.

After irrigation of the wound with normal saline, the external oblique fascia is closed with a 2–0 Dexon suture, Scarpa's fascia is reapproximated with a 3–0 chromic suture, and the skin is closed with a 4–0 Dexon running subcuticular suture reinforced with Steri-strips. If local anesthesia is being used, a total of 40 to 50 ml of lidocaine will be needed for a unilateral procedure.

After a brief stay in the recovery room, the patient who has undergone a retroperitoneal or inguinal varicocele ligation is discharged with appropriate analgesics and instructions to avoid activity for 72 hours. Thereafter, he may voluntarily increase his activity and should return for an initial postoperative visit in one week.

TESTIS BIOPSY AND VASOGRAPHY

In the azoospermic man with normal-sized testes and a serum follicle-stimu-

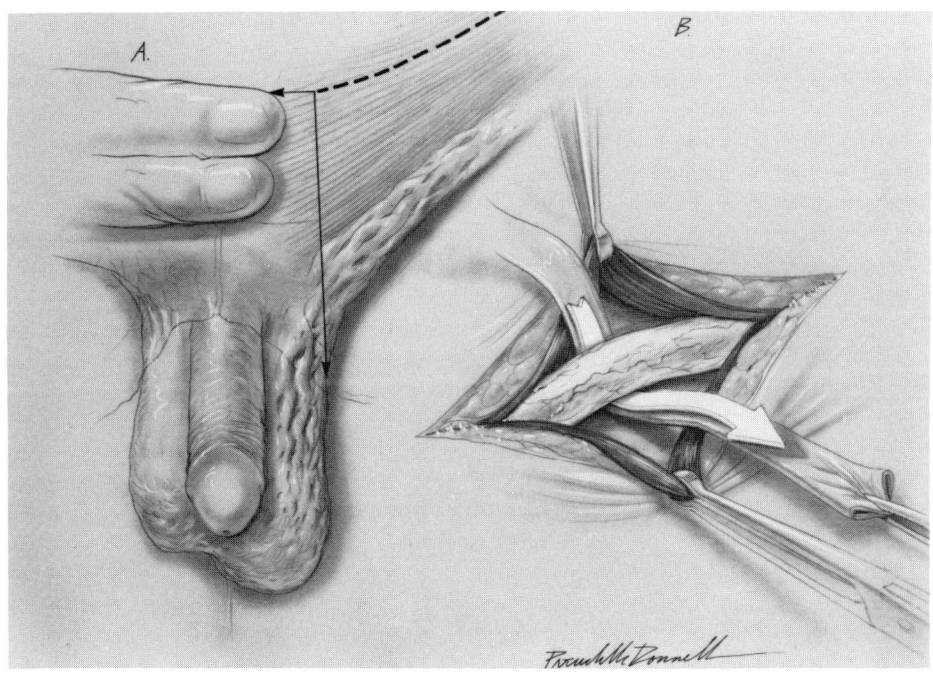

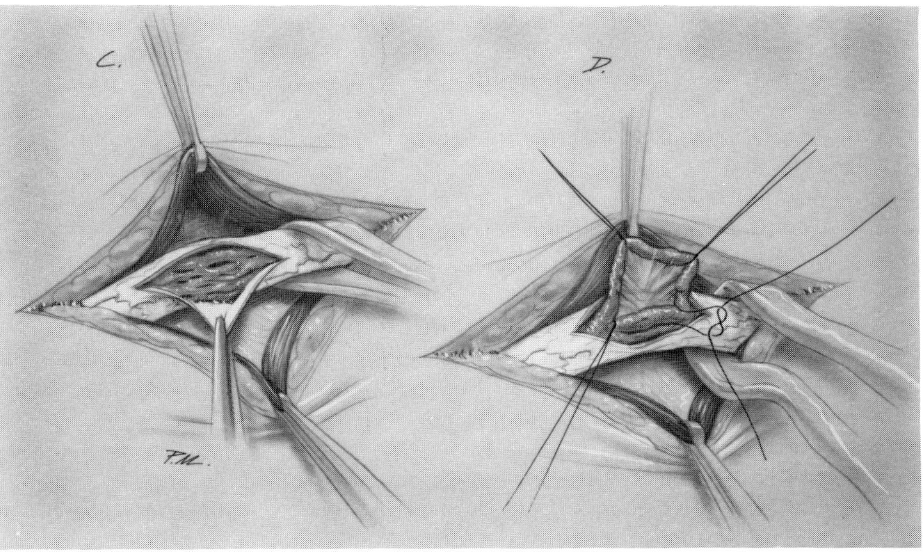

Fig. 27–3. Varicocele ligation via the inguinal approach. *(A)* Site of incision. *(B)* Spermatic cord retracted on a Penrose drain. *(C)* Opening of spermatic fascia. *(D)* Freeing and ligation of the vessels. *(E)* Incision of the vessels.

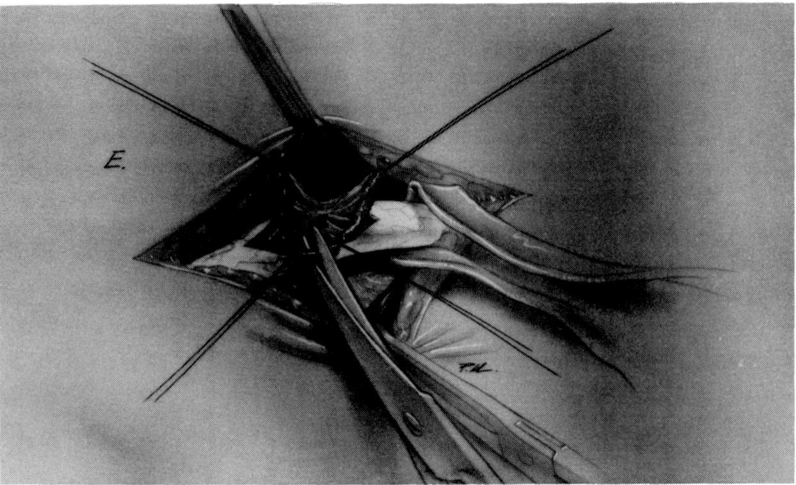

Fig. 27–3. ***continued***

lating hormone (FSH) level of less than two times normal, bilateral testicular biopsy is necessary to establish whether abnormal spermatogenesis or ductal obstruction is the cause of the sterility.[7] Much less often, testicular biopsy may be indicated in the subfertile male with abnormal testicular size and an elevated FSH level. It must be stated, however, that rarely does the pathologic result of the biopsy significantly alter the therapeutic options or prognosis in these patients.

It is the authors' bias that the surgeon should be prepared to proceed with vasography and possible microsurgical repair of ductal obstruction in the azoospermic man on the basis of the biopsy findings. Therefore, in an outpatient setting, we prefer to use either a general anesthetic or a local anesthetic (including a cord block) with general anesthesia on standby. The testis is delivered into the operative field, permitting full inspection for epididymal dilation or other abnormalities. The exceptions to such an approach are few: the patient who desires more time to consider his therapeutic options after testicular biopsy and the patient in whom there is good reason to believe the epididymis is normal. In these cases, a simple "window technique" is used with local anesthesia.

Testis Biopsy

With the patient supine and the scrotal skin stretched tightly over the anterior part of the testis, being sure that the epididymis is well posterior, a 2-cm incision is made after infiltration of the skin with 1% lidocaine without epinephrine (Fig. 27–4A). The incision is made transversely in the hemiscrotum in order to parallel the scrotal vessels and minimize bleeding and is carried down to the tunica vaginalis. With the tunica vaginalis tented between two smooth forceps, it is sharply incised, exposing the underlying testis. It is usually unnecessary to perform a cord block, as the brief abdominal discomfort upon incision of the tunica albuginea is tolerable to the conscious patient. However, the patient must be forewarned and a cord block administered if the pain becomes intolerable.

Using a No. 11 blade, the tunica albuginea is sharply incised for approximately 1 cm. Gentle pressure on the tes-

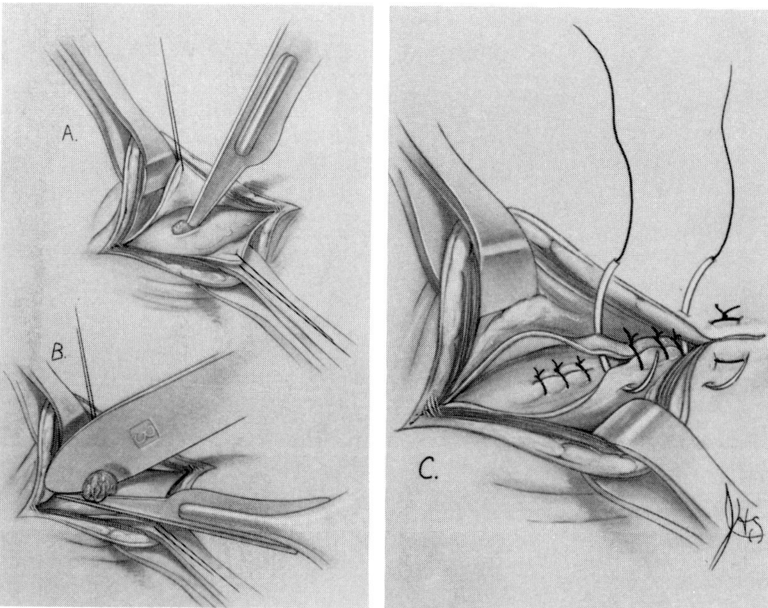

Fig. 27–4. Testis biopsy. *(A)* Incision site. *(B)* Gentle pressure to extrude stroma. *(C)* Closing of tunica vaginalis.

tis allows the testicular stroma to extrude (Fig. 27–4*B*). The biopsy specimen is excised with a "no-touch" technique, using a scalpel or scissors. The specimen is sent in Zenker's or Bouin's fixative for pathologic evaluation, since formaldehyde will make the biopsy difficult to interpret. The tunica albuginea is closed with 4–0 Dexon on a cutting needle. The tunica vaginalis is closed with a running 4–0 chromic suture and the skin with a 4–0 chromic interrupted horizontal mattress stitch (Fig. 27–4*C*).

Vasography

When exploration of the testis and epididymis is indicated, general anesthesia or local anesthesia with cord block is administered. After delivery of the entire testis and epididymis into the operative field, a testicular biopsy is performed as described above and sent for frozen section. The epididymis is inspected for any obvious abnormality. If the biopsy confirms active spermatogenesis and the epididymis looks unobstructed, vasography is clearly indicated.

We favor performing vasography with some form of optical enhancement, either an operating zoom microscope or optical loupes. A formal vasotomy is performed under direct vision with a No. 11 blade. Because the site of the vasotomy is important, the vas deferens is exposed by sharp dissection just proximal to its convoluted portion. The vasotomy incision should involve approximately one half of the circumference of the vas, easily exposing its lumen. A blunt 25-gauge cannula is inserted in the direction of the abdominal vas (Fig. 27–5). Ten milliliters of radiologic contrast material (Conray 60 diluted 1:2 with saline) is injected under gentle pressure as the film is obtained. A vasogram is not performed in the direction of a convoluted vas and epididymis, as the contrast material may cause fibrosis and secondary obstruction.

Upon completion of the vasogram, the vasotomy is closed under direct vision with the aid of the operating microscope

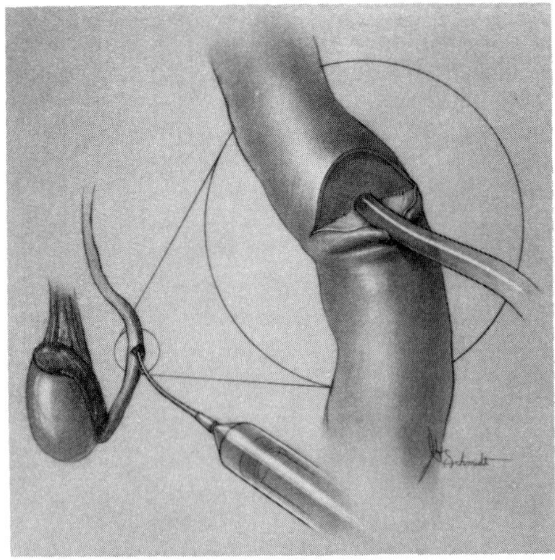

Fig. 27–5. Insertion of cannula for vasography.

or optical loupes. Two full-thickness sutures of 10–0 nylon (Ethicon 10–0 Ethelon suture on a GS-16 needle) are placed at the two o'clock and ten o'clock positions and tied (Fig. 27–6*A*). Seromuscular 8–0 nylon sutures are placed between and on either side of the 10–0 sutures (Fig. 27–6*B*). Depending on the results of the vasogram, the surgeon may proceed to microsurgical repair or closure of the incision in layers with absorbable sutures. Postoperatively, the patient is discharged with appropriate analgesics, an ice pack for the initial 24 hours, and scrotal support for one week. Sexual abstinence is suggested for two weeks.

ARTIFICIAL INSEMINATION

Artificial insemination with the husband's semen (AIH) is most successful in anatomic or psychologic conditions that preclude normal intercourse or the proper placement of seminal fluid deep within the vagina. These include hypospadias, procidentia, retrograde ejaculation, congenital anomalies, vaginismus, and impotence. It is far less successful in cases of poor semen quality. In a consenting couple, artificial insemination with donor semen (AID) is a proven alternative when the man is irreversibly infertile. It is beyond the scope of this chapter to discuss the moral, ethical, or legal aspects of donor insemination. On the contrary, it will be our purpose to

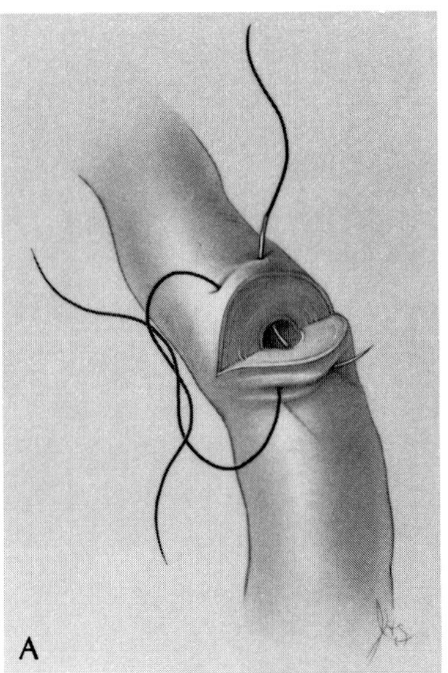

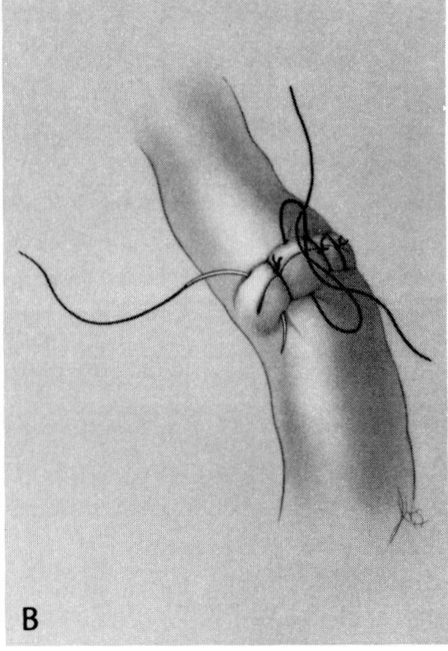

Fig. 27–6. Closure of vasostomy. *(A)* Insertion of full-thickness sutures. *(B)* Insertion of seromuscular sutures.

describe the techniques of outpatient insemination.

The most important factor in successful insemination is determining ovulation time. Therefore, it is mandatory that a basal body-temperature chart be maintained by the patient and reviewed by her physician in order to predict the time of ovulation more accurately. For example, if the woman's temperature increase consistently occurs between days 14 and 16 of a 28-day cycle, and if her cervical mucus is clear and demonstrates extensive threading when grasped with forceps (spinnbarkeit), then the patient would be inseminated optimally on days 13, 15, and 17. In a small proportion of women, unilateral pelvic pain (mittelschmerz) may also be a useful sign of ovulation. It is of utmost importance that at least two inseminations be done during each of several cycles. In this manner, the physician will be better able to time ovulations and increase the probability of success.

There are essentially three accepted methods commonly used for artificial insemination: the intrauterine, cervicovaginal, and cervical-cup techniques (Fig. 27–7).[8] Of these, the most generally used in the outpatient office setting is the cervical-cup method.

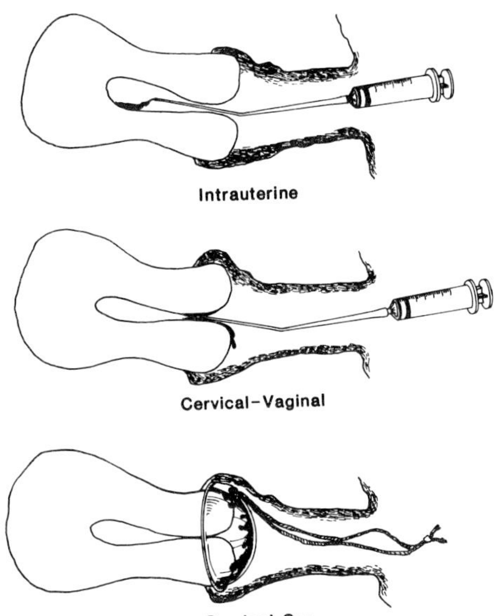

Fig. 27–7. Accepted methods of artificial insemination.

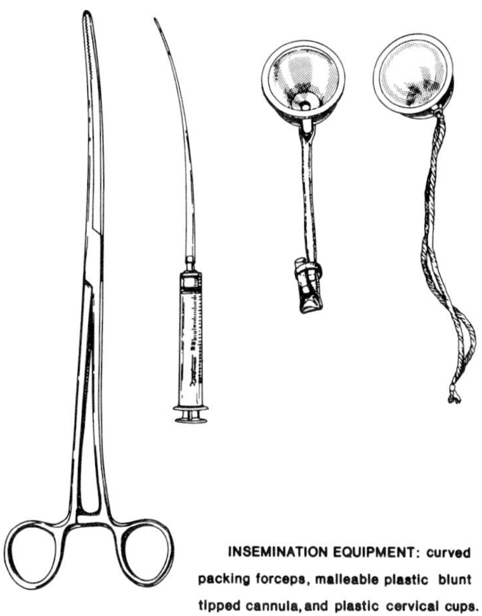

INSEMINATION EQUIPMENT: curved packing forceps, malleable plastic blunt tipped cannula, and plastic cervical cups.

Fig. 27–8. Equipment for artificial insemination.

Cervical-Cup Technique

The cervical-cup technique requires either a blunt-tipped, malleable metal cannula or plastic "tomcat" catheter (so called for its use in veterinary medicine to catheterize obstructed tomcats), curved packing forceps, and a small plastic cup with attached tubing or string (Fig. 27–8). The patient is placed in the standard lithotomy position, and an appropriate-sized speculum is inserted, using water as the only lubricant. (Other lubricants, such as K–Y Jelly, should be avoided, as they may retard sperm motility.) Under direct vision, the cervix is cleaned with a dry sponge, and a small amount of cervical mucus is aspirated using a 1-inch syringe and a plastic Intercath tip. The mucus is placed on a microscope slide and examined for consistency, cellularity, and spinnbarkeit. The semen specimen is drawn up into a 3-ml syringe, and approximately 0.5 ml is deposited in the endocervical canal. The remainder of the semen is placed within an appropriate-sized cervical cup or through the tubing attached to the cup and positioned on the cervix with the packing forceps. Because of the cervical cup, the semen remains in contact with the cervical mucus, protected from the more hostile vaginal environment. The vaginal speculum is removed, and the patient is discharged from the office with instructions to remove the cup in 4 to 5 hours. This is easily accomplished because of the attached string or tubing.

Cervicovaginal Technique

The cervicovaginal method is similar to the cervical-cup technique except that, after 0.5 ml of semen has been deposited in the endocervical canal, the remainder is placed directly in the vaginal vault near the cervix. No cervical cup is applied. This method has three principal disadvantages. First, in order for the semen to be in contact with the cervix, the patient must remain supine with her legs flexed for at least 40 to 60 minutes; this is not cost effective in a busy clinical practice. Second, the semen in the vaginal vault is not protected from the hostile vaginal acidity, resulting in the inactivation of many viable spermatozoa. Last, many patients become distraught when part of the semen sample is lost when they arise from the table.

Intrauterine Technique

The intrauterine method requires the direct placement of semen through the cervical os into the uterine cavity. Again, a blunt-tipped cannula is used. Because of the greater risks with such a procedure, its use should be reserved for those patients with abnormal (i.e., hostile) cervical mucus. Possible complications include uterine trauma with hemorrhage, uterine infection, and uterine contractions that expel the semen. The risk of uterine contractions increases greatly when more than 0.3 ml is instilled. Because of these potential complications, it is the authors' bias that this technique is best performed by skilled physicians well versed in handling problems of the female genital tract.

CONCLUSIONS

It has been emphasized that many of the procedures for the evaluation and treatment of the subfertile couple can easily be accomplished in the outpatient setting. Complications and risks are negligible, and the savings in time and cost are gratifying.

REFERENCES

1. Thomason, A.M., and Fariss, B.L.: The prevalence of varicoceles in a group of healthy young men. Milit. Med., *144*:181, 1979.
2. Charney, C.W., and Baum, S.: Varicoceles and infertility. J. Am. Med. Assoc., *204*:1165, 1968.
3. Stewart, B.H.: Varicocele in infertility: incidence and results of surgical therapy. J. Urol., *115*:222, 1974.
4. MacLeod, J.: Further observations on the role of varicocele in human male infertility. Fertil. Steril., *20*:545, 1969.
5. Palomo, A.: Radical cure of varicocele by a new technique: preliminary report. J. Urol., *61*:604, 1969.
6. Ivanissevitch, O.: Left varicocele due to reflux: experience with 4,470 operative cases in 42 years. J. Int. Coll. Surg., *34*:742, 1960.
7. Hotchkiss, R.S.: Testicular biopsy in the diagnosis and treatment of sterility in the male. Bull. N.Y. Acad. Med., *18*:600, 1942.
8. Beck, W.W.: Artificial insemination and preservation of semen. Urol. Clin. North Am., 5:593, 1978.

28

Diagnosis of Skin Lesions and Other Outpatient Operations on the Penis

VALDA N. KAYE, M.D., F.C. Path.(S.A.), ELWIN E. FRALEY, M.D., and ROBERT W. GOLTZ, M.D.

There are many times, particularly when there is a question of malignancy, that even the most expert clinician needs the help of a microscopic study to identify lesions of the penis; and thus the correct method of taking a specimen for biopsy is an essential skill for the management of many skin disorders. The method should be convenient, quick, easy, safe, inexpensive, and as pain free as possible, because these considerations are important in themselves and they encourage the performance of a biopsy. Most important, the method must produce an undamaged specimen sufficiently representative of the lesion to permit the pathologist to make the diagnosis. This chapter describes such a method, as well as minor penile operations usually performed on an outpatient basis that may be needed in the patient who requires a biopsy. Clinical features and management of the diseases are discussed only briefly.

BIOPSY AND OPERATIVE METHODS

Biopsy

Preparation of the Patient. After the patient has been told the reason for and the nature of the procedure and has been informed of the rare complications of hemorrhage and infection, he signs a consent form. He should be asked whether he is allergic to local anesthetics; but in our experience, reactions to 1% lidocaine are rare, and this drug provides adequate local anesthesia in most cases. The patient should lie down during the biopsy, because this makes the procedure easier for the operator and because patients sometimes faint.

Site Selection. The specimen of greatest value is one from the most representative part of the lesion that is not obscured by ulceration, necrosis, or secondary infection. Identification of this area requires clinical judgment. If one suspects tumor, the most indurated, thickened area is usually best. In evaluating infections, the advancing edge of the lesion is usually the most representative, and it is there that the causative organism is usually most abundant.

The old dictum that the specimen should be taken from the edge of the lesion and include normal skin is usually wrong. Few pathologists require normal skin for comparison, and in laboratory processing, the most representative part of such a specimen is likely to be trimmed away and discarded.

Techniques. Particularly for exophytic lesions, simple snipping out of a sample with curved iris scissors is often all that is needed (Fig. 28–1). Rat-toothed forceps may be useful for picking up the specimen after it has been cut out if care is taken not to squeeze, tear, or otherwise distort it. Hemostasis is obtained by light cauterization or electrodesiccation of bleeders with a hyfrecator or a Bovie unit. Some clinicians prefer agents such as ferric subsulfate (Monsel's solution) or packing the wound with Oxycel. Occasionally, tying off bleeding vessels or suturing may be necessary, so the necessary instruments and suture material should be handy.

Cutaneous punches are popular biopsy instruments, especially for a deep lesion, although they are less useful on the penis than elsewhere because the penile skin is thin and the vascularity of the organ makes hemostasis difficult. Punches are available in diameters of 2 to 8 mm, with those of 3 to 6 mm being used most often. The cutting edges should be examined to be certain they are not dented, which sometimes happens during sterilization. The punch is applied to the lesion with moderate pressure and a rotating motion to cut out a plug of appropriate depth (Fig. 28–2), which is held with forceps and cut off at its base with curved scissors.

Surgeons often prefer elliptic incisions that are closed with sutures. Although this produces specimens of adequate size, it creates problems with hemostasis when done on the penis and thus is probably best restricted to operating rooms. Because this adds considerably to the cost and inconvenience of the procedure, it may be an impediment to biopsy.

Cytology studies (Tzanck smears) are useful for bullous lesions such as herpes simplex, herpes zoster, and pemphigus. If a blister is present, it is opened; and its base and roof are scraped with a blade or ringed curette to obtain material for a smear.

Other special methods are described in appropriate sections elsewhere in this chapter.

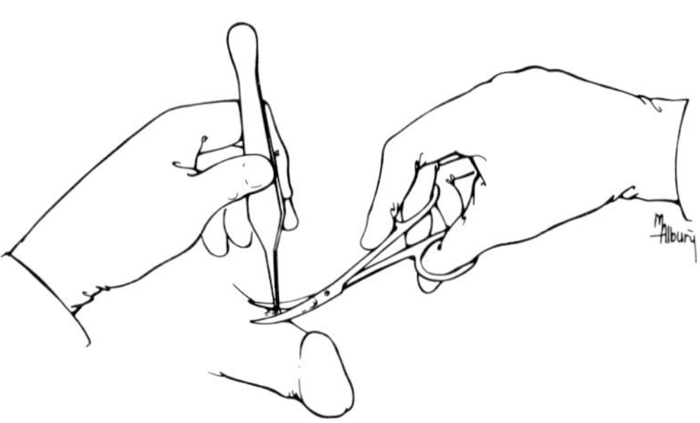

Fig. 28–1. Iris scissors and rat-toothed forceps are useful for obtaining small, especially exophytic, lesions from the skin of the penis.

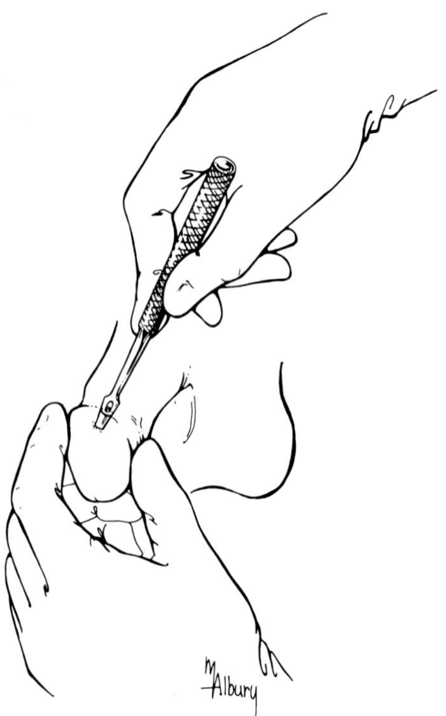

Fig. 28–2. Cutaneous punch being used to obtain a plug of tissue for biopsy of the glans.

Postprocedure Care

The wound is dressed with gauze. The patient is told to remove the dressing the next day and to begin cleansing the wound daily with 3% hydrogen peroxide until it has healed. It is all right if the area gets wet. A mild analgesic (e.g., acetaminophen), may be needed for the first day or two. The patient should immediately report persistent soreness and any redness or swelling. He should be instructed not to have sexual intercourse for two to three weeks.

Adjunctive Techniques

In many patients, operations on the foreskin prove necessary for the production of adequate biopsy specimens. The techniques described here are also suitable when no biopsy is planned.

Dorsal Slit of the Foreskin. This operation is performed after infiltration of the area of the incision with 1–2% lidocaine without epinephrine and can be used for phimosis or, with modification, paraphimosis. With care not to enter the urethral meatus, the upward-tilted lower jaw of a straight hemostat is passed under the foreskin in the dorsal midline until it meets resistance. The hemostat is then moved 1 cm distally and closed on the foreskin. It is removed, and the line of crushed tissue is cut with scissors. Bleeding vessels are controlled by electrocoagulation, and the edges are oversewn with continuous 4–0 chromic catgut (Fig. 28–3*A*,*B*). The foreskin is then separated from the glans to the extent possible, with adhesions being lysed. Topical antibiotics should be applied to infected areas. Biopsy specimens of the glans or foreskin may then be taken as described earlier.

In the patient with paraphimosis, the surgeon should attempt to free the foreskin by slow, firm squeezing of the edematous tissue so that the dorsal slit procedure can be performed as described. It is useful to perform a penile block initially (see Chapter 8), as direct infiltration of local anesthesia only increases the edema. If squeezing fails, the dorsal aspect of the constricting band of foreskin is incised with a scalpel. The dorsal slit procedure can then be performed.

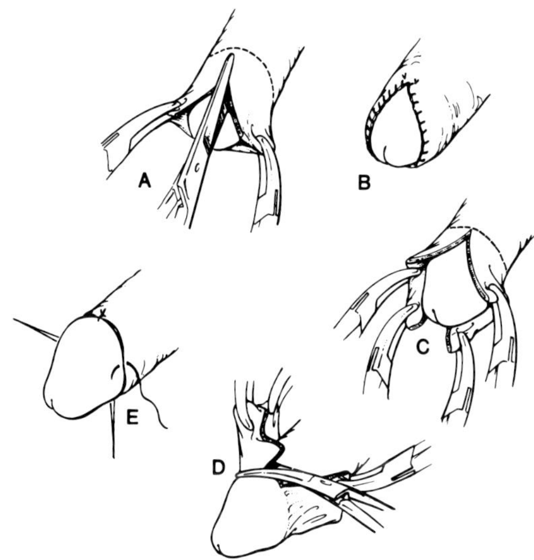

Fig. 28–3. Dorsal slit and circumcision. *(A)* Tissue is crushed and incised in the midline; hemostats holding the foreskin help prevent meatal injury. *(B)* For dorsal slit, edges of incision are oversewn. *(C)* For circumcision, a second incision is made. *(D)* Foreskin is removed, with care taken to cut inner and outer layers to the same depth. *(E)* Closure; note stay sutures to prevent misalignment.

Circumcision. In adults, this procedure is usually performed as part of the management of phimosis, recurrent paraphimosis or balanoposthitis, or chronic yeast infection (particularly in diabetics). Less common indications are the patient's wish to be circumcised or the excisional biopsy of a suspected carcinoma.

Some surgeons prefer to use general anesthesia for circumcision in adults, but a penile block (see Chapter 8) with local supplemental lidocaine is better suited to the outpatient surgery clinic. A dorsal slit is made as described, and the two cut edges are held distally with hemostats (see Fig. 28–3*A*,*C*,*D*,*E*). Clamping and incision are then repeated on the ventral side in the midline to the base of the frenulum. (If the frenulum is large, it should be excised and a new one created.) Hemostats are applied to the newly cut edges, and the most proximal aspects of the two incisions are joined on both sides with curved Mayo scissors, leaving approximately 1 cm of foreskin below the corona. The interior and exterior sides of the foreskin must be cut to the same depth.

The skin of the penile shaft is drawn cephalad, and hemostasis is obtained with electrocautery and fine ligatures. When electrocautery is used, the coagulation current should be set low and the side of the penis should be against the body to prevent a high current from passing along the penile shaft and causing necrosis. The cut edges of the skin on the shaft and the remaining rim of foreskin are then united. Stay sutures are placed at the 12, 6, 3, and 9 o'clock positions to stabilize the tissues, which are then closed with a running suture of 4–0 chromic catgut. Antibiotic ointment is applied to the suture line.

No dressing is used on the penis, as it may stick to the suture line, causing bleeding or constricting the penis. Instead, a light lower-abdominal dressing is created from which the patient can remove his penis to urinate.

Meatotomy. This operation is generally used in children, because it is rarely curative in adults. After adequate anesthesia has been obtained, the meatus is crushed in the midline with a fine hemostat, and the crushed tissue is incised. The edges of the wound are smeared with sterile petroleum jelly. In the older child, a few Dexon or 5–0 catgut sutures may be needed. The parents must keep the incision from closing by parting the edges gently every day. The most common reason for failure of this procedure is noncooperation of the parents.

Meatoplasty. This operation is better suited than meatotomy to meatal and submeatal strictures in adults, such as those caused by lichen sclerosis et atrophicus *(vide infra)*. If the patient is uncircumcised, the results will be better if a circumcision is performed at the same time. After a penile block has been performed, a soft Doyen clamp is placed on the penis to keep the field dry, and a U-shaped flap is created in the ventral skin (Fig. 28–4). The strictured area of the urethra is incised until healthy tissue is reached. The tip of the U-shaped flap is sewn to the distal part of the urethral incision, and the flap is folded into a funnel-shaped meatus. All suturing is done with 5–0 catgut or Dexon. A foam compression dressing is applied for 2 hours to control oozing. The patient should understand that his urinary stream will spray after this operation, but attempts to create a nar-

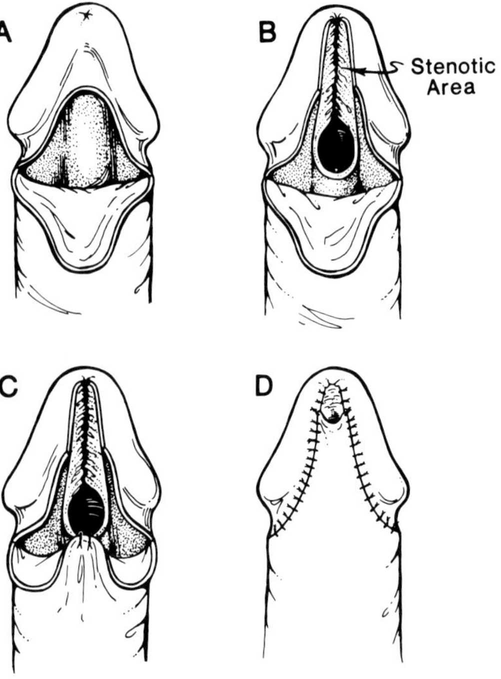

Fig. 28–4. Meatoplasty (Blandy's method). *(A)* U-shaped flap is made on the ventral surface and allowed to fold over. *(B)* Incision is made through lesion into healthy corpus spongiosum. *(C)* Tip of flap is sewn to opened urethra. *(D)* Flap is folded into a funnel and sutured in place.

row opening to prevent this will simply create another stricture.

Handling the Biopsy Specimen

All biopsy specimens should be immersed in a suitable fixative, generally a 10% buffered formaldehyde solution. The record that accompanies the specimen should contain a description of the gross features of the lesion and a list of the differential diagnoses. All too frequently, specimens are sent to the pathologist with little or no clinical information; in such cases, the surgeon should not be surprised when a vague, nonspecific histologic diagnosis is returned.

Material obtained for Tzanck smears is spread on a glass slide, allowed to dry, heat-fixed gently, and stained with Giemsa or Wright's stain. Examination under the microscope will reveal multinucleated and otherwise distorted epithelial cells when there is a virus infection (Fig. 28–5) or the characteristic acantholytic epidermal cells in pemphigus.

INFECTIONS

Yeasts and Other Fungi

Fungal infections may involve the penis, inguinal areas, or anal region. Candidiasis generally occurs in body clefts of obese individuals where the skin is macerated and presents as well-defined erythematous areas that frequently burn or itch. Genitocrural ringworm (tinea cruris) is an erythematous, scaly eruption that often has vesicular edges. It is caused by the dermatophytes *Epidermophyton floccosum*, *Trichophyton rubrum*, and *Trichophyton mentagrophytes*.

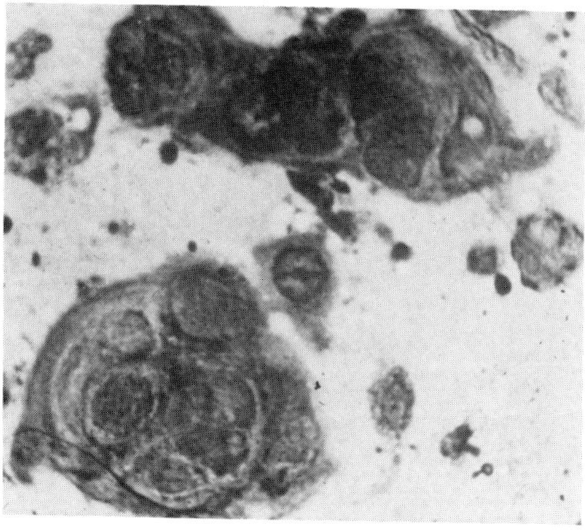

Fig. 28–5. Multinucleated epithelial giant cells in a scraping from a blister of herpes simplex.

Proper diagnosis of fungal infections requires both examination of fresh clinical specimens and isolation and identification of the organism in culture, a step for which many hospitals, and virtually all outpatient laboratories, are unprepared. Fortunately, proper direct examination is often enough for selecting treatment.

Direct Examination. Scrapings from the skin of the penis or groin are placed on a slide, and a drop of 10% potassium hydroxide (KOH) in water or dimethylsulfoxide (DMSO) is added to dissolve the skin and keratin to make the organisms more visible. Gentle heating may be necessary. A coverslip is placed over the specimen, and the slide is examined under the microscope. The lamp iris should be closed and the condenser diaphragm aperture reduced to increase the refractility of the organisms. The most productive areas to examine are generally at the periphery of the specimen, where epithelial-cell remnants and keratin are sparser and thinner.

Dermatophytes are recognizable by their long tubular, septate, sometimes branched hyphae (Fig. 28–6), whereas yeasts, such as *Candida*, are present as round or sometimes budding individual cells that sometimes form short nonseptate tubes called pseudohyphae. A possible error is mistaking the spaces between any remaining keratinocytes for hyphae, particularly when these spaces are interrupted by desmosomal "prickles" that can be mistaken for septations. True hyphae usually extend across more than one epithelial cell.

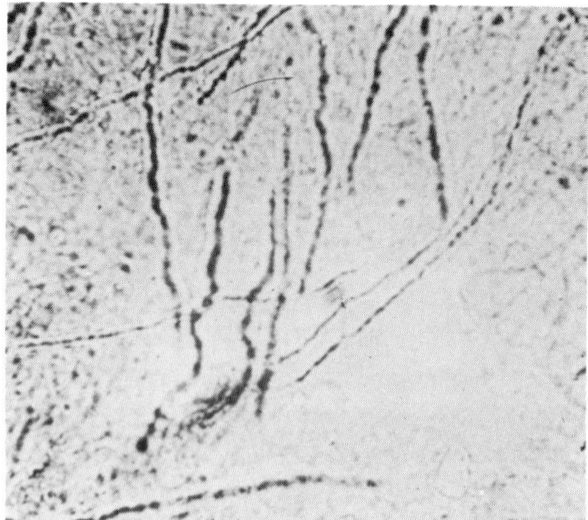

Fig. 28–6. Septate hyphae in a scraping from an inguinal lesion; specimen treated with 10% KOH in DMSO.

Culture. Initial isolation attempts are usually made on Sabouraud dextrose agar pH 5.6. For biopsy specimens or scrapings from penile lesions, addition of antibiotics to the medium may be necessary to control bacterial contaminants. In these cases, a variation of Sabouraud's medium containing less dextrose and having a higher pH is helpful (Mycosel or Mycobiotic Agar). Yeasts and molds grow slowly, the former requiring approximately a week to form evident colonies and the latter four to six weeks.

Proper identification of pathogenic fungi often requires a number of specialized methods such as the *in vitro* hair perforation test for distinguishing *Trichophyton* species.[1] These are beyond the capabilities of the typical outpatient surgery unit laboratory.

Syphilis

Clinical Picture. The old dictum that a penile ulcer is a chancre until proved otherwise is still true (Fig. 28–7). The Centers for Disease Control estimate that there are 325,000 untreated cases of syphilis in the United States, from which a resurgence in new cases is arising. Approximately half of the new cases are occurring in homosexuals and bisexuals.[2] In such patients, the primary lesion is often found in the anal area.

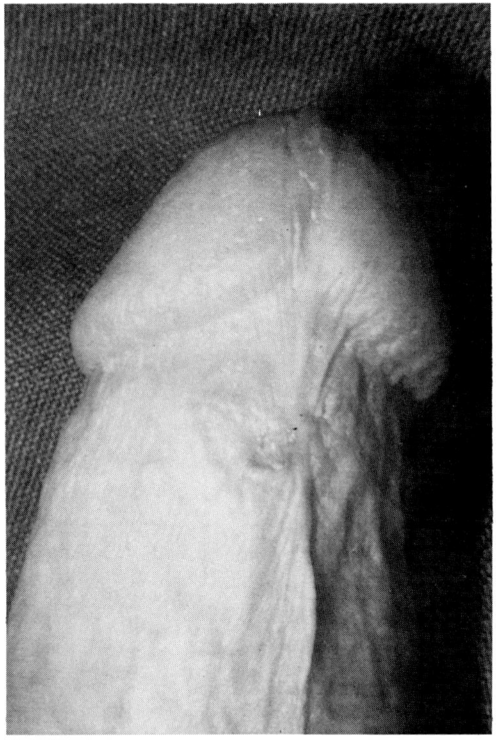

Fig. 28–7. Chancre of primary syphilis. The lesion is small and innocent-looking but teeming with spirochetes that are demonstrable by dark-field examination.

Dark-Field Examination. In primary and secondary, but not late syphilis, living spirochetes can be demonstrated in the lesions by dark-field examination. The operator should wear gloves when obtaining and handling specimens.

The lesion is cleansed of all crusts, blood, and extraneous material and squeezed gently to obtain a small drop of serum, which is picked up on a coverslip. Chancres usually are clean; and if they are not traumatized, bleeding should not be a problem. A drop of saline is applied to a slide, and the serum drop and the coverslip are laid atop it. The slide is examined immediately, as even a short period of cooling, drying, and exposure to air reduces the mobility of the fragile and obligately anaerobic spirochetes, making them more difficult to identify.

The slide is examined with an oil immersion objective on a microscope with a dark-field condenser, which must be centered properly. A drop of immersion oil is placed between the condenser and the slide and also between the slide and the objective. The spirochetes appear as bright wriggling beads or corkscrews against a black background. They are approximately one-and-one-half times the diameter of red blood cells in length.

A proper diagnosis of syphilis requires serologic confirmation, although some of these tests, such as the VDRL, are not positive in the earliest stages of primary syphilis, even after the appearance of the chancre.

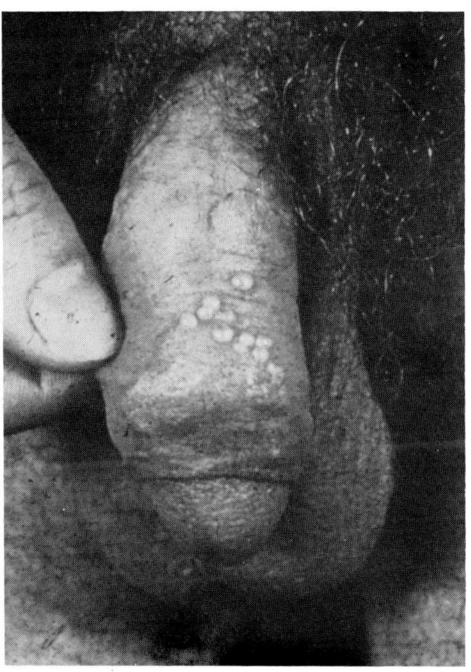

Fig. 28–8. Grouped vesicles of herpes simplex occurring as a primary infection on the shaft of the penis.

Herpesviruses

In the past, Herpes simplex type 1 was found almost exclusively in nongenital sites, whereas type 2 was confined to the anogenital region ("One above the waist, two below it"). In general, this is still true, but some cases of genital herpes are now being caused by the type 1 virus.

Clinical Picture. Primary genital herpes is a systemic as well as a local infection. Locally, there are groups of small (1–2 mm) painful or pruritic vesicles (Fig. 28–8), with tender inguinal lymphadenopathy being present in 80% of patients. Occasionally, the lesions have a zosteriform pattern. Dysuria is frequent (63%). More than half the patients have constitutional symptoms, with one third having aseptic meningitis characterized by headache, stiff neck, and mild photophobia. The symptoms are more severe in women. Secondary yeast infections afflict one patient in ten. The primary episode persists for a mean of 19 days, with a range of two to six weeks.[3,4]

Recurrences may be triggered by sexual intercourse, emotional stress, or fatigue, although often no precipitating event can be identified. In approximately half the cases, mild tingling hyperesthesia or dysesthesia precedes recurrences by one to two days. Recurrent lesions are usually smaller and less painful than primary ones and usually disappear in seven to ten days. Constitutional manifestations are uncommon.

Genital infections with Herpes simplex type 1 virus are less likely to recur than are infections with type 2.

Diagnosis. A presumptive diagnosis can be made by a Tzanck smear of material from the floor of a blister, or more accurately, if less easily, by direct immunofluorescence or direct immunoperoxidase methods, the results of which correlate with virus isolation studies in 82% of patients.[5] A dark-field examination is also advisable to rule out syphilis, and cultures or tests for the other common sexually transmitted organisms, namely *Chlamydia trachomatis* and *Neis-*

seria gonorrhoeae, also are appropriate. The laboratory diagnosis and the treatment of sexually transmitted diseases are described elsewhere.[4,6–9] Fluorescence techniques should simplify the diagnosis. Monoclonal antibodies commercially available from Ciba or Ortho permit rapid identification of the virus and distinction between type 1 and type 2 herpes infections.

SCABIES

Sites of predilection for this ectoparasitic disease are the interdigital folds, the flexor aspects of the wrists, the extensor surfaces of the elbows, the anterior axillary folds, and the areas surrounding the nipples, naval, and girdle. The penis may also be affected, but the scalp is almost always spared.

The causative mites, *Sarcoptes scabiei,* live in cutaneous burrows that appear as whitish tortuous channels with a gray speck at the end. The principal presenting feature is pruritus, which is worse at night. Definitive diagnosis depends on demonstration of the mite, which may be found in tissue sections as well as in skin scrapings.

A persistent form of scabies presents as nodular lesions on the penile glans and shaft and the scrotum. These lesions may persist for weeks or months after eradication of the mites by lindane or other miticides. Only occasionally can mites be demonstrated in biopsy material from such nodules.

SKIN AND MUCOSAL LESIONS REQUIRING HISTOLOGIC EVALUATION

Carcinoma

Epidermoid carcinoma of the penis, although rare in white men in the United States, Canada, and Europe, is a significant problem elsewhere in the world, accounting for 10% or more of the cancers in men in some countries.[10] The initial lesion often appears on the glans as a nodular ulcerated area. By the time the patient seeks medical attention, the tumor is usually fungating and invasive; and the inguinal lymph nodes are enlarged, either because of metastases or because of the infection that is virtually universal in these tumors. A foul, purulent, blood-tinged discharge is common.

Verrucous or papillary carcinomas closely resemble the giant condyloma of Buschke–Löwenstein (Fig. 28–9), and some pathologists consider these to be different stages of the same tumor.[11,12] Verrucous carcinomas can be exceptionally malignant.[13]

Uncommon malignant lesions of the penis are basal cell carcinoma, mela-

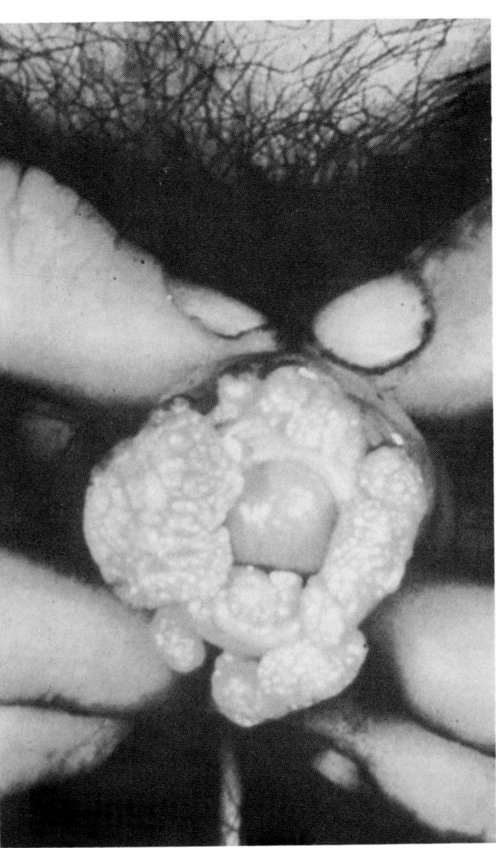

Fig. 28–9. An exaggerated verrucous lesion, which may represent a giant condyloma of Buschke–Löwenstein or a verrucous carcinoma.

noma, connective-tissue tumors such as fibrosarcoma, and metastatic tumors, most often arising from primary cancers in the bladder or prostate.[14]

Premalignant Lesions

Erythroplasia of Queyrat, carcinoma *in situ*, and Bowen's disease are probably the same lesion. Characteristically, the lesion is a solitary shiny red velvety plaque that may be ulcerated (Fig. 28–10). Invasive squamous cell carcinoma appears in 10% of patients with erythroplasia and 5% of patients with Bowen's disease. Patients with Bowen's disease are also at high risk for other dysplasias and neoplasms, including cancers of the viscera.[15–17]

Bowenoid papulosis produces multiple reddish brown or violaceous papules, primarily on the penile shaft (Fig. 28–11).[18,19] It usually affects younger men, many of whom have a history of genital viral lesions. Because the histologic features of Bowenoid papulosis and Bowen's disease may overlap, it is essential that the pathologist be given adequate clinical information with the tissue specimen. Some lesions of Bowenoid papulosis regress spontaneously, and others can be removed by excision and electrocautery or treatment with 5-fluorouracil. Although Wade et al. found carcinoma *in situ* in the lesions of all 34 of their cases,[19] the natural history of Bowenoid papulosis is unknown; and thus the appropriate management is unclear. In our series of patients, there have been no progressions of Bowenoid papulosis to frank carcinoma.

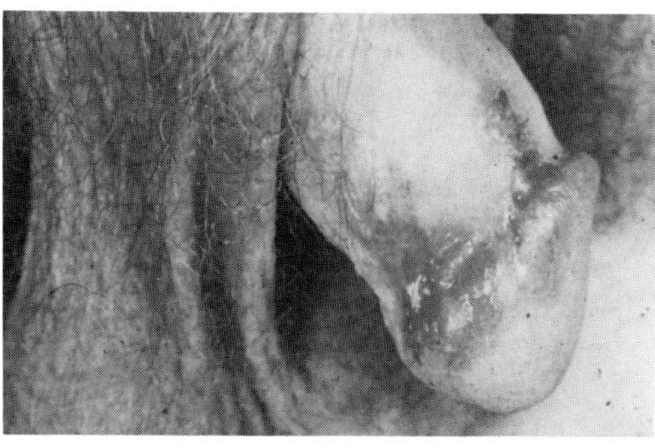

Fig. 28–10. Erythroplasia of Queyrat. These lesions, which superficially resemble dermatitis, are in fact carcinoma *in situ* of the skin.

Paget's Disease

Another form of intraepithelial carcinoma is anogenital Paget's disease, which results from the presence of an intraepidermal adenocarcinoma in the rectum, urethra, or sweat glands. Paget's disease commonly presents as a white, irregular plaque that may be eroded. In women, the labia majora are most frequently affected, but there may be involvement of the perianal and perineal skin. In men, the scrotum, perianal area, and groins are the most common sites of involvement. In approximately half the cases, deep carcinoma cannot be found; and it is postulated that the tumors in these cases originated in the intraepidermal portion of a sweat gland or from a multipotential basal cell.

Kaposi's Sarcoma

Formerly, this endothelial neoplasm was confined, in North America, to elderly men of Mediterranean or Jewish descent. Now, it has become a virtual epidemic—in the past few years, New York University alone has treated more than 140 cases—by virtue of its position as one of the end-points of the newly identified acquired immunodeficiency syndrome (AIDS).[20,21] Thus, it is important for physicians to become familiar with the clinical picture of this neoplasm.

Earlier reports of Kaposi's sarcoma in North America described solitary, irregular, bluish red or purplish brown growths on the glans or prepuce, sometimes with verrucose or telangiectatic surfaces, with long-term survival.[22–25] In the form now being seen, generalized small light purple or pink lesions are common at presentation; and extensive nodal

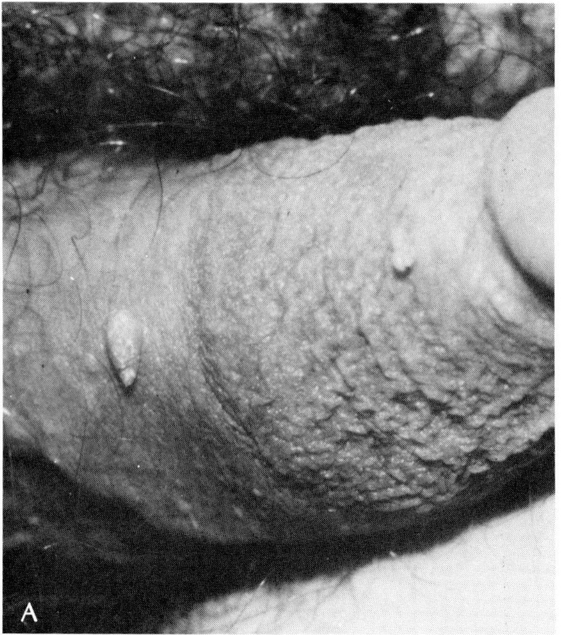

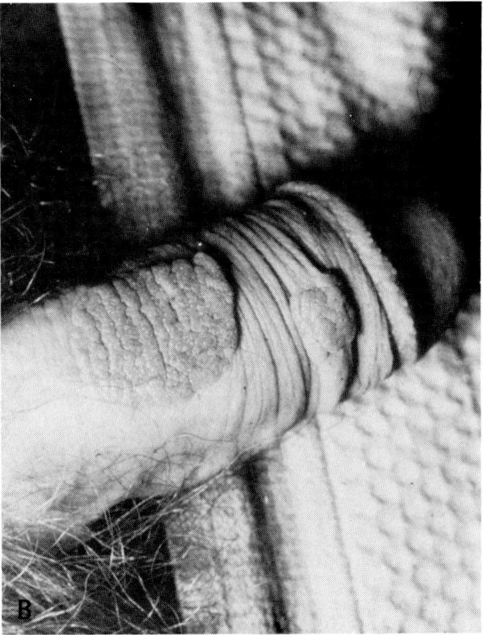

Fig. 28–11. Bowenoid papulosis. Multiple pigmented papillomatous lesions on the shaft of the penis. They may be small *(A)* or form large plaques *(B)*.

and visceral involvement may occur. Some lesions become elongated and follow lines of cutaneous cleavage. Early lesions are characterized histologically by anastomosing capillary networks and proliferating spindle cells with hyaline droplets, which later come to dominate the lesion.[25] Epidemic Kaposi's sarcoma is a systemic disease, so the local excision with or without radiation that was recommended by earlier authors is of no value. Krigel and associates have had encouraging results with VP-16 (epipodophyllin) but note that the underlying problem—a generalized immunodeficiency that leaves the patient prey to opportunistic infections—remains.[27]

Nonneoplastic Conditions

Lichen Planus. This condition is characterized by a pruritic eruption of violaceous scaling angular papules, primarily affecting the flexor surfaces and mucous membranes. In men, 25% show genital involvement; the incidence of genital involvement in women is not known. Lichen planus runs a variable course, depending on the extent and sites of involvement. The disease usually resolves within a few months but may recur.

Psoriasis. This is a chronic skin condition characterized by discrete erythematous papules and plaques covered by silvery scales (Fig. 28–12). Sites of predilection are the elbows, knees, and scalp, with variable genital involvement. There is an increased rate of epidermal turnover. The course is generally lifelong, with frequent exacerbations and remissions, sometimes as the result of known precipitating causes but often unrelated to any recognized factors.

Reiter's Disease. Many authors believe that Reiter's disease represents a severe form of psoriasis. It occurs most often in individuals with the HLA B-27 haplotype, as does severe psoriasis. Reiter's disease produces a joint disease similar to severe psoriatic arthritis, and progression of the skin lesions of Reiter's disease

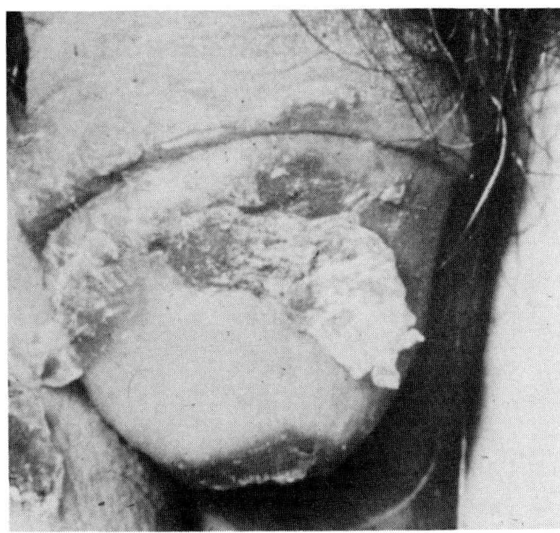

Fig. 28–12. Psoriasis of the penis is characterized by sharply marginated plaques with laminated silvery scales.

to typical psoriasis has been observed. On the penis, Reiter's disease is characterized by reddened areas that have various amounts of heaped up and lamellar scale.

Lichen Sclerosus et Atrophicus. This condition is characterized by atrophy of the epidermis with edema and inflammation of the dermis (Fig. 28–13*A*). The same lesion on the glans, surrounding the meatus, is called balanitis xerotica obliterans (Fig. 28–13*B*) and may produce marked meatal stenosis, the treatment of which was described earlier. Individual lesions are small, angulated, slightly atrophic, and ivory or porcelain white in color. Lesions may occur in sites other than the anogenital region; but when the condition occurs in the postpubertal period, it is usually anogenital. Resolution is uncommon. The association of this condition with carcinoma is controversial,[28] but according to Jeffcoate and Woodcock, there is no direct relation between lichen sclerosus et atrophicus and carcinoma of the vulva.[29]

Dermatitis. This condition, namely an inflammatory response of the skin, may

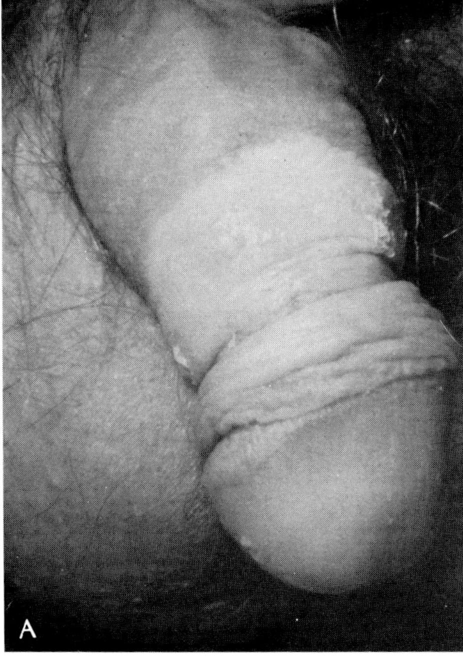

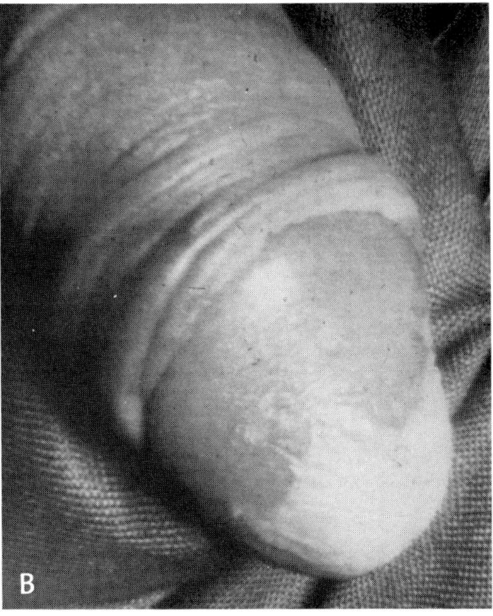

Fig. 28–13. Lichen sclerosus et atrophicus. *(A)* When the coronal sulcus and nearby skin is involved, there is atrophy and an ivory-like hardening. *(B)* When the urethral meatus is involved, this condition may result in attenuation of the urinary stream and is called balanitis xerotica obliterans.

be acute or chronic and may be a response to many exogenous or endogenous agents. Often, the cause is unknown. Contact dermatitis may result from exposure to certain fabrics, medications, or cosmetics. Drugs may result in an eczematous eruption. Genital involvement may be part of a generalized process but may be an isolated phenomenon in contact dermatitis.

CONCLUSIONS

The penile lesions one may encounter in an outpatient setting range from the minor and self-limited to the potentially lethal. To deal with them, the urologist must be an expert in the performance of a proper biopsy and be supported by an experienced laboratory.

REFERENCES

1. Cooper, B.H., et al.: Fungi. *In* Manual of Clinical Microbiology, 3rd Ed. Edited by E.H. Lennette, et al. Washington, D.C., American Society for Microbiology, 1980.
2. Sell, S., and Norris, S.J.: The biology, pathology, and immunology of syphilis. Int. Rev. Exp. Pathol., *24*:203, 1983.
3. Corey, L., et al.: Genital herpes simplex virus infections: clinical manifestations, course, and complications. Ann. Intern. Med., *98*:958, 1983.
4. Corey, L., and Holmes, K.K.: Genital herpes simplex virus infections: current concepts in diagnosis, therapy, and prevention. Ann. Intern. Med., *98*:973, 1983.
5. Schmidt, N.J., et al.: Comparison of direct immunofluorescence and direct immunoperoxidase procedures for detection of Herpes simplex virus antigen in lesion specimens. J. Clin. Microbiol., *18*:445, 1983.
6. Nev, H.C.: Centers for Disease Control: gonorrhea—recommended treatment schedules, 1979. Sex. Transm. Dis., *6* (Suppl.):89, 1979.
7. Märdh, P-A., et al.: Sampling, specimen handling, and isolation techniques in the diagnosis of chlamydial and other genital infections. Sex. Transm. Dis., *8*:280, 1981.
8. Felman, Y.M., and Nikitas, J.A.: Nongonococcal urethritis: a clinical review. JAMA, *245*:381, 1981.
9. Judson, F.N.: The importance of coexisting syphilitic, chlamydial, mycoplasmal, and trichomonal infections in the treatment of gonorrhea. Sex. Transm. Dis., *6* (Suppl.):112, 1979.
10. Persky, L.: Epidemiology of cancer of the penis. Recent Results Cancer Res., *60*:97, 1977.
11. Bulkley, G., Wendel, R., and Grayhack, J.: Buschke–Lowenstein tumor of the penis. J. Urol., *94*:731, 1967.
12. Dawson, D.F., et al.: Giant condyloma and verrucous carcinoma of the genital area. Arch. Pathol., *79*:225, 1965.
13. Kraus, F.T., and Perez-Mesa, C.: Verrucous carcinoma: clinical and pathologic study of 105 cases involving oral cavity, larynx and genitalia. Cancer, *19*:26, 1966.
14. Hoppmann, H.J., and Fraley, E.E.: Squamous cell carcinoma of the penis. J. Urol., *120*:393, 1978.
15. Graham, J.H., and Helwig, E.B.: Erythroplasia of Queyrat: a clinicopathologic and histochemical study. Cancer, *32*:1396, 1973.
16. Andersson, L., Jonsson, G., and Brehmer-Anderson, E.: Erythroplasia of Queyrat: carcinoma in situ. Scand. J. Urol. Nephrol., *1*:303, 1967.
17. Merrin, C.E.: Cancer of the penis. Cancer, *45*:1973, 1980.
18. Wade, T.R., Kopf, A.W., and Ackerman, A.B.: Bowenoid papulosis of the penis. Cancer, *42*:1890, 1978.
19. Wade, T.R., Kopf, A.W., and Ackerman, A.B.: Bowenoid papulosis of the genitalia. Arch. Dermatol., *115*:306, 1979.
20. Gottlieb, G.J., and Ackerman, A.B.: Kaposi's sarcoma: an extensively disseminated form in young homosexual men. Hum. Pathol., *13*:882, 1982.
21. Waterson, A.P.: Acquired immune deficiency syndrome. Br. Med. J., *286*:743, 1983.
22. Waugh, T.R.: Endothelioma of corpora cavernosa of penis. Arch. Pathol., *55*:98, 1953.
23. Leiter, E., and Lefkovitz, A.M.: Circumcision and penile carcinoma. NY State J. Med., *75*:1520, 1975.
24. Houston, W., et al.: Kaposi's sarcoma of the penis. Br. J. Urol., *47*:315, 1975.
25. Linker, D., Lieberman, P., and Grabstald, H.: Kaposi's sarcoma of the urogenital tract. Urology, *5*:684, 1975.
26. Hutt, M.S.R.: Pathology of Kaposi's sarcoma. Antibiot. Chemother., *29*:32, 1981.
27. Krigel, R.L.: Epidemic Kaposi's sarcoma: staging and treatment. Presented at the 19th Annual Meeting, Amer. Soc. Clin. Oncol., San Diego, May 1983.
28. Hart, W.R., Norris, H.I., and Helwig, E.B.: Relation of lichen sclerosus et atrophicus of the vulva to development of carcinoma. Obstet. Gynecol., *45*:369, 1975.
29. Jeffcoate, T.N.A., and Woodcock, A.S.: Premalignant conditions of the vulva with particular reference to chronic epithelial dystrophies. Br. Med. J., *1*:127, 1961.

29

Implantation of the Inflatable Penile Prosthesis Using Local Anesthesia

J. KEITH LIGHT, M.D., and F. BRANTLEY SCOTT, M.D.

Implantation of the inflatable penile prosthesis using local instead of general anesthesia has been evolving over the past few years since the realization that the operation causes little discomfort outside the operating field. Upwardly spiralling hospital costs created a further impetus to the development of a technique that would produce significant financial savings without jeopardizing the patient's safety.

This chapter describes our experience implanting inflatable penile prostheses* in 32 patients using local anesthesia.† Because of the need to have resuscitative equipment on hand, and because of the importance of minimizing traffic in the operating room as a precaution against infection, we perform these implantations in a hospital operating room. However, the operation could also be done in a suitably equipped ambulatory surgery center.

We prefer the penoscrotal approach because it is simple to perform, even in obese patients. In addition, it permits anchoring of the prosthesis pump to the scrotal tissues, decreasing the chances of displacement; and it makes any necessary later revisions of the prosthesis easy because the tubes and connections are easily palpable. Finally, the incidence of postoperative scrotal hematoma is lower with this approach than with the suprapubic one. In more than 1,400 cases in which the penoscrotal incision has been used for various procedures, there have been no urethral injuries.

PREOPERATIVE PREPARATION

The patient's urine must be sterile. He is admitted the day of the operation. Approximately 1 hour before the procedure, an antibiotic is given intravenously to provide time for the tissue level to reach the therapeutic range. Antibiotics are continued for 48 hours afterward. Sedation is used only as necessary.

In the operating room, the patient is positioned supine on the table with his legs apart and his knees flexed. The operative area is shaved and then scrubbed for 10 minutes with povidone–iodine solution. As a further precaution against infection, the members of the surgical team apply povidone–iodine solution to their hands before donning gloves.

*American Medical Systems, 10400 E. Bren Road, Minnetonka, MN 55343

†Evaluation of the impotent patient and the implantation of semirigid prostheses are described in Chapter 30; correction of vasculogenic impotence by transluminal angioplasty is reviewed in Chapter 21.

LOCAL ANESTHETIC

Unless the patient is allergic to amide-type local anesthetics, we use lidocaine (Xylocaine). The procedure requires a 21-gauge 1-½-inch needle, a 27-gauge 1-inch needle, an 18-gauge butterfly needle, a 60-ml syringe, and 100 ml of sterile water.

Because the drug is absorbed rapidly into the systemic circulation from the corpora cavernosa, the patient must be monitored for cardiovascular and central nervous system reactions. The former consist principally of hypotension and bradycardia and the latter of either excitation or depressant effects. We have seen no such reactions in our 32 patients.

We use two vials of 0.5% lidocaine hydrochloride without epinephrine or preservatives and dilute it to 0.25% by mixing it 1:1 with the sterile water. Dilution permits the safe use of a large volume of solution ($\leq$ 120 ml, as the maximum recommended dose of lidocaine is 300 mg or 4.5 mg/kg), thus increasing the segmental spread of the drug.

The first areas to be anesthetized are the corpora cavernosa and the glans penis. A subcutaneous bleb is raised approximately 5 mm below the corona on the lateral aspect of the shaft with diluted anesthetic injected through the 27-gauge 1-inch needle. The butterfly needle is then introduced percutaneously into one of the corpora, and the 60-ml syringe with the anesthetic is attached. A small amount of blood is aspirated to confirm the needle's placement in the cavernous tissue.

The assistant then pushes a fist against the perineum to apply pressure to both corpora simultaneously, and local anesthetic is injected (Fig. 29–1). The combination of the anesthetic solution (approximately 50–60 ml in the average man) and the perineal compression causes an erection, and it is essential that a full erection be created to ensure adequate anesthesia. After approximately two minutes, the perineal compression is released, resulting in rapid detumescence. The butterfly needle is left in position until the corpus cavernosum is dilated, both to avoid subcutaneous extravasation of blood and anesthetic and to make it easy to inject more anesthetic if it is required.

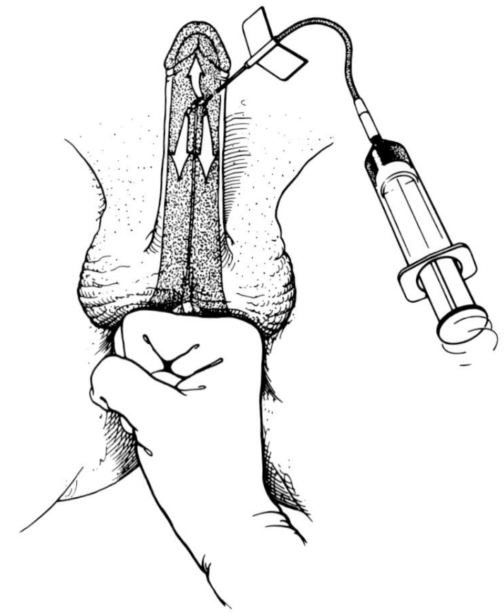

Fig. 29–1. Anesthetizing the glans and corpora. Because of the communications among the corpora cavernosa and the corpus spongiosum, a single injection anesthetizes the entire shaft of the penis.

Next, the site of the incision along the median raphe is infiltrated for 3–4 cm and for 1–2 cm on either side using a total of 3–5 ml of anesthetic solution (Fig. 29–2). The scrotal branches of the ilioinguinal nerve on the side where the prosthesis pump will be placed are then blocked where they emerge from the external inguinal ring (Fig. 29–3*A*). To do this, the external ring is palpated, and the spermatic cord structures are identified and stabilized with a finger. (If it is difficult to palpate the external ring, the scrotal skin can be invaginated.) Anesthetic is infiltrated around the ring and cord through a 21-gauge 1-½ inch needle. The needle is then introduced perpendicular

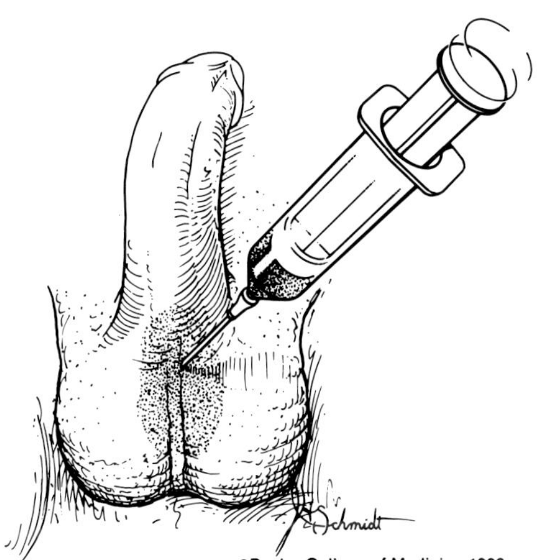

Fig. 29–2. Anesthetizing the skin and subcutaneous tissues along the median raphe. The butterfly needle, which is left in place in the shaft, is not shown.

to the fascia transversalis and advanced slowly into the retropubic space through the external ring while anesthetic is injected (Fig. 29–3*B*).

Anesthesia of the glans is confirmed by a painful stimulus such as a pinprick before the procedure is started. Additional anesthetic can be injected at any stage if required.

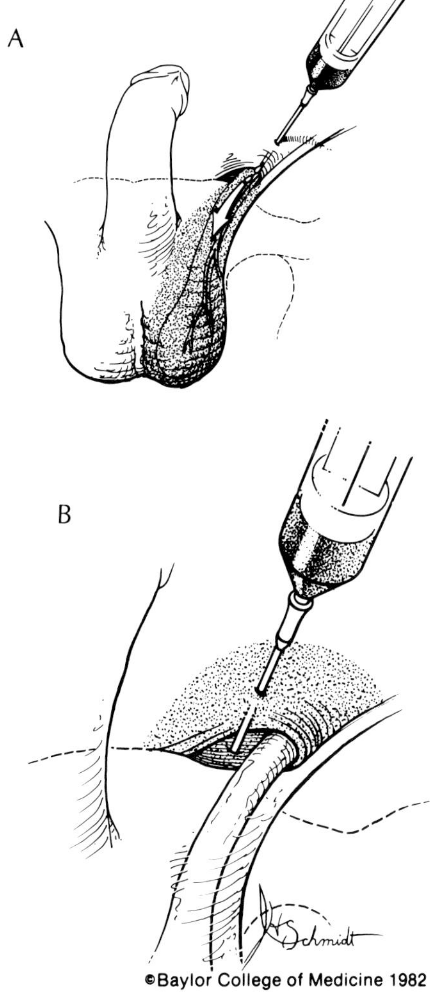

Fig. 29–3. Anesthetizing the scrotum for implantation of the prosthesis pump. *(A)* The branches of the ilioinguinal nerve are infiltrated where they emerge from the external inguinal ring. *(B)* The retropubic space is anesthetized to permit painless implantation of reservoir connectors.

OPERATIVE TECHNIQUE

Bracing and Immobilizing the Penis

A bracing tube of silicone rubber is placed in the slots of a Scott retractor in such a way as to support the base of the penis at the point where the tunica albuginea will be entered. It also provides a counterforce for full stretching of the organ. An elastic hook is anchored inside the urethral meatus and hooked into a slot as the penis is stretched toward the umbilicus (Fig. 29–4*A*). The arrangement stabilizes the penis during the operation and allows more accurate measurement of the corpora for selection of prosthesis cylinders.

Incision

A 2- to 3-cm incision is made along the median raphe in the penoscrotal angle, and the opening is deepened using blunt and sharp dissection to expose the corpus spongiosum and the junction of the tunica albuginea of the corpora cavernosa (Fig. 29–4*B*). Elastic hooks are applied to the deeper layers of soft tissue to ensure

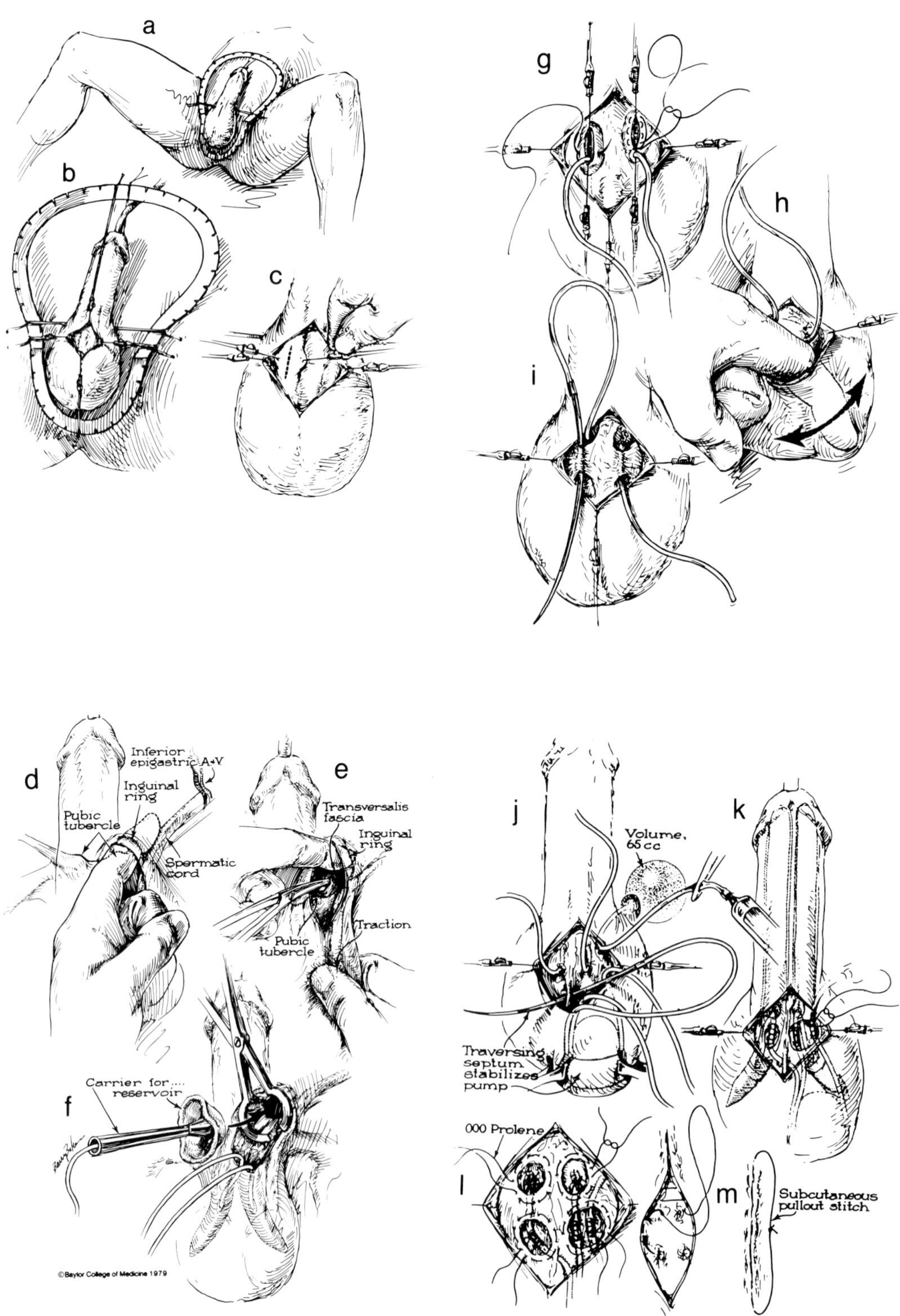

Fig. 29–4. (*A* through *M*) Technique of inflatable prosthesis implantation via penoscrotal approach.

proper exposure with gentle handling (Fig. 29–4*C*), thus reducing postoperative swelling and discomfort. The tunica albuginea is then incised vertically for 1.5 cm beginning at the point opposite the bracing tube (dotted line in Fig. 29–4*C*).

Insertion of the Inflatable Cylinders

The Dilamezinsert* has been designed specifically for simultaneous dilatation and measurement of the corpora cavernosa and implantation of the inflatable cylinders of the prosthesis (Fig. 29–5*A*). It is introduced through the corpus cavernosus adjacent to the ventral aspect of the tunica albuginea and advanced toward the tip of the penis until it can be palpated inside the glans. The penis must not be overstretched during this maneuver. The measurement of corporal length is then made between the glans and the proximal angle of the incision in the tunica albuginea, and the appropriate size prosthesis cylinder is selected.

The suture in the tip of the cylinder is threaded into a 2-inch Keith needle, which is loaded on the plastic needle carrier and dilator of the Dilamezinsert (Fig. 29–5*B*). Forcing the plastic dilator through the metal blades of this instrument serves both to dilate the corpus cavernosum and to carry the tip of the needle through the skin of the glans. The needle is then grasped with a hemostat and pulled out, and the suture is used to pull the prosthesis cylinder into place without twisting it.

The Dilamezinsert is then introduced into the proximal part of the corpus until the resistance of the pelvic bone is felt. The distance from the bone to the proximal angle of the incision in the tunica albuginea is measured to determine the proper length for the rear tip extender. Accurate measurement is essential to prevent backward migration of the cylinder when the prosthesis is inflated, as this increases the wear on the input tube. Again, care is taken not to twist the cylinder while the proximal portion is being inserted. After the cylinder is seated, it is inflated gently, and the point of exit of the input tube is inspected in relation to the tunica albuginea: the tube should exit from the proximal angle of the incision to minimize wear. The incision in the tunica is then closed with a running horizontal mattress suture of 3–0 Prolene, with care not to damage the cylinder.

After both cylinders have been implanted, they are dilated hydraulically with sterile fluid until the tunica albuginea is palpably tense. If the results are satisfactory, the fluid is evacuated until the penis is flaccid.

Implantation of the Reservoir

To place the reservoir intraabdominally via the external inguinal ring, the index finger is introduced through the incision along the spermatic cord (Fig. 29–4*D*). The cord can be displaced laterally by applying pressure across the pubis. If one suspects that the bladder is distended, it should be drained before dissection begins in the prevesical space. With the finger in the external inguinal ring, Metzenbaum scissors are introduced between the finger and the pubis and spread to puncture the transversalis fascia (Fig. 29–4*E*). The finger is then introduced between the blades into the prevesical space, and the proper location of the dissection is confirmed by palpating the posterior aspect of the pubic symphysis and the rectus muscle. A space is created for the reservoir with gentle blunt dissection with the finger. An elongated speculum is then introduced alongside the finger to inspect for bleeding (Fig. 29–4*F*).

The reservoir inserter* containing the

*Lone Star Medical Products, Houston TX 77001

*Lone Star Medical Products, Houston, TX 77001

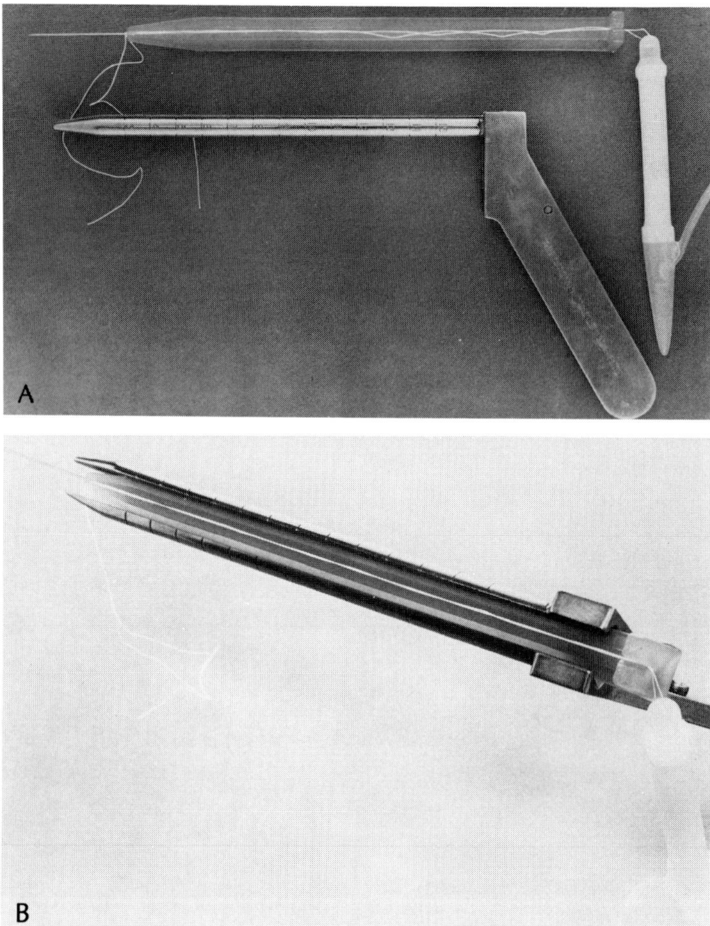

Fig. 29–5. The Dilamezinsert. *(A) Above,* the plastic needle holder and dilator with Keith needle and prosthesis cylinder with rear tip in place. *Below,* the calibrated metal blades and the handle. *(B)* Dilator loaded for cylinder insertion.

reservoir is then introduced through the defect created in the transversalis fascia; this instrument allows placement of the reservoir in the prevesical space with minimal dilatation of the external inguinal ring (Fig. 29–6). The reservoir is filled with 65 ml of Cysto-Conray 2 solution and checked with the examining finger to be sure that the tubing is not kinked. The nipple should be easily palpable at the external ring. The tubing to be connected to the contralateral prosthesis cylinder is then introduced by means of blunt dissection through the intrascrotal septum in order to anchor the pump, with the tubing from both cylinders being routed through the soft tissues in order to place the connections in the anterior scrotal compartment (Fig. 29–4*G*,*H*, and *I*).

A subdartos pouch is created for the pump by blunt dissection (see Fig. 29–4*H*). Excess tubing is cut off, and the connections are made using stainless steel connectors doubly ligated with 3–0 Prolene sutures. The pump is anchored in the scrotum with bilateral Babcock forceps during this procedure to prevent

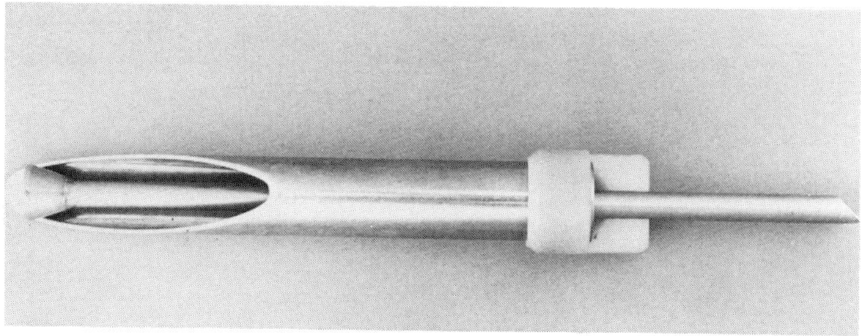

Fig. 29–6. Reservoir inserter.

displacement (Fig. 29–4*J*,*K* and *L*). The wound is inspected for bleeding, and the function of the prosthesis checked by alternately inflating and deflating it. The erection should be palpated to be certain it is firm to verify that there is enough fluid in the device. The deeper soft tissues of the scrotum and penis are then closed with a running suture of 3–0 Prolene, and the more superficial soft tissues are closed with a running suture of 3–0 plain catgut. Finally, the skin is closed with a running subcuticular suture of 3–0 Dermalon and the skin sealed with collodion (Fig. 29–4*M*). A Foley catheter is inserted to provide continuous urinary drainage and thus decrease the chance of retention, and the penis is left partially erect for the first 24 hours in order to minimize intracorporeal hematoma.

Approach in Patients with Previous Surgery

In the event that the patient has undergone any form of retropubic surgery or bilateral inguinal herniorrhaphies, a separate incision is made in the lower anterior abdominal wall and the reservoir inserted in the submuscular tissue plane under direct vision. The tubing is passed subcutaneously to exit through the original penoscrotal incision for connection to the pump as previously described.

RESULTS

Our 32 patients ranged in age from 29 to 77 years, with a mean of 58 years. Most were impotent as a result of vascular lesions or diabetes (20 cases), while two had Peyronie's disease, three had psychogenic impotence, and the remaining seven various other diseases.

In 24 patients, local anesthesia was used for financial reasons, but in the others there were medical problems that made general anesthesia too risky. Four patients had cardiac problems, two had tracheal stenosis, one had respiratory problems, and the other had uremia. The presence of these patients with additional medical problems accounts for the variability of the hospital stay, which was as long as 10 days with an average of 3.5 days. However, almost half the patients (15) spent only one day in the hospital.

There were complications in seven patients. Two patients complained of significant pain and swelling, but neither desired hospital admission. Another patient had urinary retention that required admission and an indwelling catheter overnight. Three patients had hematomas surrounding the prosthesis pump, but aspiration was needed in only one. The only serious complication was an enterococcal infection in one patient that necessitated removal of the prosthesis; it is unlikely that the use of local rather than general anesthesia contributed to the problem in any way.

CONCLUSIONS

In comparing our results in the 32 patients with those in our larger series of cases done using general anesthesia, we found no difference in the frequency of immediate and delayed complications. As a result, the technique described here is being recommended more frequently at our institution.

30

Insertion of the Semirigid Penile Prosthesis

PAUL H. LANGE, M.D., and KEITH W. KAYE, M.D., F.C.S.(S.A.), F.R.C.S.

With the introduction of effective penile prostheses and the greater understanding recently gained of the causes of erectile impotence, correction of this distressing condition has become commonplace. The remaining challenge is to make the evaluation and treatment more cost-effective without increasing the risk. Part of this challenge has been met by inserting the penile prosthesis in an outpatient setting, often under local anesthesia. This approach is particularly appropriate for semirigid prostheses but also can be used for the inflatable device (see Chapter 29).

EVALUATION OF THE PATIENT

If treatment of the impotent patient is to succeed, he must be thoroughly evaluated so that the proper mode of management can be selected. In most patients, the evaluation should encompass the medical and sexual history, physical and psychologic examinations, and endocrine studies.[1] The exceptions are patients in whom the cause of impotence is clear; for example, those with spinal-cord injuries or those who have undergone radical prostatectomy, in whom some of the studies can be dispensed with. The discussion that follows emphasizes the aspects of the evaluation that facilitate outpatient care.

Medical and Sexual History

If is often more efficient if these initial steps are done by a physician's assistant or nurse practitioner with the aid of standardized forms and audiovisual programs. Of course, the physician must develop a rapport with the patient; but with experience, paramedical staff can easily obtain the essential data, answer the common questions, and decide which basic tests are appropriate. The physician, therefore, needs only to ask a few questions and perform the physical examination to make the diagnosis and be ready to discuss therapeutic options with the patient.

Obtaining a medical history is facilitated by having the patient complete one of the available standard questionnaires[2,3] before the interview. In obtaining a sexual history, we have found that many patients do not understand the distinction between erection, orgasm, and ejaculation, so a preliminary orientation is helpful. This can be accomplished with one of the several brochures available from the prosthesis manufacturers or one created in house, but we have been most satisfied with a videocassette program we developed.* This program, which each patient sees at the beginning of his evaluation, helps him understand impotence in general and gain insight into his own problem and provides him with an overview of the treatment options, including the various types of penile prostheses.

Physical Examination and Studies

In most patients, the appropriate physical studies are measurements of penile blood flow, urodynamics, and nocturnal penile tumescence (NPT) monitoring.

Penile vascular competence is assessed from the history, palpation of peripheral pulses, and measurement of the penile blood pressure by Doppler ultrasound, using a brachial:penile flow ratio of ≤ 0.7 as the criterion of probable vascular insufficiency. Arteriography is performed only when we strongly suspect significant insufficiency that might be correctable by transluminal angioplasty; in such cases, diagnosis and treatment can be carried out in a single procedure with a short hospital stay (see Chapter 21).

Our only routine urodynamics test is uroflowmetry. If voiding is impaired, other studies, including cystoscopy, may be performed. Cystometry and measurements of the sacral latency response are performed in patients with known relevant neurologic deficits or impaired voiding (see Chapter 13).

Despite the routine requirement by the Veterans Administration and many insurance companies for NPT monitoring in impotent patients, this is a troublesome and controversial test that is more often informative than diagnostic, because the traditional procedure is subject to artifact, malfunction, and diverse interpretation. These problems have been reduced, although not abolished, by a device that incorporates three thin-film plastic snap elements, each of which is calibrated to break at a different specific pressure.[4]* The device is placed around the base of the penis at night. None of the elements will break if there is no significant erectile activity; all will break if sufficient rigidity is achieved for intercourse. More complicated NPT studies may be required if only one or two elements break.

Psychologic Evaluation

We believe that a psychologic interview by a professional experienced in sexual counselling is essential even in patients with obviously organic impotence. Most impotent men have some psychologic problems, and many will require postoperative sexual counselling. This evaluation also is advisable from a medicolegal viewpoint. We do not require the partner's participation in this, but we strongly encourage it.

Endocrine Evaluation

The definition of "appropriate" in this context is changing rapidly as the introduction of exquisitely sensitive assays reveals an unexpectedly high incidence of endocrine dysfunction in impotent patients.[5] Traditional wisdom states that impotent patients should have a blood-glucose study and assays for serum follicle-stimulating hormone (FSH), luteinizing hormone (LH), and testosterone and perhaps for prolactin. Because the yield of significant findings in the hormone assays is low, it is tempting to reduce the cost by eliminating these studies. However, we recently found FSH, LH, or testosterone abnormalities in 19% of a large series of impotent patients and

---

*Available through the National Medical Audiovisual Center, National Library of Medicine, Bethesda, MD 20209. We also participated in the development of a 12-minute videotape, complemented by a 13-minute version for professionals, that can be borrowed for three weeks free of charge from Dācomed Corporation, 1701 E. 79th St., Minneapolis, MN 55420.

*Snap-Gauge Impotence Testing Device, Dācomed Corp., Minneapolis, MN 55420

so continue to use these assays plus blood-glucose determinations in patients who complain of impotence for which no cause is apparent. The presence of libido does not justify bypassing these studies.[6]

CHOICE OF PROSTHESIS AND OPERATION

Once the physician and patient have elected penile prosthesis implantation, the next question is, which device? We have conducted two studies of the results with semirigid and inflatable prostheses and have found no clear advantage of one over the other for most patients.[7,8] Therefore, unless the patient has some problem that would make one type of device inappropriate—for example, a patient with limited manual dexterity who would have [illegible] e in- [illegible] n of [illegible] f the [illegible] ice. [illegible] rigid [illegible] r op- [illegible] e ex- [illegible] e di- [illegible] lical [illegible] from [illegible] ance [illegible] hese [illegible] nce.

[illegible] N

[illegible] idea [illegible] have [illegible] re it [illegible] o ex- [illegible] nt is [illegible] cov-

[illegible] ions. [illegible] Beta- [illegible] wice [illegible] e the [illegible] the [illegible] e had [illegible] the

night before the operation;[9] Surgex* is generally well tolerated.

(2) Prescriptions. Before coming to the surgery unit, the patient should obtain the oral analgesic and the antibiotic he will take postoperatively. We usually prescribe oxycodone hydrochloride (Percodan) and a cephalosporin.

(3) Clothing. The patient should bring a bathrobe with him, because street clothes will be too uncomfortable and revealing immediately after the operation.

(4) Companion. A responsible adult should accompany the patient.

(5) Food. A light breakfast is allowed.

OPERATIVE TECHNIQUE

Position and Anesthesia

The patient is placed in a frog-leg position, and residual hair is shaved off. An intravenous line is inserted, and an aminoglycoside and a cephalosporin are given intravenously. A penile block is then performed with 0.5% bupivacaine hydrochloride (Marcaine) (see Chapter 8). The subcutaneous tissues at the base of the penis are infiltrated circumferentially with the same anesthetic, and the site of the skin incision is infiltrated with 0.25% bupivacaine. Approximately 5 ml of 0.25% bupivacaine is then injected into each corpus cavernosum with a 25-gauge needle (see Chapter 29).

A small urethral catheter is usually inserted as a landmark and to delay postoperative voiding.

Incision

Several incisions, all suitable for use with local anesthesia, have been used: perineal, penoscrotal[10] (see Chapter 29), circumcision,[11] dorsal penile, and infrapubic.[12,13] We prefer the infrapubic,

*Sparta Instrument Corp., 26602 Capade Ave., Hayward, CA 94545

which provides excellent exposure of the corpora cavernosa at the base of the penis, making dilatation easy. Certainly, incisions on the penile shaft also offer excellent exposure; but in our experience, some patients, particularly those with diabetes mellitus, have significant long-term pain or irritation from these incisions. We use the circumcision incision only when circumcision is necessary, because this approach, with its sleeving of the penile skin along the shaft intraoperatively, can produce considerable distal edema and pain, and wound healing may be troublesome.*

The infrapubic incision is made at the base of the penis without transecting the subcutaneous tissue in the midline. This approach preserves the superficial dorsal penile vein and lymphatics and thus reduces postoperative penile edema and the risk of venous thrombosis. Each corpus cavernosum is identified and marked with two parallel stay sutures 5 mm apart (Fig. 30–1*A*). Placement of these sutures too laterally hinders exposure, however, and may impede corporal dilatation (Fig. 30–1*B*).

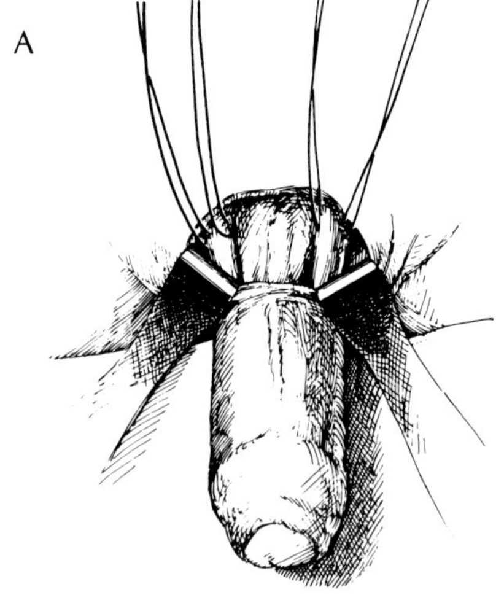

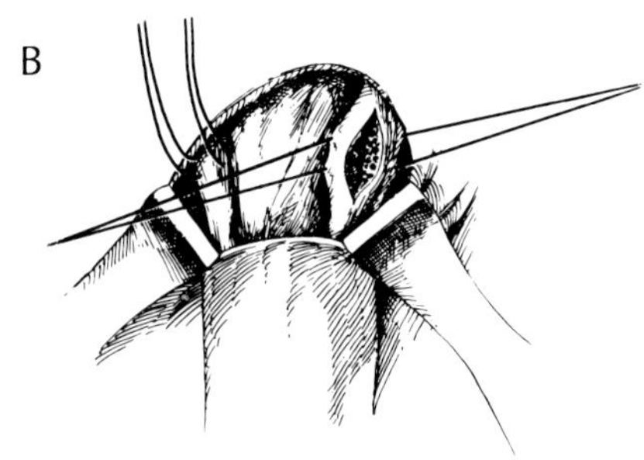

Fig. 30–1. Exposure and opening of the corpora cavernosa. Midline subcutaneous tissue should be left intact. *(A)* Position of stabilizing sutures in corpora. *(B)* Opening corpus. Note position and use of sutures.

Procedure[14]

The tunica albuginea of one corpus is incised, and a plane is created in the spongy tissue with dissecting scissors. A common error is to make this incision too small; it should be approximately 4 cm long so the prosthesis cylinders can be inserted easily and should extend only a minimal distance onto the penile shaft (Fig. 30–1*B*). The corpus is then dilated proximally and distally with Hegar dilators starting with a No. 9 and usually continuing to a No. 12 (Fig. 30–2). When dilating distally, it is important to keep the penis stretched and untwisted; a common error is to press the penis down over the dilator rather than passing the dilator through the corpus. Such inappropriate "concertina" action may injure the urethra.

Selection of the correct size of prosthesis is essential to the patient's satisfaction and requires some experience. If too short a prosthesis is inserted, the result will be the aptly named "SST" deformity, in which the glans penis drops down from the shaft like the front of the Concorde airplane. However, if the cylinders are too long, the result will be penile bowing and pain. The width of the

*This incision is also useful in patients with significant deformity caused by Peyronie's disease, as it permits the surgeon to make relaxing incisions in the corpora. However, we do not perform such operations on outpatients or under local anesthesia.

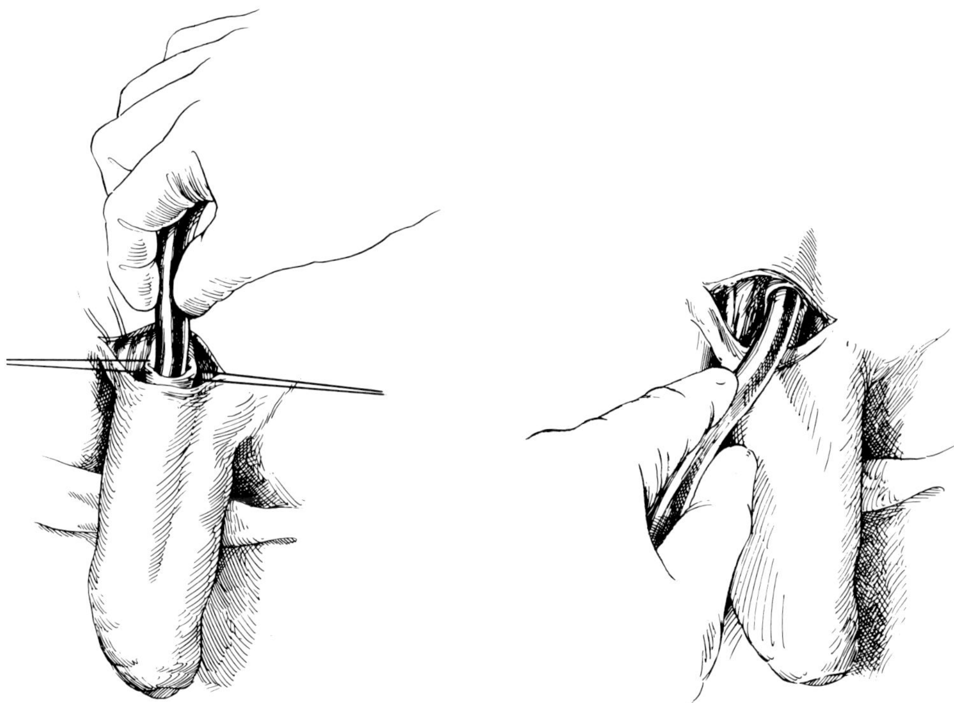

Fig. 30–2. Distal *(A)* and proximal *(B)* dilatation of the corpora.

cylinder is also important: if possible, the ≥ 1.1 cm sizes should be used (Fig. 30–3).

After the cylinder has been inserted, the corpus is closed with a running 3–0 Vicryl suture (Fig. 30–4). After the second cylinder has been inserted in a similar fashion, the skin incision is closed with 4–0 chromic catgut subcutaneous sutures and 4–0 Vicryl subcuticular sutures. The urethral catheter is removed, and a moderate pressure dressing is applied circumferentially to the penile base and the incision and left for 24 hours.

POSTOPERATIVE CARE AND FOLLOWUP

Patients are given a clearly written instruction sheet that includes the following points:

(1) Bed rest is suggested for much of the first three to five days;
(2) The names, doses, and possible side effects of the analgesic and antibiotic prescribed are listed;
(3) The surgeon's day and nighttime telephone numbers;
(4) Instructions to call if there is fever, increasing pain, bleeding, or voiding problems;
(5) Instructions to remove the pressure dressing after 24 hours.

Patients are seen on the third, seventh, and thirtieth days after the operation. At the first visit, it is helpful to discuss the ways of positioning the penis when wearing street clothes. At first, the organ is easily irritated by movement, and this can cause significant stress if the patient is not prepared for it.

CONCLUSIONS

Despite the occasional complexity of the evaluation of an impotent patient, it can be organized into an efficient, accurate, cost-effective outpatient procedure.

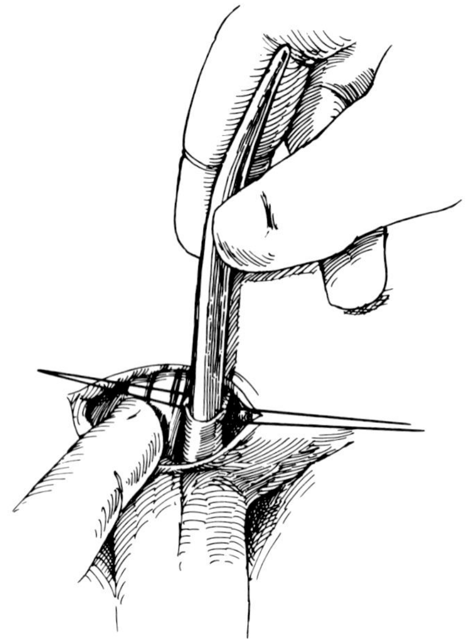

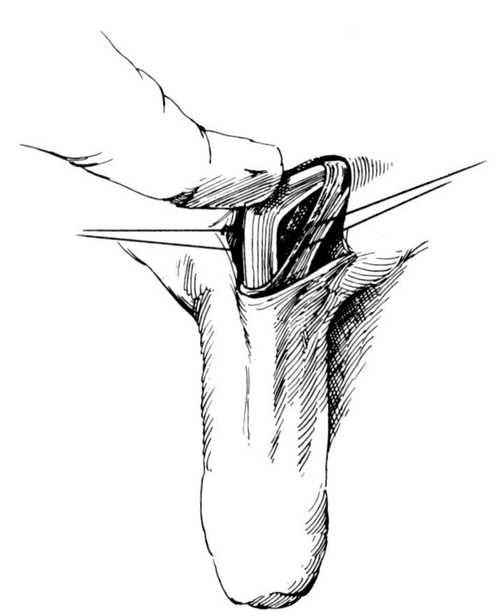

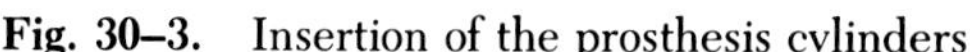

Fig. 30–3. Insertion of the prosthesis cylinders.

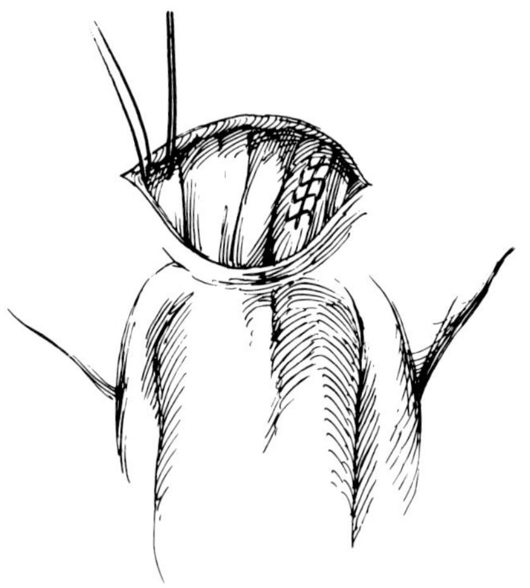

Fig. 30–4. Closure of the corpus cavernosum.

Further, in most patients, a penile prosthesis, especially a semirigid one, can be implanted to the patient's satisfaction in an outpatient unit under local anesthesia. The savings are significant: at our hospitals, the difference in the costs of implanting a semirigid prosthesis on an outpatient and on an inpatient basis with a two-day hospital stay (assuming a 1-hour operating time in both cases) is approximately $800. Clearly, then, impotence is another disorder that can be evaluated and treated on an outpatient basis in most cases.

REFERENCES

1. Montague, D.K.: Clinical evaluation of impotence. Urol. Clin. North Am., *8*:130, 1981.
2. Smith, A.D., and Lange, P.H.: Impotence—pathogenesis and evaluation. Minn. Med., *63*:701, 1980.
3. Mallory, T.R., and Wein, A.J.: The etiology, diagnosis and surgical treatment of erectile impotence. J. Reprod. Med., *20*:183, 1978.
4. Ek, A., Bradley, W.E., and Krane, R.J.: Nocturnal penile rigidity measured by the snap-gauge band. J. Urol., *129*:964, 1983.
5. Sparks, S.R.F., White, R.A., and Connolly, P.B.: Impotence is not always psychogenic. JAMA, *243*:750, 1980.
6. Slag, M.F., et al.: Impotence as an organic disease in medical clinic outpatients. (in press.)
7. Lange, P.H., and Smith, A.D.: A comparison of two types of penile prosthesis used in the surgical treatment of male impotence. Sex. Disabil., *1*:307, 1978.
8. Smith, A.D., Lange, P.H., and Fraley, E.E.: A comparison of the Small–Carrion and Scott–Bradley penile prostheses. J. Urol., *121*:609, 1979.
9. Seropian, R., and Reynolds, B.M.: Wound infections after preoperative dipilatory versus razor. Am. J. Surg., *121*:251, 1971.
10. Barry, J.M., and Seifert, A.: Penoscrotal approach for placement of paired penile implants for impotence. J. Urol., *122*:325, 1979.

11. Smith, A.D.: Circumcision incision for insertion of semi-rigid penile prostheses. Urology, *18*:609, 1981.
12. Kelami, A.: "Infrapubic" approach in operative andrology. Urology, *12*:580, 1978.
13. Kaye, K.W., Reddy, P., and Suryanarayanan, V.: Infrapubic incision in operative andrology. Urology, *21*:524, 1983.
14. Narayan, P., and Lange, P.H.: Semirigid penile prostheses in the management of erectile impotence. Urol. Clin. North Am., *8*:169, 1981.

31

Needle Suspension for Stress Incontinence in the Female

GARY E. LEACH, M.D., and SHLOMO RAZ, M.D.

The introduction of the Pereyra needle-suspension procedure in 1959[1] revolutionized the surgical treatment of female stress urinary incontinence. Since this original description, numerous modifications have been proposed;[2–4] herein, we describe the Raz modification,[5] which has been used in approximately 300 females, both as a primary procedure and after multiple unsuccessful bladder-neck suspensions.

At present, this operation is not being done on an outpatient basis. However, the length of hospitalization is greatly reduced in comparison with that of other incontinence procedures and local anesthesia may be used. Thus, it is possible that the procedure will eventually prove feasible for outpatient surgery or at least for operation with only an overnight hospital stay. Therefore, this discussion is included in this book.

SELECTION OF PATIENTS

A thorough history is essential to the proper selection of patients for surgical treatment of stress incontinence. Predisposing factors include multiple vaginal deliveries, pelvic operations, and declining estrogen levels. A history of urine escape during coughing, laughing, sneezing, or change of position that is exacerbated by a full bladder should be obtained, and the presence of urgency (with or without incontinence) and frequency must be noted.

As part of the physical examination, objective demonstration of incontinence during coughing or other maneuvers that raise the intraabdominal pressure is paramount. A common finding is prolapse of the urethra to a low, poorly supported position with hypermobility of the proximal portion and bladder neck during stress. The vagina also must be examined to assess its ability to provide adequate exposure for an anterior incision; a markedly contracted vagina secondary to atrophic vaginitis can present significant technical problems for a needle-suspension procedure. A careful search must be made to rule out ureterovaginal or vesicovaginal fistulas as a cause of incontinence. Finally, a neurologic examination is performed to rule out gross abnormalities.

URODYNAMIC, ENDOSCOPIC, AND RADIOLOGIC EVALUATION

If the history and physical examination confirm the presence of stress urinary incontinence, a urodynamic evaluation may be indicated. The evaluation we perform in the research setting is more extensive than that usually required in the office setting; however, we will outline our protocol, as it may help to explain some aspects of the pathophysiology of female stress urinary incontinence.

Initially, rapid water-filling cystometry is performed via two urethral catheters, an 8F red Robinson catheter used for bladder filling and an 8F feeding tube used for pressure monitoring. Intravesical pressure, intraabdominal pressure, and true detrusor pressure (intravesical minus intraabdominal pressure) are recorded simultaneously on a strip chart recorder. The study is performed with the patient in the supine, sitting, and standing positions and using various provocative maneuvers (coughing, heel jouncing, etc.) in an attempt to elicit an uninhibited detrusor contraction. In general, the patient with significant bladder instability in combination with stress incontinence is best treated initially with anticholinergic drugs, with bladder-neck suspension performed later if significant stress urinary incontinence persists.

In some instances, the loss of urine may be delayed until 1 to 2 seconds after the cough. In this situation, we have frequently been able to document uninhibited detrusor contractions stimulated by coughing but occurring 1 to 2 seconds later. This phenomenon, known as stress hyperreflexia, is best treated by anticholinergic drugs before proceeding with bladder-neck suspension.

The remainder of the urodynamic evaluation includes a voiding uroflow study and urethral-pressure profilometry. An integral part of the former study is documentation of stress incontinence without change in the true detrusor pressure as monitored by the 8F feeding tube. When incontinence is demonstrated during stress without a change in true detrusor pressure, a satisfactory operative result can be expected in most cases.

After the urodynamic evaluation is completed, cystourethroscopy is performed. The position and configuration of the urethra and bladder neck are noted at rest and during straining. As mentioned, the patient with stress incontinence typically has a low, poorly supported urethra during straining, with persistent patency and incompetence of the bladder neck. The bladder is thoroughly inspected also. A voiding cystourethrogram is then performed with the patient standing for radiographic documentation of urethral prolapse and loss of contrast material during stress.

PREOPERATIVE PREPARATION

The patient is prepared with lower abdominal cleansing and a vaginal douche with a povidone–iodine solution the night before and the morning of surgery. Parenteral broad-spectrum antibiotics (usually an aminoglycoside and ampicillin) are also administered the night before and the morning of surgery.

OPERATIVE PROCEDURE

Anesthesia

The modified Pereyra bladder-neck suspension can be performed under general, spinal, or local anesthesia. When local anesthesia is used, lidocaine is injected in three places. First, a bilateral pudendal nerve block is obtained by bilateral injection medial to the ischial tuberosities. Second, the anterior vaginal wall is anesthetized in the area where the inverted U-shaped incision will be made; and third, an area 1 cm above the pubis is anesthetized where the 2-cm transverse suprapubic incision will be made.

Technique

After the patient has been placed in the lithotomy position, the vagina and suprapubic area are prepared and draped, with careful exclusion of the rectum from the operative field. A weighted posterior vaginal retractor is inserted, and the labia minora are sewn laterally to provide ad-

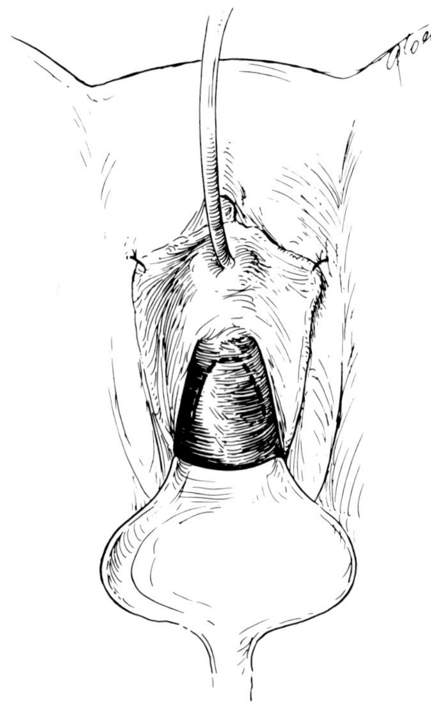

Fig. 31–1. Position of inverted U-shaped incision in anterior vaginal wall. Note sewing of labia away from the field.

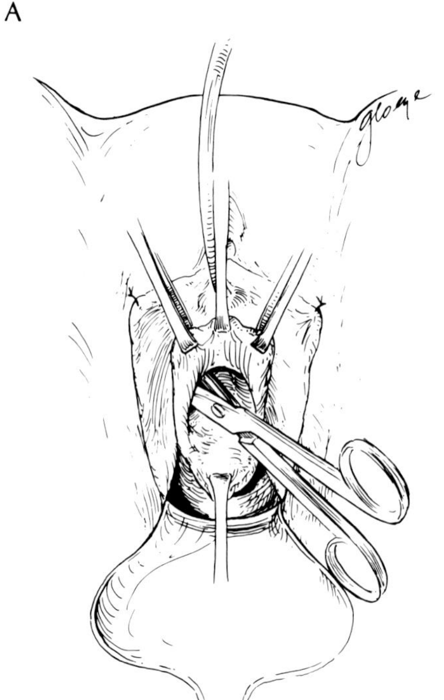

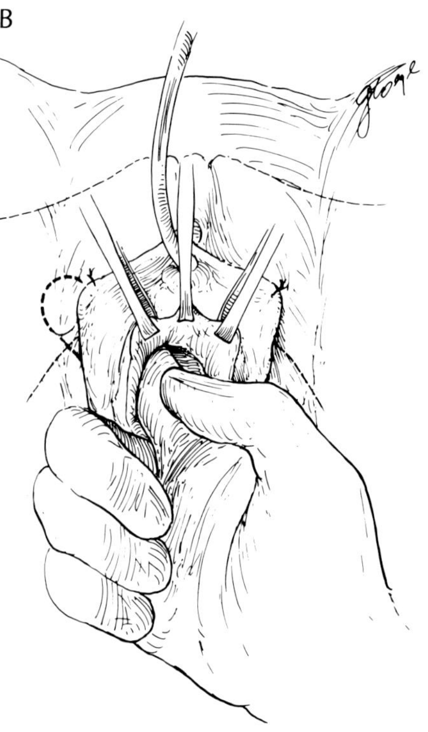

Fig. 31–2. Approach to the retropubic space. *(A)* Sharp lateral dissection beneath the vaginal mucosa to the pubic bone. Medial dissection is avoided to prevent entry into bladder or urethra. *(B)* Finger in retropubic space after perforation of deep endopelvic fascia.

equate exposure of the anterior vaginal wall. An 18F urethral Foley catheter is inserted, and the catheter balloon is inflated to aid in the identification of the bladder neck.

After saline is injected beneath the vaginal mucosa, an inverted U-shaped incision is made in the anterior vaginal wall, with the apex of the U midway between the bladder neck and the urethral meatus (Fig. 31–1). Sharp dissection is then performed bilaterally, moving beneath the vaginal mucosa laterally to the pubic bone on each side (Fig. 31–2*A*). After the pubic bone is reached, the deep endopelvic fascia is perforated at the level of the pubic bone on each side with sharp or blunt (finger) dissection. It is important that the deep endopelvic fascia be perforated laterally, in the direction of the pubic bone, rather than medially, so as to avoid entry into the bladder or urethra.

After the deep endopelvic fascia has been perforated, the finger enters the retropubic space (Fig. 31–2*B*). Blunt finger dissection is used to sweep any tissue off the posterior aspect of the superior pubic rami and thus better define the retropubic space on each side. If there have been previous attempts at bladder-neck suspension, it is essential to mobilize the urethra and anterior vaginal wall completely from surrounding adhesions so that these structures can be properly suspended.

A helical suture of No. 1 polypropylene is then placed bilaterally at the level of the bladder neck; each suture incorporates three bites of both the deep endopelvic fascia and the full thickness of the anterior vaginal wall but excludes the vaginal mucosa (Fig. 31–3). The mucosal tissue acts as an anchor for the suture, which will be used to elevate the bladder neck and proximal urethra. We believe that avoiding periurethral suture placement decreases the risk of periurethral fibrosis, recurrent incontinence, or urethral obstruction.

After the sutures have been placed, a 2-cm skin incision is made 1 cm above the pubis through the skin and subcutaneous tissue only. A finger is then inserted through the vaginal incision to the

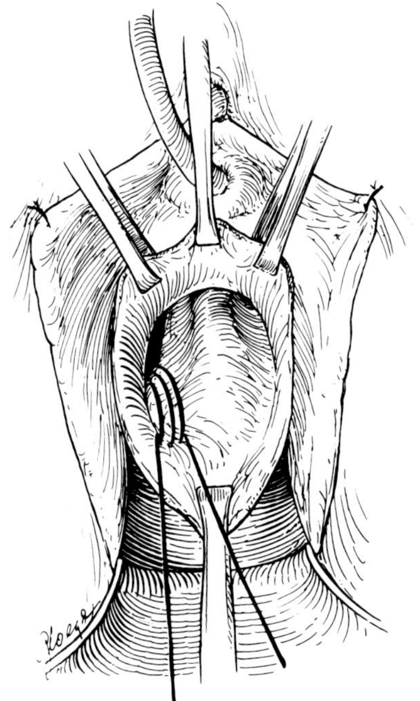

Fig. 31–3. Helical No. 1 polypropylene suture incorporating three bites of the deep endopelvic fascia and anterior vaginal wall but excluding vaginal mucosa.

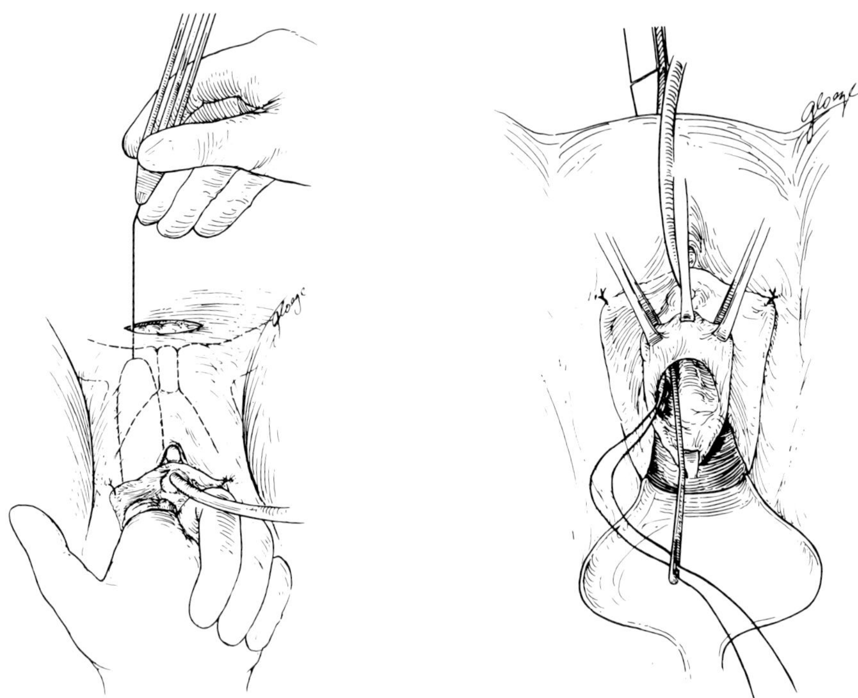

Fig. 31–4. *(A)* Passage of ligature carrier through retropubic space with constant finger control. *(B)* Ends of ipsilateral polypropylene suture threaded through eye of ligature carrier.

retropubic space. Under constant finger control (Fig. 31–4*A*), the ligature carrier is passed from the lateral aspect of the suprapubic incision through the retropubic space and out through the vaginal incision (Fig. 31–4*B*). After the suture on the opposite side has been transferred in similar fashion, 5 ml of indigo carmine is administered intravenously.

Cystoscopy is performed at this point for three reasons: (1) to make certain there has been no perforation or suture entry into the bladder or urethra, (2) to confirm ureteral patency by observing efflux of the indigo carmine from both ureteral orifices, and (3) to confirm adequate elevation of the bladder neck and proximal urethra when traction is applied to the suprapubic sutures. After the endoscopy is completed, the urethral Foley catheter is reinserted; and the incision in the anterior vaginal wall is closed with absorbable running sutures. The weighted posterior retractor is removed, and the suprapubic sutures are tied individually and then together over the rectus fascia so as to provide adequate elevation of the bladder neck and proximal urethra (Fig. 31–5). The suprapubic incision is then closed with a subcuticular absorbable suture, and antibiotic-soaked vaginal packing is inserted.

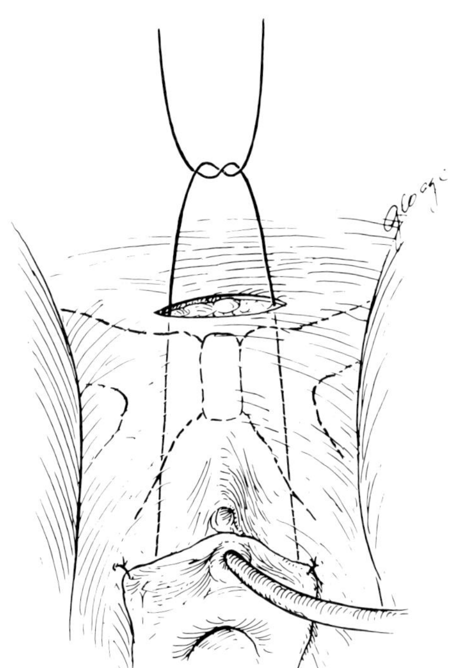

Fig. 31–5. Polypropylene sutures are tied across the midline over the rectus fascia to elevate the bladder neck and proximal urethra.

POSTOPERATIVE CARE

Parenteral antibiotics are continued for 24 hours, and the vaginal pack is removed on the first postoperative day. The urethral catheter is removed on the second postoperative day; and if the patient is unable to empty her bladder adequately, a program of clean intermittent self-catheterization is begun. No medication is given to facilitate bladder emptying. Fifty-five percent of our patients have required temporary self-catheterization, with the longest period of postoperative retention being eight weeks; 70% resumed normal voiding within the first two weeks.

RESULTS AND COMPLICATIONS

In almost 300 cases of female stress urinary incontinence managed with the modified Pereyra bladder-neck suspension procedure, the success rate was 96% with postoperative followup ranging from 6 months to 5 years. In the 54 patients who had undergone between 1 and 9 previous unsuccessful bladder-neck procedures, 94% had their stress urinary incontinence cured.

In addition to the temporary urinary retention already described, the complications included bleeding from anterior vaginal-wall varices in one patient, perforation of the urethra or bladder in three patients, and rupture of the polypropylene sutures from the anchoring tissue in two patients. Although there were no retropubic infections, two patients had superficial skin infections. One patient died of a cerebral vascular accident one month after the procedure.

CONCLUSIONS

The modified Pereyra bladder-neck suspension is a simple, effective operation for the management of female stress urinary incontinence. It is applicable both to the patient who has undergone unsuccessful bladder-neck suspensions and to those who have not had previous surgical treatment. With the proper selection of patients, an excellent success rate can be obtained with minimal morbidity.

REFERENCES

1. Pereyra, A.J.: A simplified surgical procedure for the correction of stress incontinence in women. West. J. Surg., *67*:223, 1959.
2. Pereyra, A.J., and Lebherz, T.B.: Combined urethral vesical suspension vaginal urethroplasty for correction of urinary stress incontinence. Obstet. Gynecol., *30*:37, 1967.
3. Stamey, T.A.: Cystoscopic suspension of the vesical neck for urinary incontinence. Surg. Gynecol. Obstet., *136*:547, 1973.
4. Cobb, O.E., and Ragde, H.: Correction of female stress incontinence. J. Urol., *20*:418, 1978.
5. Raz, S.: Modified bladder neck suspension for female stress incontinence. Urology, *18*:82, 1981.

32

Female Urethrotomy and Kollmann Dilatation Under Local Anesthesia

AHMAD ORANDI, M.D., F.A.C.S.

Internal urethrotomy and Kollmann dilatation of the urethra as a means of treating chronic bladder and urethral problems in females continue to be controversial. Proponents cite many occasions when these procedures proved successful,[1–5] whereas opponents document contrary instances.[6,7] Recently, urodynamic studies have unveiled different etiologic factors, resulting in new treatment methods;[8–11] but female patients with chronic bladder and urethral symptoms of obscure origin that often resist treatment are still a significant proportion of a urologic practice. Distressed and disturbed by their refractory problem, these patients often go to one urologist after another, traveling to distant cities in search of relief.

The purpose of this chapter is to demonstrate that internal urethrotomy and Kollmann dilatation of the urethra are made simpler and safer by local anesthesia and that in many cases the patient's symptoms abate afterward. As Kerr has pointed out,[3] either procedure can be combined inexpensively with the outpatient cystoscopic evaluation, with no need for an extensive work-up or hospitalization. Over a 5-year period, I have used this method on 120 women, ages 15 to 94 years, who suffered recurrent urinary-tract infections, nocturia, frequency, urgency, burning, and slow stream; that is, the urethral syndrome. The use of local anesthesia reduced the cost 75% in comparison with the cost of the same procedure done under general anesthesia.

TECHNIQUES

Selection and Preparation of Patients

Any female patient with a possibly stenotic urethra and persistent bladder problems unresponsive to conservative treatment can be managed by this approach if she is old enough to handle the apprehension of an operation under local anesthesia and does not have a history of allergy to the drugs. She is given an analgesic and a sedative (usually meperidine hydrochloride and sodium pentobarbital), and cystoscopy and urethral calibration are performed after topical anesthesia has been obtained by instillation of 2% lidocaine hydrochloride.

Anesthesia

A few milliliters of 1% lidocaine hydrochloride is injected around the external urethral meatus with a fine needle. A 22-gauge, 3-inch spinal needle is then used to instill approximately 20 ml of the drug parallel to the urethra up to the bladder, the needle being guided with a finger in the vagina (Fig. 32–1).

Internal Urethrotomy

The urethra is gradually stretched and cut to 45F at the 12 o'clock position with an Otis urethrotome. A 30F Foley catheter is left in the bladder and snugly taped over the pubis to secure hemostasis and urinary drainage. The patient is observed for a few hours before being discharged with an analgesic such as acetaminophen with codeine sulfate (Tylenol No. 3) tablets. Apprehensive patients, those unable to care for themselves, and those with bleeding potential are admitted to the hospital and observed for 24 hours. Patients are instructed to remove the catheter after 24 hours, to take sitz baths, and to avoid exertion for a few days.

RESULTS

Patients feel the initial needle puncture and the infiltration of lidocaine as the needle advances above the urethra. Adequate anesthesia often lasts for several hours and greatly reduces postoperative discomfort, such that many patients require no analgesics.

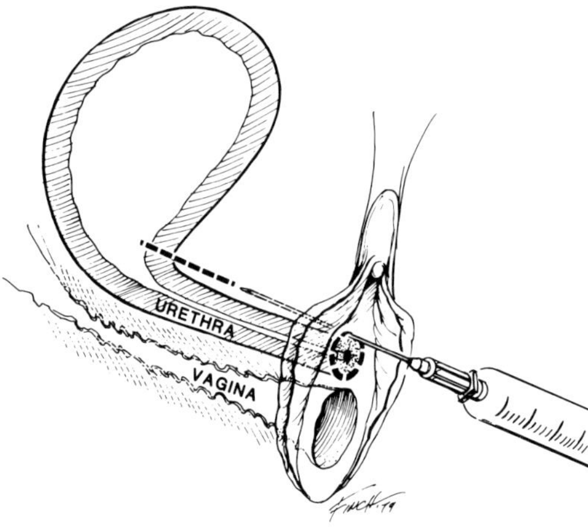

Fig. 32–1. Lidocaine is injected around the external meatus and above the urethra up to the bladder.

The author's experience with 590 patients treated chiefly by internal urethrotomy since 1967 (470 under general and 120 under local anesthesia) encompasses a broad range of results. For some patients, the treatment failed to reduce their symptoms. However, for many others, including such sophisticated and critical patients as doctors' wives and nurses, the procedure prevented recurrent infections and cured vesicoureteral reflux and chronic bladder symptoms. Patients with idiopathic urinary retention requiring an indwelling catheter also responded well to a simple internal urethrotomy under local anesthesia.

For the past 20 months, no drugs or other treatment have been used after internal urethrotomy, even in patients with documented active urinary infection. Postoperatively, the infection subsided and, frequently, sustained relief was achieved from both chronic symptoms and the need for medication.

COMPLICATIONS

Of the 120 patients who underwent urethrotomy or Kollmann dilatation under local anesthesia, five complained of tinnitus and two experienced slight hypotension during the injection of lidocaine. No treatment was necessary. Nonetheless, the possibility of lidocaine side effects and the appropriate precautions were kept in mind. Two patients bled postoperatively, necessitating hospitalization but not transfusion. No urinary incontinence was encountered.

CONCLUSIONS

Female internal urethrotomy and Kollmann dilatation of urethra can be performed safely and satisfactorily under local rather than general anesthesia, eliminating many risks and complications as well as an extensive work-up and hospitalization.

REFERENCES

1. Lyon, R.P., and Smith, D.R.: Distal urethral stenosis. J. Urol., *89*:414, 1963.
2. Halverstadt, D.B., and Leadbetter, G.W.: Internal urethrotomy and recurrent urinary tract infection in female children: results in the management of infection. J. Urol., *100*:297, 1968.
3. Kerr, W.: Results of internal urethrotomy in female patients for urethral stenosis. J. Urol., *102*:449, 1969.
4. McLean, P., and Emmett, J.L.: Internal urethrotomy in women for recurrent chronic urethritis. J. Urol., *101*:724, 1969.
5. Keitzer, W.A., and Allen, J.S.: Operative treatment of chronic cystitis by urethrotomy: ten years of experience. J. Urol., *100*:429, 1970.
6. Carson, C.C., Segura, J.W., and Osborne, D.M.: Evaluation and treatment of the female urethral syndrome. J. Urol., *124*:609, 1980.
7. Marbry, E.W., Carson, C.C., and Older, R.A.: Evaluation of women with chronic voiding discomfort. Urology, *18*:244, 1981.
8. Lipsky, H.: Urodynamic assessment of women with urethral syndrome. Eur. Urol., *3*:202, 1977.
9. Kaplan, W.E., Firlit, C.F., and Schoenberg, H.W.: The female urethral syndrome: external sphincter spasm as etiology. J. Urol., *124*:48, 1980.
10. Frewen, W.K.: The management of urgency and frequency of micturition. Br. J. Urol., *52*:267, 1980.
11. Godec, C.J., Esho, J., and Cass, A.S.: Correlation among cystometry, urethral pressure profilometry and pelvic floor electromyography in the evaluation of female patients with voiding dysfunction symptoms. J. Urol., *124*:678, 1980.

33

Needle and Aspiration Biopsy of the Prostate

P.J.P. VAN BLERK, B.Sc. (Med.), M.B.B.Ch., DIP. SURG., and
NAOMI A. EPSTEIN, M.D., M.B.B.Ch., B.Sc., F.I.A.C.

Definitive diagnosis of prostatic cancer still requires pathologic study of representative tissue from suspicious areas within the gland.[1] Essentially, there are four routes by which such tissue may be obtained: open biopsy, transurethral resection, and transperineal or transrectal needle biopsy.

Although some transurethral resections are being performed on an outpatient basis (see Chapter 15), both this and open biopsy are generally thought to require hospital admission and, accordingly, shall not be discussed further. The mainstay of diagnosis, rather, is needle biopsy; and this has been considered an outpatient procedure for more than two decades.[2,3] Three methods need to be discussed: transperineal and transrectal needle biopsy for histologic assessment and fine-needle aspiration biopsy for cytologic examination.

Although the safety and efficacy of these procedures has been clearly substantiated,[4-6] prostatic biopsy is by no means an innocuous undertaking; and there is a formidable list of complications. This chapter emphasizes the selection of patients and the contraindications and precautions. If these measures are observed, we believe that prostatic biopsy can be done on an outpatient basis in most cases with minimal risk while providing specimens suitable for accurate diagnosis.

ADVANTAGES AND DISADVANTAGES OF VARIOUS METHODS

Transperineal Needle Biopsy

Proponents of this approach claim a lower incidence of infectious complications in comparison with the transrectal route,[7] although the use of prophylactic antibiotics has brought the infection rate well within acceptable limits for all routes.[8] Further, there appears to be no significant difference in the rates of noninfectious complications with the transperineal and transrectal routes.[9]

The disadvantages of the transperineal method are the greater pain and discomfort it causes and its lower accuracy, with false-negative results being obtained in 16.2–27% of cases.[9-11] The explanation for these errors may lie in the greater difficulty one has in placing the needle in the desired area in comparison with the more direct transrectal approach. Rarely, tumor cells are implanted along the needle tract.[12] Overall, complications occur in approximately 7% of cases of transperineal biopsy.[11]

Transrectal Needle Biospy

Twenty years ago, Anderson showed that transrectal needle biopsy of the prostate could be performed safely on an outpatient basis without anesthesia. Indeed, virtually all patients tolerated the procedure as easily as they did a venipuncture, and the complications were less serious than those in hospitalized patients.[2] These advantages remain, and the wide acceptance of this method has meant that most urology residents learn it during their training. The tissue specimen usually is easily interpretable by any experienced anatomic pathologist.

The disadvantages of the transrectal method are that small nodules, which are often the most worrisome, may be difficult to locate and that adequate sampling requires several cores, yet the incidence of complications rises in tandem with the number of cores obtained. Also, traumatic or infectious complications occur in 15–33% of cases.[7,13] The former results from needle damage to the bladder, urethra, seminal vesicles, or prostate and are expressed as hematuria, hematospermia, or hematomas of the perineal, retropubic, or pelvic regions.[14] Urinary retention may occur as the result of hematoma or edema. The infectious complications include transient bacteremia, which is common immediately after the biopsy and poses an obvious threat to the patient with valvular heart disease, as well as cystitis, prostatitis, epididymitis, local abscess, pyelonephritis, fever, and rarely, septicemia or osteomyelitis.[15–17] Infections may involve anaerobic organisms.[18,19]

Recently, the incidence of infectious complications after transrectal biopsy has been significantly reduced by prophylactic antibiotics.[2,8,20] For example, 80 mg of trimethoprim and 400 mg of sulfamethoxazole (Septra DS; Bactrim DS) given every 12 hours beginning 24 hours before the biopsy and continuing for 72 hours afterward led to a reduction in the rate of bacteriuria from 21% in the untreated group to 0 and a reduction in the rate of bacteremia in blood samples obtained 15 to 25 minutes after the biopsy from 59% in the untreated group to 24%.[20] In another study, two tablets of carbenicillin indanyl sodium (Geocillin) given four times daily for the 24 hours preceding and following the biopsy reduced the rate of bacteriuria from 36% in the untreated group to 8.6% and reduced the incidence of postbiopsy fever. However, there was no significant reduction in the frequency of bacteremia 15 minutes after the procedure.[8] Other authors have suggested using cleansing enemas and instilling povidone–iodine solutions into the rectum immediately before the biopsy,[21] but the value of these measures has not been proved.

Fine-Needle Aspiration Biopsy

This technique, popularized in Scandinavian countries in the 1960s and 1970s, has only recently become popular in the United States.[5,22] Because it is done transrectally, it causes little discomfort; and because no preoperative antibiotic or bowel preparation is used, it can be done during the patient's initial visit if there are no feces in the rectum. The examiner's finger is placed directly over the lesion, and the needle is inserted at the fingertip, with aspiration beginning as soon as the needle has penetrated the prostatic capsule. This approach, plus the ability to obtain liberal samples by moving the needle to and fro while aspirating, may make the technique more accurate for evaluating small lesions, which may be missed with the standard cutting-needle biopsy technique. The procedure is safe, with one clinical hematoma, one case of pneumothorax, and three episodes of syncope being the only complications in one series of more than 1,000 thin-needle aspiration biopsies at all sites.[5] Further, there have been no reports of implantation of cancer cells along the needle track. The results can be obtained rapidly, usually in less than 1 hour. Finally, the results are accurate.[22–24] For example, in our series of 118 patients, aspiration biopsy was accurate in 86.6% of cases (six false-negative results) and cutting needle biopsy was accurate in 85.6% of cases (five false-negative results). When the results of both methods were considered, the accuracy rate was 95.8%.[23] In our first 34 cases, we described 8 cases of atypia as being malignant, but when followup proved that these were benign lesions, we revised our criteria for malignancy; and there were no false-positive results in our remaining 84 cases. Likewise, Esposti had no false-positive results in his large series.[24]

The principal disadvantage of fine-needle aspiration biopsy is the need for an expert cytopathologist experienced in prostate cytology if the interpretation is to be reliable and accurate. Such a person will be unavailable in some outpatient surgery units. A lesser disadvantage is the unfamiliarity of most urologists with the technique, but this can be expected to change as its advantages become clear.

CONTRAINDICATIONS

Patients with various prostheses, valvular heart disease, diabetes, debilitation, urinary tract infection, or severe obstructive voiding symptoms should not have prostatic biopsies on a true outpatient basis. Even in some of these patients, however, the patient can begin antibiotics and bowel cleansing at home, be admitted early in the morning for the biopsy, remain under observation for the rest of the day, and be discharged late in the afternoon if he is voiding easily and has no evidence of infection.

PREOPERATIVE PREPARATION

Patients are informed of the nature of the procedure and warned of the possible complications, particularly fever and urinary symptoms, and their consent is obtained. A regimen of two tablets of trimethoprim–sulfamethoxazole DS is started 24 hours before the procedure and continued for 48 hours afterward. Immediately before the procedure, the rectum is irrigated with 20 ml of full-strength povidone–iodine solution, although this probably is not necessary for needle aspiration biopsy.[3,5,22]

TECHNIQUE

Transperineal Biopsy

The patient is placed in the lithotomy position, and the perineum is thoroughly cleaned with a povidone–iodine solution. An assistant lifts the scrotum out of the way, and the surgeon locates the area to be biopsied with a gloved index finger in the rectum. Local anesthetic is infiltrated along the expected route of the needle on either side of the midline approximately two fingerbreadths anterior to the rectum. (It is better to create two routes rather than to cross the midline, as this may cause urethral injury.) The guiding index finger remains in the rectum until the anesthetic has taken effect.

A nick is made in the skin with a scalpel blade, and a Tru-Cut needle* is passed into the prostate to obtain a core of tissue (Fig. 33–1). Usually, a core is obtained from both sides of the midline. Pressure is maintained on the prostate with the intrarectal finger for 1–2 minutes to minimize bleeding.

Transrectal Biopsy

This route necessitates no anesthesia and can be done without an assistant. The patient is placed in the lithotomy position, and a rectal examination is per-

*Travenol Laboratories, Deerfield, IL 60015.

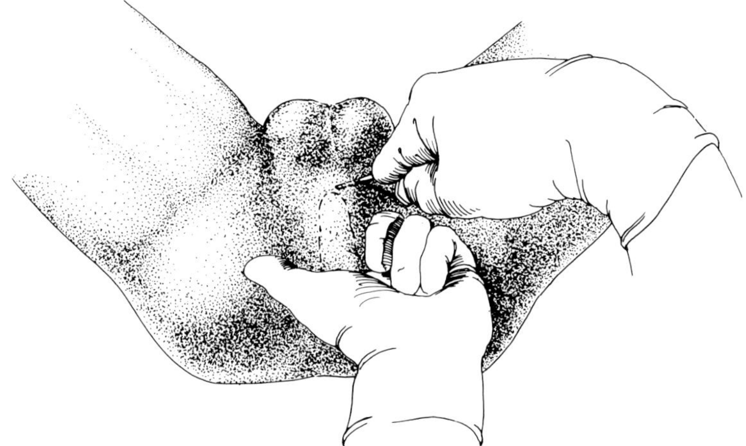

Fig. 33–1. Transperineal needle biopsy. Finger in rectum marks position of lesion.

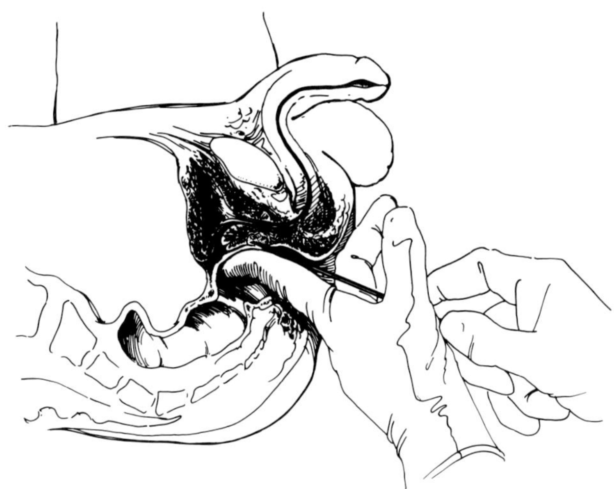

Fig. 33–2. Transrectal needle biopsy. Finger in rectum marks position of lesion.

formed with the index finger of the non-dominant hand, which is covered with one or two gloves. The finger is with-drawn, and the bevelled side of the Tru-Cut needle is pressed firmly into the pulpy tip of the finger. If the surgeon is wearing two gloves, the needle point can be caught in the outer one as a further precaution against inadvertent pricking of the patient.

The finger and needle are passed into the rectum, and the obturator is retracted so that the specimen notch is covered by the sheath. The finger guides the needle to the area to be biopsied, the needle is advanced, and the finger is withdrawn (Fig. 33–2).

The recommended technique for use of the Tru-Cut needle is to advance the closed assembly into the chosen area with the obturator notch covered (Fig. 33–3*A*). The cannula handle is then pulled outward until it stops while the obturator is held still (Fig. 33–3*B*), thus opening the specimen notch. The tissue is pressed into the notch with the right index finger (for right-handed surgeons), and the cannula handle is advanced quickly without moving the obturator (Fig. 33–3*C*). The assembly is then withdrawn from the rectum with the cannula still covering the obturator. This technique is safer than the one originally recommended, in which the obturator needle was rapidly shot into the area to be biopsied. It permits more accurate location of the needle tip by palpation, and there is less chance of damaging the bladder and urethra.[25]

Needle Aspiration Biopsy

This technique can be performed using Franzen's device[3] (Fig. 33–4), the disposable prostatic biopsy kit,* or a 10-ml syringe with a 22-gauge spinal needle and a short piece of plastic tubing.

Franzen Method. The patient is placed in the lithotomy position, and the suspicious area is palpated with the index finger of the nondominant hand. The needle, with the plunger down, is advanced into the prostate. As the needle moves through the suspicious area, the plunger is pulled back as far as possible, creating a vacuum that sucks prostate cells into the needle. The needle is moved back and forth 3–5 times with the plunger out. It is advisable to sample several areas. When this is complete, the pressure is allowed to equalize and the needle is pulled up into the guide. The finger is withdrawn from the rectum.

The syringe is disconnected from the needle, filled with air, and reconnected.

*Cook Urological, P.O. Box 227, Spencer, IN 47460.

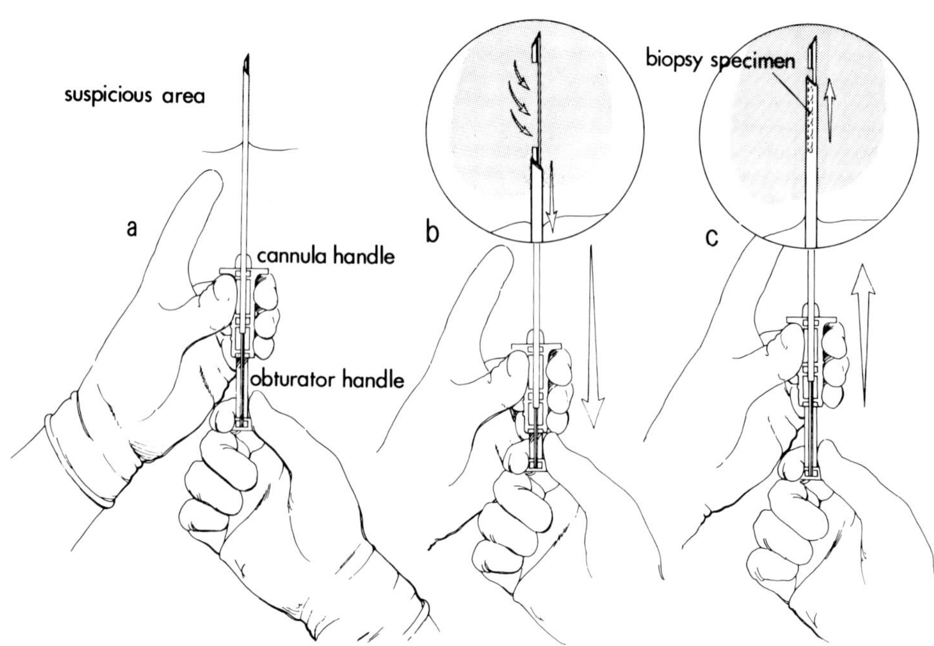

Fig. 33–3. Tru-Cut needle. *(A)* Assembly is advanced closed into lesion. *(B)* Opening device in lesion. *(C)* Withdrawal of specimen.

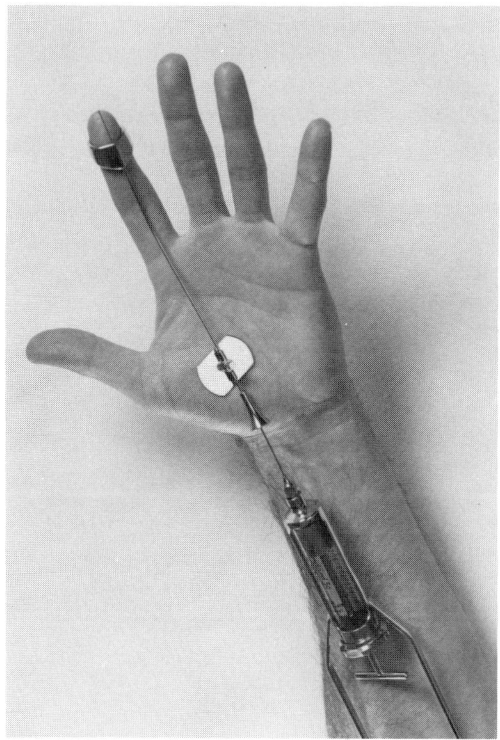

Fig. 33–4. Franzen needle for fine-needle aspiration biopsy.

The material in the needle is expressed gently onto two glass slides and spread as in a blood smear. The larger fragments that collect at the end are squeezed gently by pressing the surfaces of the two slides firmly together. The needle of this reusable system is then rinsed immediately to prevent blockage.

A simple technique is to tape a short piece of plastic tubing to the index finger, insert the finger into the rectum, and pass a syringe with a standard 22-gauge spinal needle through the tubing. It is helpful to have a piece of tape around the needle just below the syringe so that one will know when the needle is about to emerge from the plastic tubing. The aspiration is then performed as described.

POSTPROCEDURE CARE

After a biopsy, patients should remain in the observation area and have their vital signs checked regularly until they have voided. Provided they do not have marked hematuria or other untoward signs, they then can be discharged with detailed instructions on whom to contact should problems arise and on the need to continue taking the antibiotic for two days. With high-risk patients, longer monitoring, and occasionally hospital admission, may be advisable.

After a needle aspiration, it probably is unnecessary to wait until the patient has voided before discharging him.

PREPARATION AND EXAMINATION OF TISSUE

Fixation

The cores of tissue obtained by needle biopsy are usually fixed in 10% formol–saline. One of the slides from the aspiration biopsy is fixed with a cytologic spray fixative or immersed in 90% ethanol for half an hour, dried, and stained with hematoxylin–eosin or by the Papanicolaou method. The second slide is air-dried and stained by the May–Grünwald–Giemsa method. Before the slides are sent to the laboratory for staining, they should be marked to show which stain is to be used.

Examination

Needle biopsy is an accepted histologic technique for the diagnosis of prostate cancer. However, false-negative results occur with sufficient frequency to mandate rebiopsy of a clinically suspicious lesion if no tumor is found in the specimen.[26]

Histologic (Gleason) grading of tumors found in biopsy specimens is subject to both undergrading and overgrading. For example, in one series of 72 cases, the combined Gleason grade of the resected tumor differed from that of the biopsy specimen in 53% of cases, being higher in 39% and lower in 14%, despite participation of experienced pathologists.[27] A

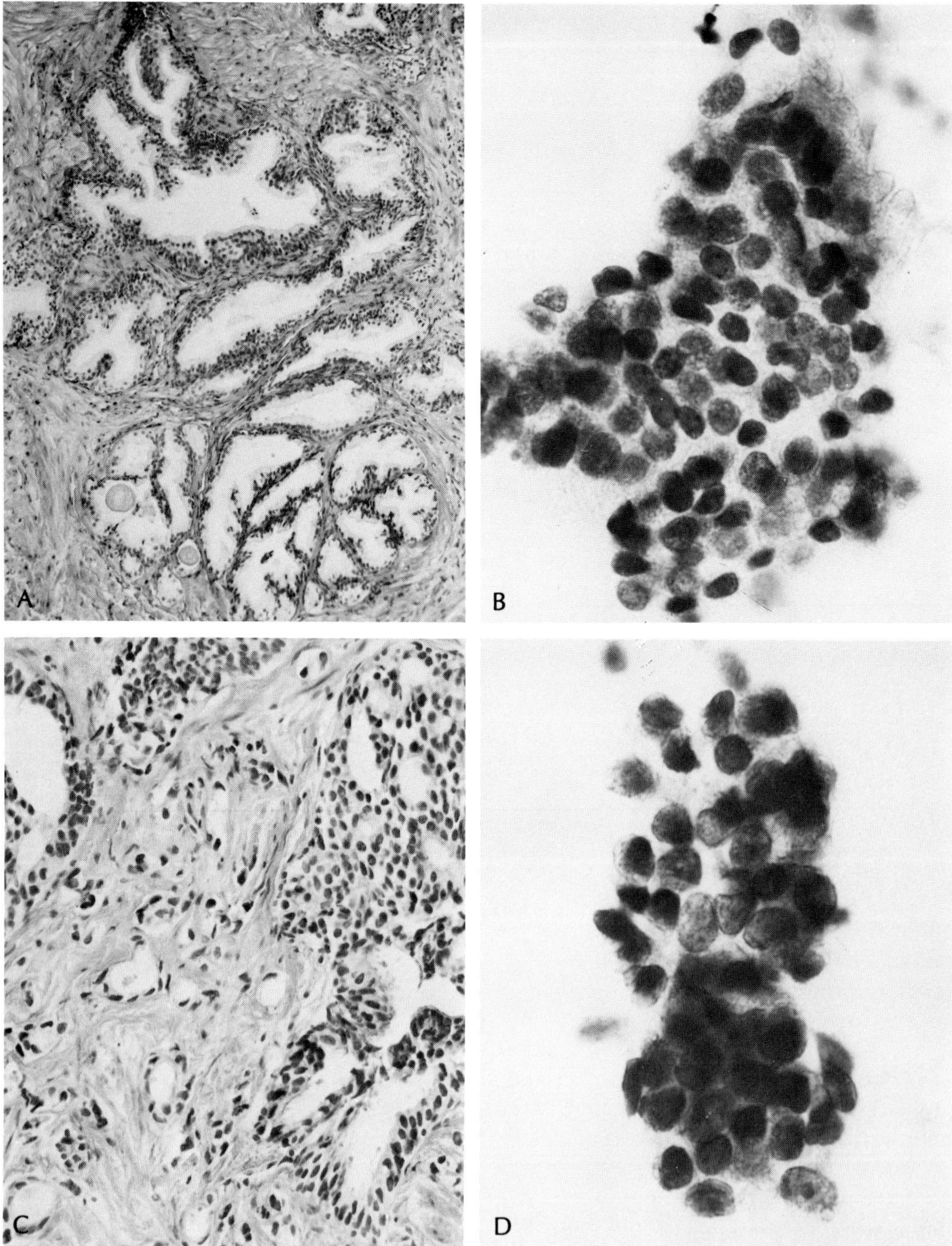

Fig. 33–5. Prostatic Pathology. *(A)* Histology of normal prostate (× 120). *(B)* Cytology of normal prostate. Note cohesive, polarized sheet, small cells, regular nuclei, moderate cytoplasmic volume (× 1200). *(C)* Histology of adenocarcinoma, Gleason grade 3–3 (× 300). *(D)* Cytology specimen from same patient. Note lack of adhesion and focal crowding, scanty cytoplasm, variable shape of the nuclei, and prominent nucleoli. Cells are larger than in normal specimen (× 1200). (Courtesy of Irene Posalaky, M.D.)

report of high-grade (less-differentiated) tumor in a biopsy specimen is more reliable than is a report of low-grade tumor.

CONCLUSIONS

Provided adequate precautions are taken against infection, biopsy of the prostate is usually a simple and safe procedure in the outpatient setting, especially if it is not accompanied by cystoscopy, which increases the risk of infection even if antibiotics are given.[28] However, even without antibiotics or bowel preparation, the frequency of hospital admission for complications after transrectal needle biopsy was only 6%.[4]

There has been a rebirth of interest in fine-needle aspiration biopsy; and, provided an experienced cytopathologist is available to examine the specimen, the method is at least as reliable as the standard needle biopsy.[5,22,23] At times, an unequivocal diagnosis of carcinoma can be made by this method alone (Fig. 33–5), and some authorities begin treatment on the basis of aspiration cytology even if the standard needle biopsy specimen is negative for tumor.[22] Nevertheless, there are some borderline cases in which it is difficult or impossible to distinguish between a well-differentiated carcinoma and atypia caused by a benign (usually inflammatory) condition, and these cases require histologic study. While one is gaining experience in the performance and interpretation of aspiration biopsies, a standard needle biopsy also should be performed. The two are complementary, with an accuracy rate of more than 95% when used together.[23]

It may well be that needle aspiration biopsy will become the method of choice for outpatient evaluation of prostatic lesions. Certainly, it is ideal for sampling the small, irregular mass that one is almost certain is not carcinoma, because a cutting-needle biopsy may easily miss the lesion. Outpatient needle aspiration biopsy without anesthesia is a safe and cost-effective way to resolve this dilemma.[5]

REFERENCES

1. Grayhack, J.T., and Bockrath, J.M.: Diagnosis of carcinoma of the prostate. Urology, *17*:54, 1981.
2. Anderson, M.J.: Transrectal needle biopsy as an outpatient procedure. Dis. Colon Rectum, 7:23, 1964.
3. Franzen, S., Giertz, G., and Zajicek, J.: Cytological diagnosis of prostatic tumors by transrectal aspiration biopsy: a preliminary report. Br. J. Urol., *32*:193, 1960.
4. Eaton, A.C.: The safety of transrectal biopsy of the prostate as an outpatient investigation. Br. J. Urol., *53*:144, 1981.
5. Howards, S.S., and Feldman, P.: Needle aspiration permits speedy, low risk diagnosis of prostatic lesions. Urol. Times, June 1982, p. 3.
6. Blath, R.A., and Fair, W.R.: Urology. *In* Outpatient Surgery. 2nd Ed. Edited by G.J. Hill, Philadelphia, W.B. Saunders, 1980.
7. Derlen, L.W., Jr., Block, N.L., and Politano, V.A.: Complications of transrectal biopsy examination of the prostate gland. South. Med. J., *67*:1453, 1974.
8. Crawford, E.D., et al.: Prevention of urinary tract infection and sepsis following transrectal prostatic biopsy. J. Urol., *127*:449, 1982.
9. Bissada, N.K., Rountree, G.A., and Sulieman, J.S.: Factors affecting accuracy and morbidity in transrectal biopsy of the prostate. Surg. Gynecol. Obstet., *145*:869, 1977.
10. Fortunoff, S.: Needle biopsy of the prostate: a review of 346 biopsies. J. Urol., *87*:159, 1962.
11. Kaufman, J.J., and Schultz, J.I.: Needle biopsy of the prostate: a re-evaluation. J. Urol., *87*:164, 1962.
12. Burkholder, G.V., and Kaufman, J.J.: Local implantation of carcinoma of the prostate with percutaneous needle biopsy. J. Urol., *95*:801, 1966.
13. Barnes, R.W.: Carcinoma of the prostate: biopsy and conservative therapy. J. Urol., *108*:897, 1972.
14. Hanafy, H.M.: Massive pelvic hematoma complicating perineal prostatic biopsy. Urology, *13*:416, 1979.
15. Thompson, P.M., et al.: Transrectal biopsy of the prostate and bacteremia. Br. J. Urol., *67*:127, 1980.
16. Edson, R.S., Van Scoy, R.E., and Leary, F.J.: Gram-negative bacteremia after transrectal needle biopsy of the prostate. Mayo Clin. Proc., *55*:489, 1980.
17. Brown, R.W., et al.: Bacteremia and bacteriuria after transrectal prostatic biopsy. Arch. Intern. Med., *138*:393, 1978.
19. Breslin, J.A., et al.: Anaerobic infection as a consequence of transrectal prostatic biopsy. J. Urol., *120*:502, 1978.
20. Ruebush, T.K., II, McConville, J.H., and Calia, F.M.: A double-blind study of trimethoprim–sulfamethoxazole prophylaxis in patients having transrectal needle biopsy of the prostate. J. Urol., *122*:492, 1979.
21. Sharpe, J.R., et al.: Urinary tract infection after

transrectal needle biopsy of the prostate. J. Urol., *127*:255, 1982.
22. Kaufman, J.J., et al.: Aspiration biopsy of the prostate. Urology, *19*:587, 1982.
23. Epstein, N.A.: Prostatic biopsy: a morphologic correlation of aspiration cytology with needle biopsy histology. Cancer, *38*:2078, 1976.
24. Esposti, P.L.: Cytologic malignancy grading for prostatic carcinoma or transurethral aspiration biopsy. Scand. J. Urol. Nephrol., *5*:199, 1971.
25. Engel, R.M.E.: Prostatic needle biopsy: comparison of needles. J. Urol., *115*:715, 1976.
26. Zincke, H., et al.: Confidence in the negative transrectal needle biopsy. Surg. Gynecol. Obstet., *136*:78, 1973.
27. Lange, P.H., and Narayan, P.: Understaging and undergrading of prostate cancer: an argument for postoperative radiation as adjuvant therapy. Urology, *21*:113, 1983.
28. Nesi, M.H., et al.: A comparison of morbidity following transurethral and transperineal prostatic needle biopsy. Surg. Gynecol. Obstet., *156*:464, 1983.

34

Establishment and Maintenance of Angioaccess for Hemodialysis

ANTHONY D. WHITTEMORE, M.D., and DAVID H. GORDON, M.D.

Care of the patient in chronic renal failure, one of the greatest challenges in medicine, mandates replacement of the complex functions of the normal kidney, control of the underlying disease process, and prevention or management of the complications of therapy. Of equal importance, comprehensive management must involve extensive patient education, strict dietary guidance, and sustained psychologic and rehabilitative therapy.

It is understandable, then, that hospitals were long the center of care for these patients. It has become apparent, however, that hospital-centered care of the dialysis patient has two serious shortcomings. First, it increases the already prodigious cost of dialysis. Second, it handicaps the patient's psychologic adjustment by emphasizing "illness" and "disease." Therefore, efforts are increasingly directed toward minimizing hospital time by means of home dialysis, the new local self-care hemodialysis centers,[1] continuous ambulatory peritoneal dialysis,[2,3] and outpatient hemodialysis. The potential savings can be significant. For example, according to a 1979 estimate, inpatient hemodialysis costs $25,000 per patient per year, whereas the same procedure can be performed for $15,000 to $22,000 in an outpatient unit, $15,750 in a self-care unit,* and $8,000 to $11,000 in the patient's home.[7] These figures become of critical importance with the recent regulations of the Health Care Financing Administration, which severely curtail the maximum weekly reimbursement for patients in dialysis units.

The establishment of a hemodialysis unit in an outpatient center is a topic well beyond the scope of this book. Certain aspects are, however, pertinent: a significant reduction in both the financial and the emotional cost for these patients may be achieved with expeditious management of their angioaccess. We will therefore confine our discussion to two common outpatient procedures for the patient in chronic renal failure: the establishment of angioaccess for hemodialysis and the options available for correction of access failure.

ANGIOACCESS

There are three basic approaches to the creation of access for hemodialysis: percutaneous catheterization; external pros-

*Figure based on the assumption that the same percentage reduction in cost could be obtained in the United States as in Switzerland.[1]

thetic devices (usually called shunts), such as the Quinton–Scribner, Buselmeier, Kauffman, Thomas appliqué, and Allen–Brown devices; and internal arteriovenous fistulas utilizing either the Brescia–Cimino or the prosthetic graft technique. At present, the first two approaches generally are considered suitable for emergency dialysis, such as in the patient with a drug overdose, postoperative acute renal failure, unanticipated acceleration of chronic renal failure, and in those with a failed access who must wait two to four weeks after the creation or revision of a permanent internal access. Also, external shunts are often preferred for long-term hemodialysis in carriers of hepatitis B, because the risk of transmission of the virus to the staff is lower with this approach than with an internal fistula.[5] For most patients in chronic renal failure, however, an internal fistula is the angioaccess of choice and thus becomes the focus of our discussion.

Because an internal arteriovenous fistula cannot be used for dialysis for at least 10 days, and preferably not for 2 to 6 months after its creation, the timing of the angioaccess operation becomes important. Ideally, the fistula is created 3 to 6 months before it is expected to be needed. Thus, for patients in whom rapid kidney shutdown is expected, such as those with rapidly progressive glomerulonephritis or diabetes, the operation is usually performed when the creatinine clearance reaches 25 ml/min. In most other patients, a creatinine clearance of 15 ml/min or a serum creatinine concentration of 7–9 mg/dl usually indicates the need for operation.

If one misjudges the rate of renal deterioration, inpatient hemodialysis should be performed temporarily via bilateral Shaldon femoral catheters. This approach not only conserves blood vessels that will be needed later for more permanent angioaccess but has the advantage of minimizing the cardiac workload. In patients with iliofemoral thrombosis, groin sepsis, or recent vascular procedures, the groin vessels may be inaccessible, and the external shunt should be placed on the wrist of the dominant arm, although this approach carries the potential risk of shunt dislodgment, with possibly fatal exsanguination.

As soon as it is clear that a patient is going to require long-term hemodialysis, the surgeon must select the most appropriate site so that further venipuncture and vessel trauma can be avoided at that site. The most common site is the nondominant forearm. Bresia–Cimino fistulas between the radial artery and the cephalic vein, either in the "anatomic snuffbox" or, more commonly, just above the wrist, have been the most popular and provide 3-year patency rates of 50–78%, with some fistulas lasting 12 years.[6] The advantages of this site are several. First, the risk of infection is lower than when the angioaccess is created in the leg. Second, if an arterial steal syndrome results from the fistula, the consequences are less devastating in the arm than in the leg. Third, placement of the fistula in the nondominant arm facilitates self-dialysis. Finally, use of the most-distal site preserves the maximum length of blood vessel for future revisions. Popular alternatives may be constructed between the radial or brachial artery and the median cubital vein near the antecubital fossa, and between the brachial artery and the cephalic vein above the elbow.

The competence of the radial and ulnar arteries can be assessed preoperatively by the Allen test. Both arteries are compressed while the patient clenches the fist to induce blanching. One of the arteries is released while the hand is observed for the return of color. The compression, blanching, and release process is then repeated for the other artery. If skin color returns at the same rate after release of each artery, either artery can be sacrificed without risking the viability of the hand. The adequacy of the venous runoff in the forearm also should be assessed by inflating a blood pressure cuff on the upper arm to 40 mm Hg to distend the veins. Phlebography may be appropriate in patients who have had several previous angioaccess operations, as the vessels may have occlusions that will compromise a proposed access site.

ENDOGENOUS ARTERIOVENOUS FISTULAS

It is essential that all angioaccess operations be performed by experienced vascular surgeons, as a failed operation wastes needed blood vessels. The entire forearm is scrubbed and draped, and local anesthesia is provided with lidocaine (Xylocaine) 1–2%. A single skin incision is used to avoid creating a strip of devascularized tissue between the vessels.

Side-to-Side Anastomosis (Fig. 34–1)

Usually, this is preferred for anastomoses in the anatomic snuffbox, but it also can be used in the wrist.[5] A 3-cm longitudinal incision is made between the artery and vein, and the cephalic vein is mobilized for approximately 3–5 cm, with its two terminal tributaries and any other large veins being preserved. Subcutaneous tissues and the deep fascia are then incised medially to expose the radial artery, which is gently skeletonized for approximately 3 cm with division of the branches between double 5–0 or 6–0 ligatures. Proximal and distal control of the artery and vein is obtained with Silastic vessel loops or microvascular clamps; and the two vessels are positioned side-by-side without tension. The lumens are appropriately occluded, and precisely corresponding 1-cm incisions are made in the apposing sides of the vessels. The opened lumens may be irrigated with 0.9% saline. If there is any question about venous patency, a 5F or, better, an 8F pediatric feeding tube may be inserted through the open lumen to gauge the ease with which heparinized saline can be injected. Alternatively, a 3F or 4F Fogarty balloon catheter can be inserted and delicately withdrawn with the balloon inflated slightly. Such dilatation of the vein maximizes the rate of blood flow postoperatively and thus may reduce the likelihood of early fistula failure.[5,6]

Beginning on the posterior wall, the fistula is created with double-armed 7–0 monofilament polypropylene or nylon, with the knot placed outside the vessels. Topical 10% papaverine or hydrodilation with isotonic heparinized saline may be helpful in the event of vasospasm. The anastomosis is then constructed with a continuous suture technique, with the bites approximately 2 mm apart.

When the anastomosis is complete, venous control is released, and blood from the distal radial artery is allowed to flow through the fistula. Oxidized regenerated cellulose (Surgicel Absorbable Hemostat) may be placed temporarily around the suture line to reduce suture-line bleeding, and the proximal radial artery is released. In most patients, a thrill will be palpable; and in virtually all there will be an audible bruit. If there is a palpable pulse in the vein without a thrill or bruit, obstruction of the fistula may well be imminent.

The management of the distal radial artery and cephalic vein remains controversial. Some surgeons prefer to ligate the cephalic vein distal to the fistula to minimize the possibility of subsequent painful and disabling venous hypertension in the hand. Similarly, some surgeons prefer to ligate the distal radial artery in the belief that an arterial steal syndrome will be less likely. After perfect hemostasis has been obtained, the wound is meticulously closed with 4–0 or 5–0 monofilament nylon mattress sutures.

End-to-Side Anastomosis (Fig. 34–2)

Because of its hemodynamic characteristics, an end-to-side vein-to-artery

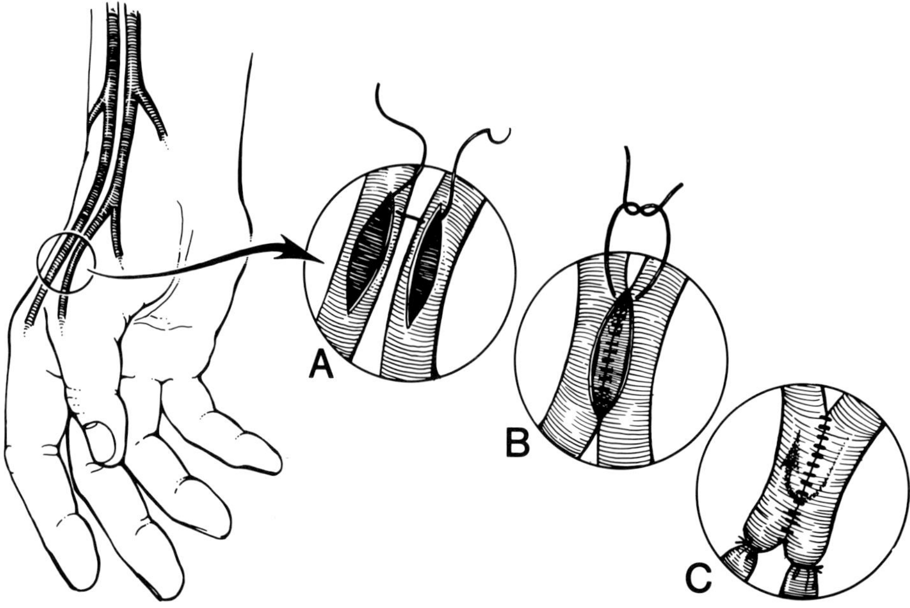

Fig. 34–1. Technique of side-to-side anastomosis in the anatomic snuffbox. *(A)* 1-cm incisions in apposing sides of artery and vein. *(B)* Creation of fistula beginning on posterior wall, with knot outside vessels. *(C)* Completed fistula.

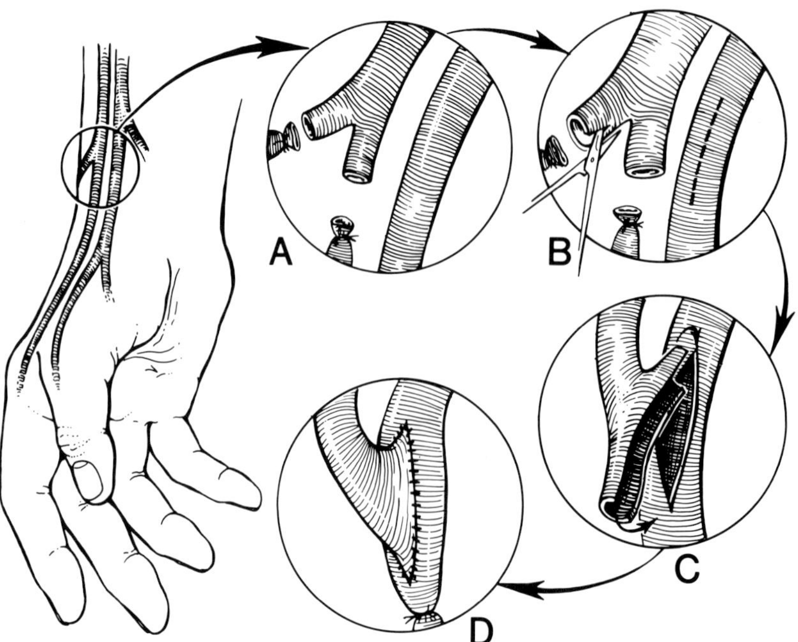

Fig. 34–2. Technique of end-to-side anastomosis in the wrist. *(A)* Ligation of terminal tributaries of cephalic vein. *(B)* Opening of vein. *(C)* Fitting of vein to arteriotomy (radial artery). *(D)* Completed fistula.

anastomosis is often preferred for fistulas at the wrist. A curvilinear incision is made over the radial aspect of the wrist, and the cephalic vein is exposed and isolated distal to the confluence of its two major terminal tributaries. Each branch is ligated and divided approximately 0.5 cm from the confluence, and the vein is opened as illustrated. Patency and suitability of the vein may be assessed as described earlier.

A longitudinal incision is made in the deep fascia to expose the radial artery, which is gently freed from the surrounding tissues with care not to avulse its delicate tributaries. Vessel loops are placed proximal and distal to the site chosen for anastomosis, and the artery is occluded. Alternatively, the artery can be ligated distal to the site to minimize arterial steal. An arteriotomy is then created in the proximal region of the incision so that the cephalic vein will curve gently without kinking after the anastomosis is made. The corners of the opened vein are trimmed to create a suitably elliptical patch, and the end-to-side anastomosis is made with continuous 6–0 or 7–0 monofilament suture. After completion of the anastomosis, the loop occluding the proximal arterial segment is released, and the anastomosis is inspected for hemostasis and patency. It is usually necessary to mobilize an additional 2–3 cm of vein distal to the fistula to optimize the blood flow and prevent significant kinking of the vein. Again, the incision is closed with interrupted 5–0 or 6–0 nylon mattress sutures after hemostasis has been secured.

Postoperative Care

A light, noncircumferential sterile dressing is applied. The arm should be kept elevated for 2–3 days, and the patient should take care not to lie on it. Any excessive induration or a decrease in the thrill over the fistula should be reported immediately and may indicate a need for an early revision.

After the incision has healed, the patient should squeeze a rubber ball for several minutes at intervals every day to promote dilatation and "arterialization" of the venous limb. Alternatively, a tourniquet may be applied proximal to the fistula for short intervals to create partial occlusion resulting in progressive dilatation of the vein. No tight jewelry or clothing should be worn over the access site.

PROSTHETIC ARTERIOVENOUS FISTULAS

Use of graft material to create a fistula is most often necessary because the native vessels have been damaged by repeated punctures or because all suitable endogenous sites have been utilized. Grafts also may be required in cachectic patients, in whom repeated venipuncture often causes subcutaneous hemorrhage, and in morbidly obese patients, in whom repeated venipuncture is often difficult. Finally, prosthetic grafts may be used in patients whose kidneys fail suddenly, as they can be used two weeks after insertion, whereas the endogenous fistula usually requires several weeks for suitable development. It is desirable to avoid using grafts, as the rates of infection and occlusion are higher than those associated with endogenous fistulas.

Materials

No perfect material is currently available. Bovine carotid artery has been preferred by some authors,[5] but the rate of infection is high; and when infection does occur, these grafts may degenerate, with subsequent formation of an aneurysm. Other authors prefer grafts of expanded polytetrafluoroethylene; e.g., Gore-Tex, Impra.[6] Autogenous or homologous saphenous vein, cadaver arteries, and Dacron velour have also been used. Human umbilical vein has recently been shown to provide yet another alternative with acceptable preliminary results.

Site Selection

The same principles described for the placement of endogenous fistulas are applicable to the selection of a site for a graft fistula: the more distal site should be used first. However, the technical problems that make a graft necessary often make vessels at the wrist unusable. A common solution is to create a loop with graft between the distal brachial or proximal radial artery and the largest, most accessible vein in the antecubital fossa. Only the loop technique will be described here; details of other methods are available elsewhere.[6,7]

Technique (Fig. 34–3)

Regional axillary block, supplemented with local anesthesia when necessary, is established; and a 4-cm transverse incision is made 1–2 cm below the antecubital crease. The proximal radial and distal brachial arteries and a suitable vein (basilic, cephalic, or median antecubital) are identified and gently mobilized. The graft is placed on the skin in a gently curved loop, free of twists or kinks, to select the site of the subdermal or subcutaneous tunnel, which is then created with a full-length Kelly clamp or curved spongestick. An alternative preferred by some surgeons is to create the tunnel after the arterial anastomosis has been made. The graft must then be decompressed with a forefinger passed along its length or with suction before it is placed in the tunnel.[7] The tunnel should be deep enough to prevent devascularization of the overlying skin yet shallow enough not to interfere with palpation and cannulation. It should be just large enough to permit passage of the graft with minimal dead space. One or more small counterincisions may be needed at the distal end of the loop to permit precise creation of the tunnel. The graft must be drawn through the tunnel with exceptional care to avoid twisting or kinking.

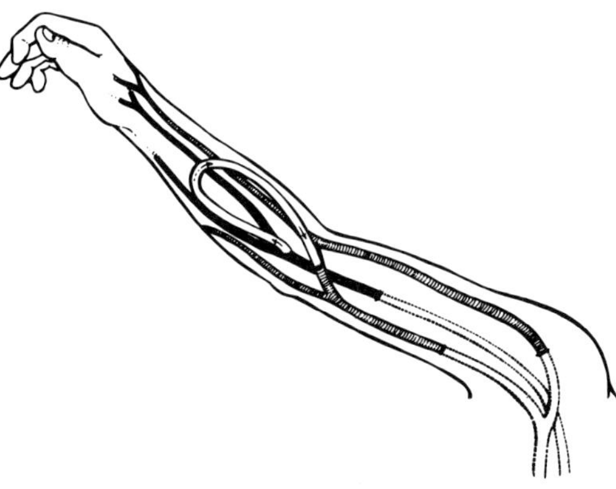

Fig. 34–3. Forearm loop with a prosthetic graft.

The arterial anastomosis is then constructed after systemic or regional heparinization has been instilled proximally and distally through the subsequently created arteriotomy. In either case, the artery is isolated between soft-jaw atraumatic vascular clamps, and an arteriotomy is made that is approximately 1.5 times the diameter of the graft selected. The arterial lumen may be irrigated with heparinized saline. The graft is trimmed obliquely such that the subsequent anastomosis approaches the ideal 30° angle of entry. An end-to-side anastomosis is made between the graft and the artery with continuous 5–0 to 6–0 monofilament suture. Just prior to completion of the anastomosis, a rubber-shod or soft-jaw clamp should be placed across the graft just distal to the anastomosis and the native vessels copiously flushed. After completion of the anastomosis, the occluding arterial clamps are removed and native arterial flow restored.

Proximal and distal clamps or Silastic vessel loops are then secured on the chosen vein and a venotomy is made, again for a distance of approximately 1.5 times the diameter of the graft. The graft is appropriately trimmed and bevelled and an end-to-side anastomosis constructed. The intima of the vein must be handled with extreme care, as it will not tolerate injury as well as arterial intima. Just prior to completion of the venous anastomosis, the graft is thoroughly flushed with heparinized saline and all residual thrombus meticulously removed.

After completion of the anastomosis, the occluding rubber-shod clamp is removed from the proximal graft, allowing flow through the fistula. The anastomoses are then inspected for hemostasis. Both pulsatile flow and a thrill should be readily palpable, since a bounding pulse in the absence of a thrill again suggests venous obstruction. It may be helpful to mobilize the vein for 2–3 cm proximal to the anastomosis to improve the hemodynamics.

The wound is irrigated with antibiotic solution and closed with interrupted vertical mattress sutures. The arm should be elevated and immobilized for two to three days to minimize edema and to promote incorporation of the graft into the subcutaneous tissue.

SECONDARY INTERVENTIONS

The most common serious complication of arteriovenous fistulas is thrombosis, which is responsible for 87% of fistula failures.[8] Often, especially if the thrombus is fresh, it can be removed in the outpatient unit under local anesthesia. Through a small incision over the distal aspect of the loop, the graft is isolated, and a 3F or 4F Fogarty embolectomy catheter is passed into the vessel. The incision in the graft can be closed with a single horizontal monofilament suture and the skin with two or three interrupted vertical mattress nylon sutures. The graft can be used immediately for dialysis.

Thrombosis is almost always associated with a progressive venostenotic lesion, and therefore the patient should undergo angiography of the angioaccess system after declotting. Rarely, an arterioanastomotic stenosis is responsible for fistula or graft thrombosis. Venous stenosis usually occurs at, or within a few centimeters of, the anastomosis and is usually characterized by fibrous intimal hyperplasia.[9] It may be caused by surgical trauma or be a consequence of the shear stresses and turbulence created in the vein by the high-pressure flow of arterial blood. In unusual cases, stenosis is caused by hypertrophic fibrosis of a residual valve.

In the past, these stenoses often necessitated the creation of a new fistula. It has become apparent recently, however, that many of these fistulas, including those involving grafts, can be salvaged by transluminal angioplasty or surgical revision.[6,10–12] The results of such procedures are significantly better if diagnosis and intervention take place before total occlusion has occurred.

Diagnosis

The usual indications for evaluation are problems during dialysis such as difficulty cannulating the fistula, inadequate blood flow with high venous resistance, or clinical signs and symptoms such as diminished pulsations, edema, varicosities, ischemia, or pulsatile or nonpulsatile masses. Angiography is often diagnostic and can be performed on an outpatient basis.[9]

If a diagnostic study without therapeutic angioplasty is planned, we proceed as follows. The brachial artery is cannulated with a 5F Teflon sheath, through which is injected (5–8 ml/second) 10–20 ml of diatrizoate meglumine and diatrizoate sodium solution, USP (Renografin-60) to which has been added 1 mg of lidocaine per milliliter. With the patient's arm abducted to avoid compression of the axillary vein that can mimic stenosis, films are made at the rate of two per second for 4 seconds and one per second for 4 seconds. The venous system is studied to the axilla or until normal veins without backflow indicate no proximal obstruction. Stenoses ≤ 4 cm long are suitable for angioplasty.

If venous stenosis is suspected and angioplasty is planned, the venous side of the graft or vein is catheterized with a 5F Teflon sheath. A pressure cuff is applied to the upper arm and inflated above the systolic pressure, and 10 ml of Renografin plus lidocaine is injected at the rate of 5–6 ml/second. The cuff is then released, and another 10 ml of the contrast medium anesthetic mixture is injected at the same rate. The cuff should not remain inflated for more than 30 seconds, as this may cause thrombosis in the fistula. This maneuver permits examination of both the arterial and venous ends of the system and allows the operator to proceed directly with angioplasty without an additional puncture.

Percutaneous Transluminal Angioplasty

Transluminal angioplasty is a minimally invasive technique that stretches and cracks the intima of the blood vessel, causing it to heal with a larger lumen.[13] Although originally used primarily for arterial lesions, it is now apparent that the method is applicable to many venous lesions, including those of angioaccess fistulas and grafts.

Angioplasty of venous stenosis is often considerably more painful than the same procedure performed on arteries, and therefore a systemic sedative and an analgesic are used to supplement locally infiltrated 2% lidocaine. A guide wire is passed through the stenotic region via a Teflon sheath in the usual manner, and the pressure gradient across the lesion is determined with a 5F catheter by measuring the pressures in the artery and vein separately if there is a question about the hemodynamic significance of the stenosis. A series of dilators are passed over the guide wire to enlarge the lumen to 8F so that the lesion will admit an 8-mm or 9-mm, 1.5-cm Grüntzig balloon catheter. (A 6-mm balloon may be better for small veins.) An intravenous injection of 6,000 units of heparin, 50 mg of lidocaine, and 50 mg of priscoline is then given. The catheter balloon is inflated under fluoroscopic observation in the usual way. As many as ten inflations may be necessary to correct the morphologic appearance of the lesion. Alternatively, the newer large, high-pressure Olbert balloons and the reinforced polyethylene "enforcer" balloons* have produced more rapid and better results.

After removal of the balloon, we compress the puncture site gently for 10 minutes with a Surgicel pad. A 4 × 4-inch gauze is then placed over the pad and fastened with a circumferential wrap of elastic Kerlix gauze. The patient is instructed to remove this dressing at the next dialysis. This method has prevented puncture-site problems after use of large angioplasty balloons.

Most of the failures of transluminal angioplasty occurred early in our series and were attributable to inappropriate selection of patients or equipment. Our more recent results have encouraged us to regard the technique as the approach of choice, because it does not jeopardize other vessels that may be needed for angioaccess in the future, as may be the case with surgical revision. Even if transluminal angioplasty fails, nothing has been lost except the time required for the procedure; and the vascular surgeon can proceed with the operation the patient would otherwise have needed.

Surgical Revision

In those cases where transluminal angioplasty either failed or is inappropriate, or if initial thrombectomy is required, surgical revision procedures must be utilized for access salvage and may be carried out, for the most part, on an outpatient basis (Figs. 34–4 and 34–5). Patch

*Cook, Inc., 925 Curry Pike, Bloomington, IN 47402

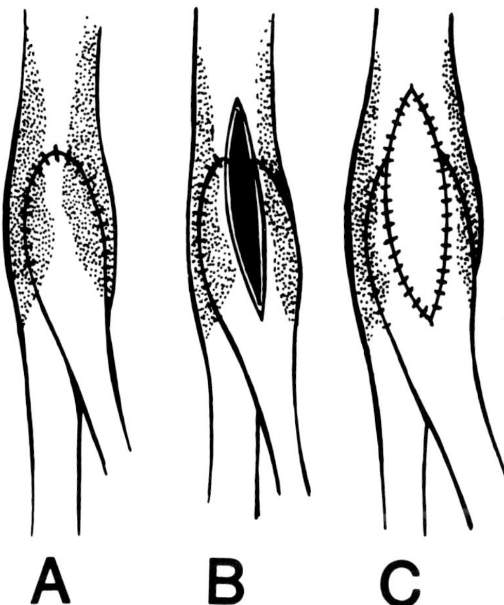

Fig. 34–4. Surgical revision of stenotic area (shaded) at venous anastomosis *(A)*. Incision in fistula *(B)* and interposition of a patch *(C)* to enlarge the vessel.

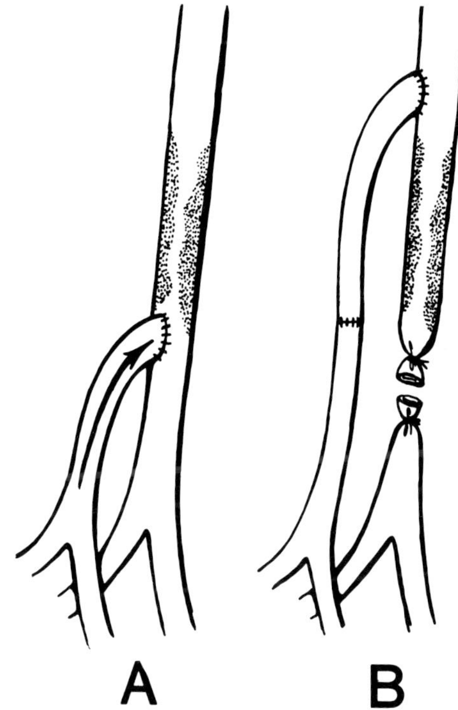

Fig. 34–5. Diffuse stenosis (shaded area in *A*) is corrected with a jump graft from the original prosthesis to a more proximal portion of the vein *(B)*.

angioplasty, interposition grafts, and "jump" grafts are all feasible alternatives and may be carried out under regional axillary block with minimal interruption of the dialysis schedule.[6]

With the knowledge that most grafts fail because of stenosis at the venous anastomosis, the previously created incision overlying this distal anastomosis is reopened and control of the graft and proximal vein secured with vessel loops. Through a short longitudinal incision in the hood of the graft, the fistula may be thrombectomized with a 3F or 4F Fogarty embolectomy catheter and adequate inflow assured. This should be carried out in the presence of established systemic anticoagulation. The venous anastomosis may then be calibrated, and if stenosis is confirmed, the graft incision is merely extended proximally through the anastomosis until normal caliber distal vein is encountered (see Fig. 34–4). The incision is then patched open with an elliptical prosthetic patch of appropriate material as illustrated.

If the stenotic process involves a longer segment of vein proximally, such that patch angioplasty over a distance of 5–10 cm would be required, it may be more appropriate to employ a "jump graft." In this case, the incision in the graft is enlarged to 1.5 cm, and a new section of prosthesis is anastomosed at this site and tunnelled to a more suitable proximal venous location where the venous anastomosis is created (see Fig. 34–5).

Finally, the access failure may involve aneurysmal degeneration or luminal stenosis because of an accumulation of excessive pseudointima at a frequently used puncture site in the midportion of the graft. In this case, the appropriate segment of graft limb may be excised and a new piece of similar material inserted as an interposition graft.

In any event, most of these basic secondary procedures can be carried out on an outpatient basis without serious interruption of subsequent dialysis. Initial concern regarding anastomotic suture-line bleeding or infection of the recently inserted prosthetic material has not been borne out in our experience. We routinely use prophylactic perioperative antibiotics with these procedures, and as long as the puncture sites utilized after revision do not traverse the recently inserted prosthetic material, we have encountered no unusual difficulties.

Secondary intervention with either percutaneous transluminal angioplasty or surgical revision has resulted in significant salvage of failed primary angioaccess and has contributed substantially toward minimizing both cost and inconvenience to the already confined lifestyle of dialysis patients. Thoughtful and timely intervention has already extended the anticipated patency rates associated with angioaccess in dialysis patients.

CONCLUSIONS

We can expect the continued pressure to reduce the cost of caring for the patient in end-stage renal failure to lead to greater use of outpatient units by these patients. The techniques described in this chapter have proved themselves in outpatient practice and should help satisfy the sometimes conflicting demands for outstanding health care and lowered costs.

REFERENCES

1. Wauters, J-P., Hunziker, A., and Brunner, H.F.: Regionalized self-care hemodialysis: a solution to the increasing cost. JAMA, *250*:59, 1983.
2. Popovich, R.P., et al.: Continuous ambulatory peritoneal dialysis. Ann. Intern. Med., *88*:449, 1978.
3. Salusky, I.B., et al.: Continuous ambulatory peritoneal dialysis in children. Pediatr. Clin. North Am., *29*:1005, 1982.
4. Manis, T., and Friedman, E.A.: Dialytic therapy for irreversible uremia. N. Engl. J. Med., *301*:1260 and 1321, 1979.
5. Butt, K.M.H., Friedman, E.A., and Kountz, S.L.: Angioaccess. Curr. Probl. Surg., *13(9)*:6, 1976.
6. Whittemore, A.D.: Vascular access for hemodialysis. *In* Surgical Care of the Patient with Renal Failure. Edited by N.L. Tilneg and J.M. Lazarus. Philadelphia, W.B. Saunders Co., 1982, p. 49.
7. Rubio, P.A., and Farrell, E.M.: Atlas of Angioaccess Surgery. Chicago, Year Book Medical Publishers, 1983.
8. Kinnaert, P., et al.: Nine years' experience with internal arteriovenous fistulas for haemodialysis: a study of some factors influencing the results. Br. J. Surg., *64*:242, 1977.
9. Glanz, S., et al.: Angiography of upper extremity access fistulas for dialysis. Radiology, *143*:45, 1982.
10. Gordon, D.H., et al.: Treatment of stenotic lesions in dialysis access fistulas and shunts by transluminal angioplasty. Radiology, *143*:53, 1982.
11. Gordon, D.H., and Glanz, S.: Balloon dilatation of arteriovenous shunts in the chronically hemodialyzed patient. *In* Transluminal Angioplasty. Edited by W.R. Castañeda-Zuñiga. New York, Thieme-Stratton, 1983, p. 172.
12. Probst, P., et al.: Percutaneous transluminal dilatation for restoration of angioaccess in chronic hemodialysis patients. Cardiovasc. Intervent. Radiol., *5*:257, 1982.
13. Castañeda-Zuñiga, W.R., and Amplatz, K.: The mechanism of transluminal angioplasty. *In* Transluminal Angioplasty. Edited by W.R. Castañeda-Zuñiga. New York, Thieme-Stratton, 1983, p. 11.

Index

Page numbers in *italics* indicate figures; page numbers followed by "t" indicate tables.